Department of Health

Report on Health and Social Subjects

48

Nutritional Aspects of the Development of Cancer

Report of the Working Group on Diet and Cancer of the
Committee on Medical Aspects of Food and Nutrition Policy

The Stationery Office

ISBN 0 11 322089 8

Printed in the United Kingdom for The Stationery Office
J27150 C35 3/98 10170

Preface

This is the first Report from COMA focusing exclusively on the influence of nutritional factors on the development of cancer. This important Report is based on a thorough review undertaken by the Working Group, who sought and received written submissions of evidence, as well as undertaking systematic reviews.

The Report accepts and exposes the uncertainties in the data, and is explicit about the judgements it has been necessary to make. The result is a prudent set of conclusions and recommendations, based on an open and clearly presented assessment.

The recommendations are generally set in the context of the public health, and provide a challenge to health professionals, including health educators, as well as the professional and lay media, to translate them into meaningful advice for individuals.

The conclusions are—happily—consistent with COMA's other recommendations, but they highlight the need for further research to increase understanding of the mechanisms and relationships involved. They are based on the best data currently available. Inevitably this will mean that firmer conclusions may well be able to be drawn in the future.

I am most grateful to the Chairman and Members of the Working Group who have toiled hard to draw robust conclusions from an incomplete and sometimes inconsistent database and I welcome their Report.

Sir Kenneth Calman

Chairman, Committee on Medical Aspects of Food and Nutrition Policy.

Contents

Committee on Medical Aspects of Food and Nutrition Policy: Working Group on Diet and Cancer

Chairman

Professor A A Jackson

Department of Human Nutrition, University of Southampton.

Members

Dr S A Bingham

MRC Dunn Clinical Nutrition Centre, Cambridge

Professor N E Day (until 1994)

Department of Community Medicine, Institute of Public Health, University of Cambridge.

Professor A D Dayan

DH Department of Toxicology, St Bartholomew's Hospital Medical College, London.

Dr B Margetts

Institute of Public Health, University of Southampton.

Dr C Muir*

Scottish Cancer Intelligence Unit

Professor J Parry

Department of Genetics, University College of Swansea.

Dr S Venitt

Haddow Laboratories, Institute of Cancer Research, Sutton.

Professor C Williams

Department of Food Science and Technology, University of Reading

Observers

Dr G Avery

Welsh Office, Cardiff.

Mrs A McDonald (until 1994)

Department of Health, London.

Dr J Battershill

Department of Health, London

---

*d. 20 June 1995

Dr K Binysh (from May 1996)	Department of Health, London
Dr C Hall	Department of Health and Social Services (Northern Ireland), Belfast.
Dr M Kemp	Medical Research Council, London.
Dr E Riboli	International Agency for Research into Cancer, Lyon, France
Dr R Skinner	Scottish Office Home and Health Department, Edinburgh.
Ms J Lewis (until 1994)	Ministry of Agriculture, Fisheries and Food, London
Dr R J Harding (1994-1995)	Ministry of Agriculture, Fisheries and Food, London
Dr D Kennedy (from 1994)	Ministry of Agriculture, Fisheries and Food, London
Professor M J Wiseman	Department of Health, London.
Mrs M Fry (until Sept 1996)	Department of Health, London.

Secretariat

Dr S Lader (Medical) (until December 1995)	Department of Health, London.
Mr R W Wenlock (Scientific) (until 1994)	Department of Health, London.
Mrs A de la Hunty (Scientific) (until March 1996)	Department of Health, London.
Dr S Martin (Administrative) (until November 1994)	Department of Health, London.
Mrs E Lohani (Administrative) (until August 1995)	Department of Health, London.
Dr J Hughes (Scientific) (from May 1996)	Department of Health, London
Dr A Redfern (Scientific) (from May 1996)	Department of Health, London

Committee on Medical Aspects of Food and Nutrition Policy

Chairman

Sir Kenneth Calman — Chief Medical Officer, Department of Health

Members

Professor P Aggett	Head of Department of Nutrition, Diet and Health, BBSRC Institute of Food Research, Norwich
Professor K G M M Alberti*	Dean of Medicine, University of Newcastle-upon-Tyne
Dr S A Bingham	Head, Diet and Cancer, MRC Dunn Clinical Nutrition Centre, Cambridge
Dr H Campbell* (from July '95)	Chief Medical Officer, DHSS Northern Ireland
Professor Sir David Carter* (from Nov '96)	Chief Medical Officer, Scottish Office
Professor F Cockburn (until Dec '96)	Samson Gemmell Professor of Child Health, University of Glasgow
Dr H Denner* (until July '95)	Chief Scientist (Food), Ministry of Agriculture, Fisheries and Food
Mr B Dickinson* (Aug '95—Sept '96)	Ministry of Agriculture, Fisheries and Food
Mr G Podger* (from Oct '96)	Ministry of Agriculture, Fisheries and Food
Professor J Grimley Evans	Division of Geriatric Medicine, Nuffield Department of Clinical Medicine, University of Oxford
Ms A Foster	Director, Scottish Consumer Council
Professor G Fowler	Professor of General Practice, Department of Public Health & Primary Care, University of Oxford
Dame Deidre Hine*	Chief Medical Officer, Welsh Office

*ex officio

Professor A A Jackson	Professor of Human Nutrition, University of Southampton
Professor W P T James	Director, Rowett Research Institute, Aberdeen
Dr M Kemp* (until Sept '96)	Medical Research Council
Dr R Kendell* (until Sept '96)	Chief Medical Officer, Scottish Office
Professor M Marmot	Professor of Epidemiology and Public Health, University College Medical School, London
Dr J McKenna* (until July '95)	Chief Medical Officer, DHSS Northern Ireland
Professor D P Richardson	Nestlé UK Limited
Ms L Stockley*	Health Education Authority
Dr P Troop (from Jan '97)	Regional Director of Public Health, Anglia and Oxford
Dr A Williams (from Jan '97)	St George's Hospital, London

*ex officio

Acknowledgements

The Working Group is grateful to the following who responded to an open invitation to make submissions to the Working Group

Cancer Research Campaign	London
Dr Andrew Collins	Rowett Research Institute, Aberdeen
Dr Leslie Davis	Maharishi Ayur-Veda College of Natural Medicine
Food and Drink Federation	London
National Dairy Council	London
Dr Kathryn O'Sullivan	Manchester
Unilever	Holland
World Cancer Research Fund	London.

The Working Group is grateful to the following who provided contributions at the request of the Working Group.

Mrs Ann Allan	Scottish Cancer Intelligence Unit, Edinburgh.
Dr V Burley	Leeds
Dr A Cassidy	MRC Dunn Clinical Nutrition Centre, Cambridge
Dr M Clifford	School of Biological Sciences. University of Surrey
Professor M P Coleman	Office for National Statistics
Mr A Finlayson	Scottish Cancer Intelligence Unit, Edinburgh
Dr R Fitzpatrick	Wales Cancer Registry, Cardiff
Professor David Forman*	Yorkshire Cancer Registry, Leeds.

*attended discussion meetings with the Panel.

Mr Allan Hackshaw	Wolfson Institute of Preventive Medicine, London
Dr Ian Johnson*	Institute of Food Research, Norwich.
Dr Tim Key*	Imperial Cancer Research Fund, Oxford.
Dr Stephen Musk	Institute of Food Research, Norwich
Nutritional Epidemiology Group	The Nutrition Society, London.
Dr Mike Quinn	National Cancer Registration Bureau, ONS, London
Dr Michel Smans	IARC, Lyon.
Dr Rachel Thompson	Institute of Public Health, University of Southampton.
Dr Gary Williamson	Institute of Food Research, Norwich.

The Working Group is grateful to the following who offered valuable comments during the preparation of the Report.

Professor N Day	MRC Biostatistics Unit, Cambridge
Professor M Gibney	Trinity College, University of Dublin
Professor R L Carter	The Royal Marsden NHS Trust

---

*attended discussion meetings with the Panel.

Summary

S.1 Introduction

S.1.1 *Background* Public and professional interest in the possible links between diet and cancer is increasing. Influential commentators have estimated that diet might contribute to the development of around one third of all cancers (see 1.4.3). Work on possible mechanisms for an influence of diet on the development of cancers has led to a perception that diet can play an important role in influencing risk of a number of common cancers in Europe, and in the UK. This Working Group was convened to examine the evidence for specific nutritional links underlying this perception.

S.1.2 *Perspectives* The Working Group recognised that the term "cancer" describes a wide variety of malignant tumours. However, a reasonable *prima facie* case for a link with nutrition has been made only for some. For instance, the development of tumours of the haemopoietic system (e.g. leukaemia) has not been proposed to be related to diet. The Working Group focused attention on those tumours for which a relationship had been suggested. In general, they are the most common cancers in the UK, though for specific groups, other cancers are more important (e.g. leukaemia in children) (see 1.4.1).

S.1.3. There is a multitude of substances in foods and drinks, many of which can modify biological processes in consumers. In addition to the essential nutrients, many other substances are natural constituents of food (see Chapter 8). Increasingly these compounds, and their biological functions, are being identified. However, many such substances in food remain to be characterized. Potentially beneficial or adverse effects of individual food components have been used as a basis for ascribing such effects to the foods which contain them. However, individual foods contain complex mixtures of potentially active substances. The nature of many of these substances is unknown and their functions unclear; some might be beneficial and others adverse; and the balance between them might be of particular importance (see 1.5.6). Consequently it is not possible to extrapolate from an effect of one particular food component to a similar effect of the food as a whole. Beyond natural constituents, foods may contain other components either from contamination, chemical or microbiological, or from purposeful addition. The Working Group considered that the presence of additives (for technical purposes in food) and contaminants, all of which fall within the remit of other expert groups, fell outside its terms of reference. In addition the Working Group did not consider the links between alcohol and cancer, because this issue had been addressed by another expert committee (see 1.4.4).

1

S.1.4. The Working Group considered a wide range of evidence although the main focus was on evidence as it relates to humans. A formal review of the epidemiology relating diet to the development of cancers was commissioned (see Chapter 5) and a scoring system to provide a systematic basis for the assessment of the scientific quality of information from case-control and cohort studies was developed (see Annex 1). In addition experimental data from *in vitro* and *in vivo* studies were considered, especially in humans, but not all the wealth of data derived from animal studies where the data are often not directly relevant to usual human exposure.

S.1.5 The Working Group concentrated on defining the nature of any possible links between nutritional factors and cancer in the UK and was concerned with direct evidence for particular factors influencing risk of specific cancers in the UK. Others have attempted by different means to assess the potential overall contribution that diet might make to the overall burden of cancer in the USA. Similar estimates specific to the UK have not been made. No attempt has been made by the Working Group to estimate the relative contributions of diet to cancer in the UK. The Working Group was not aware of evidence challenging previous such estimates, and did not examine the wider body of evidence necessary to make such an estimate themselves (see 1.4.3). The Working Group recognised that the emerging evidence on the multi-stage processes involved in carcinogenesis and the wide variety of dietary factors which could influence each stage of the process means that the dietary contributors to the stages of carcinogenesis a decade or more before a cancer becomes apparent are difficult to identify even in detailed prospective studies which form the major basis of the analyses in this report (see 1.5.5).

S.1.6 The Working Group examined both the epidemiological evidence and the evidence from mechanistic studies and assessed how likely the observed associations are to be causal relationships, based on widely accepted criteria (see Chapter 9). The complexity of the evidence required the development of a terminology to categorise the evidence (see Annex 2). In the event, the evidence for any links between specific dietary factors and cancer was insufficient to establish causality with absolute confidence although there was moderate or strong evidence for some. Particular problems apply to identifying critical dietary exposures and characterising them in detail in humans (see section 1.5). The fact that we have not been able to prove causal links does not mean that they do not exist, and where the degree of evidence for some links was sufficient, we have made recommendations (see Chapter 9).

S.2 Diet and cancers

S.2.1 The epidemiological associations are described in terms of their consistency (strongly, moderately, weakly, inconsistent or insufficient); the evidence for mechanisms is described in terms of the extent of its existence (no/little/some/ substantial, exists in animals/in vitro, operates in humans) and in terms of its strength (convincing, equivocal, unconvincing, lacking/no evidence); and the overall conclusion in terms of the strength of evidence (strong, moderate, weak, not enough) (see Annex 2). The overall conclusion might differ from that in relation to, say, the epidemiology alone, for instance, because of a lack of evidence for mechanisms (see Chapter 9). The following cancers are listed in order of greatest prevalence in either sex.

S.2.2 *Breast cancer* The evidence that greater adiposity, particularly central adiposity, and weight gain during adulthood, increase the risk of post-menopausal breast cancer is strong. Greater height and earlier menarche, which may also be influenced by diet, are both associated with higher risk of post-menopausal breast cancer (see 6.2.7). Greater lifetime exposure to circulating oestrogens probably accounts for the effects of obesity and early menarche (see section 7.13).

S.2.3 Epidemiological data revealed moderately consistent evidence that higher meat consumption, particularly red and fried meat, is associated with higher risk of breast cancer (see section 5.2.2); and weakly consistent evidence that higher intakes of fruits and moderately consistent evidence that higher intakes of vegetables are associated with lower risk of breast cancer (see section 5.2.5). Mechanisms for both these effects have been postulated, though evidence for their operation in humans is lacking (see 7.13.2). The evidence from epidemiological studies for an association between the risk of breast cancer and higher total and saturated fat consumption in adult life within the range of fat intakes found in Western populations and independent of BMI is inconsistent. It remains possible that dietary fat intake during childhood and adolescence may affect breast cancer risk several decades later. There is moderately consistent evidence for a lack of association between intakes of mono- and polyunsaturated fatty acids and the risk of breast cancer (see section 5.2.4).

S.2.4 There is weakly consistent evidence that higher intakes of vitamin A, either total, pre-formed retinol or carotenoids, are associated with a reduced risk of breast cancer, but vitamin A supplements are unlikely to influence the risk of breast cancer among women whose dietary intake of vitamin A is not low (see 5.2.7). There is insufficient epidemiological evidence to draw conclusions on vitamins C and E (see 5.2.7), and phytoestrogens (see 5.2.8) on risk of breast cancer and inconsistent evidence that intakes of dietary fibre are associated with risk of breast cancer (see 5.2.6).

S.2.5 *Lung cancer* Cigarette smoking is the most important cause of lung cancer. The potential for confounding by smoking is great, in particular as it is difficult to characterise precisely exposure to tobacco smoke. There is weakly consistent evidence for a weak association between higher total meat consumption and increased risk of lung cancer (see section 5.3.5). No specific mechanism has been proposed to account for this association. There is moderately consistent evidence that higher fruit consumption, and weakly consistent evidence that higher vegetable consumption, are associated with lower risk of lung cancer (see section 5.3.2). The suggestion for a possible protective effect of fruits and vegetables through the antioxidant capacity of components of fruits and vegetables in protecting against free-radical induced DNA damage remains plausible (see section 7.6.4). However β-carotene and α-tocopherol appear unlikely to be the mediators of any effect. The strongly consistent negative association between

3

serum β-carotene and lung cancer has not been confirmed as causal by intervention studies (see section 5.3.3). Nevertheless, if these nutrients have an effect at an early stage in the carcinogenic process, these trials might not be capable of demonstrating a protective effect.

S.2.6 *Colorectal cancer* There is moderately consistent evidence that diets with less red and processed meat and more vegetables are associated with reduced risk of colorectal cancer (see section 5.4.2). There are preliminary data from humans for possible mechanisms to explain such associations. The importance in human cancer of nitrogenous residues, e.g. ammonia and N-nitrosocompounds from meat and other protein containing foods, and heterocyclic aromatic amines from cooked meats, is uncertain and there is no direct evidence that they are involved in human colorectal carcinogenesis (see 7.13.4). There is weakly consistent evidence that higher total fat intakes are associated with a higher risk of colorectal cancer although the increased risk is small (see section 5.4.3). Possible mechanisms have been suggested, for example through the action of secondary bile acids (see 7.13.4) but the evidence that these operate in humans is equivocal.

S.2.7 The evidence from epidemiological studies that higher intakes of vegetables are associated with lower risk of colorectal cancer is moderately consistent but there is only limited and inconsistent evidence of an effect of consumption of fruits (see 5.4.4). Evidence is inconsistent that this can be attributed to vitamins A, C and E, and β-carotene, though higher fibre intakes may play a role (see 5.4.5 and 5.4.6). Plausible mechanisms for the association of dietary fibre and colorectal cancer through colonic fermentation and increasing stool weight have been suggested, and there is some direct evidence that they operate in humans (see 7.13.4).

S.2.8 The evidence for a positive association between higher BMI (obesity) and risk of colon cancer in men is strongly consistent, but is less so in women.

S.2.9 *Prostate cancer* There is moderately consistent evidence that higher red meat consumption and weakly consistent evidence that higher total meat and total fat consumption are associated with increased risk of prostate cancer (see 5.5.2 and 5.5.3). Conversely, there is moderately consistent evidence that higher vegetable consumption, especially raw and salad vegetables, is associated with reduced risk of prostate cancer but the evidence that consumption of fruits, and intakes of vitamin A, C and E and β-carotene, are associated with prostate cancer is inconsistent (see sections 5.5.4 and 5.5.5). Data in support of mechanisms operating in humans are lacking.

S.2.10 *Bladder cancer* The major human environmental risk factor for bladder cancer is smoking. There is moderately consistent evidence from limited data that consumption of fruits and vegetables is inversely associated with risk of bladder cancer but there is insufficient evidence to associate other dietary factors with risk of bladder cancer.

4

S.2.11 *Gastric cancer* Infection with *Helicobacter pylori* is now thought to be the major determining cause of gastric cancer (see 5.7.1). Smoking is also accepted as a risk factor. There is moderately consistent evidence that diets rich in salted meats and fish and salted and pickled vegetables are associated with increased risk of gastric cancer but these foods are not characteristic of the UK diet (see 5.7.2). It has been proposed that high salt intakes initiate the process of chronic injury and repair postulated as the precursor of gastric carcinogenesis (see 7.13.6).

S.2.12 There is moderately consistent evidence that higher intakes of fruits and vegetables are associated with lower risk of gastric cancer (see 5.7.3) and this is reinforced by the strongly consistent evidence that higher dietary intakes of vit-amin C and moderately consistent evidence that higher dietary intakes of carote-noids are associated with lower risk of gastric cancer. Any effects of supplementation with vitamins C and E, β-carotene and selenium appears to be limited to those with initial intakes lower than those usually encountered in the UK (see 5.7.4). Although it is possible that confounding by *H. pylori* infection may account for these findings, the strength and consistency and dose response relationship argue against this. A plausible mechanism via vitamin C has been proposed (see 7.13.6) but the evidence that it operates in human gastric carcino-genesis is equivocal.

S.2.13 *Cervical and ovarian cancers* There are few studies, especially cohort studies, which have looked at diet and cervical cancer. The limited evidence is strongly consistent that higher intakes of fruits and vegetables are associated with reduced risk of cervical cancer, which is reinforced by the limited evidence showing that higher intakes and/or blood levels of vitamin A and/or carotenoids, vitamins C and E and folate are associated with reduced risk (see 5.8.2 and 5.8.3). There is insufficient evidence to draw conclusions on the association between consumption of fat, meat, dairy products, fruits and vegetables and risk of ovarian cancer (see section 5.9).

S.2.14 *Endometrial cancer* There is no evidence of links between specific dietary factors and endometrial cancer (see 5.10.3), though the evidence is strong that higher body weight and higher BMI (obesity) are associated with higher risk, and for greater lifetime exposure to circulating oestrogens as a mechanism to explain such an effect (see 6.5).

S.2.15 *Pancreatic cancer* Cigarette smoking is the only well documented risk factor for pancreatic cancer (see 5.11.1). There is moderately consistent evidence that higher total and red meat consumption (see 5.11.2) and high levels of coffee consumption are associated with increased risk of pancreatic cancer (see 5.11.6). The evidence for an association with total fat and fatty acid intakes is insuffi-cient to draw conclusions (see 5.11.3). There is moderately consistent evidence that higher intakes of fruits and vegetables, vitamin C and dietary fibre are associated with lower risk of pancreatic cancer but the evidence for intakes of β-carotene is inconsistent (see sections 5.11.4, and 5.11.5). However there is inadequate evidence for any mechanism for these dietary components operating in humans.

S.2.16 *Oesophageal cancer* There is a clear link between alcohol and tobacco consumption and risk of oesophageal cancer. There is strongly consistent evidence from case-control studies that higher intakes of fruits and vegetables are associated with lower risk of oesophageal cancer but what prospective data exist cannot directly be exptrapolated to the UK (see 5.12.3). Higher dietary intakes of antioxidant nutrients are also associated with lower risk of oesophageal cancer. However, results from intervention trials of supplementation with various micronutrients have not demonstrated a reduction in risk (see 5.12.4). The evidence relating meat consumption to oesophageal cancer is inconsistent (see 5.12.5).

S.2.17 *Laryngeal cancer* The major risk factors of laryngeal cancer are smoking and alcohol consumption. There is limited, moderately consistent evidence that higher intakes of fruits and vegetables are associated with reduced risk of laryngeal cancer. There is not enough evidence to draw conclusions about other dietary factors (see 5.14.3).

S.2.18 *Oral and pharyngeal cancer* The effects of diet appear to be modest when compared with those for smoking and alcohol consumption. There is weakly consistent evidence that higher consumption of fruits is associated with a reduced risk of oral and pharyngeal cancers but the evidence for vegetables is inconsistent (see 5.15.5).

S.2.19 *Testicular cancer and melanoma* There is not enough evidence to reach any conclusions about the relationship between dietary factors and risk of testicular cancer or of melanoma (see 5.13 and 5.16).

S.3   Conclusions and Recommendations

S.3.1 *General*   The Working Group found the body of evidence complex and that potential for reaching conclusions was hampered by two principal deficiencies in the data. Firstly, the epidemiological evidence was very diverse in nature, encompassing studies with different designs, and with different classifications of foods and/or nutrients. Measurement error—a particular problem in characterizing dietary exposure—was a key problem in many studies which would tend to obscure positive relationships, especially where relative risks are small. Secondly, the evidence relating to actual or possible mechanisms in humans was often inadequate. Consequently causal inferences could not be ascribed with confidence to observed associations in all instances. For the reasons outlined in S.1.6 however, this cannot be taken as excluding such links. Nevertheless the overall evidence linking a number of nutritional factors with risk of certain cancers was strong or moderately strong, and these form the basis of the recommendations.

S.3.2   The cautious conclusions reflect a consideration of the specific links between nutritional factors and particular cancers in the UK and differ from those of some commentators, and from a wide general perception. The main reason for this was that the Working Group placed less weight on case-control studies. For many diet/cancer relationships, positive links are primarily found in case-control rather than prospective studies, but there is evidence that dietary data from such studies can be inherently biased (see 4.1.4.1). Using evidence pooled from large numbers of biased studies does not mitigate bias, and may even exacerbate it.

S.3.3   Though the conclusions of the Working Group on the links between nutrition and the development of cancer form the basis of the Recommendations, the latter also take into account other possible effects on health (see Chapter 9). The Working Group has not reviewed data pertaining to this wider context, but in order to address it, has set its current recommendations in the framework of COMA's previous recommendations in their Reports on Dietary Reference Values[1] and on Nutritional Aspects of Cardiovascular Disease[2].

S.3.4   *Conclusions and Recommendations*

S.3.4.1   Fruits and Vegetables   Overall, the evidence is moderately consistent that higher vegetable consumption would reduce the risk of colorectal cancer, and that higher fruit and vegetable consumption would reduce the risk of gastric cancer. There is weakly consistent evidence, based on fewer data, that higher fruit and vegetable consumption would reduce the risk of breast cancer. These cancers combined represent about 18% of the cancer burden in men and about 39% of the cancer burden in women in the UK. Even a small reduction in relative risk would have important public health benefits in terms of the reduction in the absolute numbers of people affected. In addition, the data are generally consistent with a graded reduction in risk for higher fruit and vegetable consumption and no cancer consistently shows a higher risk with higher fruit and vegetable consumption. The overall picture, therefore, is consistent and supports the hypothesis that the consumption of fruits and vegetables protects against the development of some cancers. **The Working Group recommends that fruit and vegetable consumption in the UK should increase** (See 9.2.8).

S.3.4.2   There is insufficient evidence to quantify the optimum level of fruit and vegetable consumption associated with the lowest cancer risk. There is some suggestion from observational studies that there might be a level of consumption above which no further benefit is seen, but this is well above the current average consumption in the UK. Advice from the COMA Working Group on Nutritional Aspects of Cardiovascular Disease[2] to increase fruit and vegetable consumption by 50%, to at least 5 portions per person per day on average, is a potentially achievable goal and is likely to be conducive to better health in general and a lower risk of cancer in particular. The Working Group considers that any increase in fruit and vegetable consumption would be expected to confer benefit.

S.3.4.3   Meat and fish, and their products   There is moderate evidence of a relationship between red and processed meat consumption and colorectal cancer. Colorectal cancers represent about 12% of all cancers. The evidence indicates that the risk of colorectal cancer is greatest in people with the highest intakes of red and processed meat. (Note: The definition of red meat and processed meat was not the same in all epidemiological studies but in general red meat referred to beef, lamb or pork in main dishes and processed meat referred to bacon, ham and sausages). Overall, therefore, there is moderate evidence that lower red meat or processed meat consumption would reduce the risk of colorectal cancer. The overall evidence that lower meat consumption would reduce risk of breast cancer, lung cancer, prostate cancer and pancreatic cancer is weak. There is insufficient evidence that lower consumption of preserved (salted) meat as eaten in the UK would reduce the risk of gastric cancer. The nature and mechanisms of the observed associations between meat consumption and the risk of cancers, should be the subject of research. It is feasible that the observed epidemiological associations between meat consumption and the risk of various cancers could be explained by confounding due to other dietary or lifestyle factors, for example low fruit and vegetable consumption, such confounding is difficult to disentangle (see 9.3.9).

S.3.4.4 Besides any potential effect meat and meat products have on cancers, they are a valuable source of a number of nutrients, including iron, whose average intake in some sectors of the population is low. Total meat and meat product consumption, as measured by the National Food Survey, has been falling since 1980. However, consumption of poultry and meat products has risen whilst that of carcase (red) meats has fallen. **The Working Group concluded that lower consumption of red and processed meat would probably reduce the risk of colorectal cancer.** However, the Working Group are aware of the possible associated adverse implications of a reduction in meat consumption on other aspects of health, particularly iron status, and **recommend that this should be the subject of review**. The Working Group was concerned that any general recommendations regarding red or processed meat should not compromise those for whom an intake of red meat, in moderation, is making an important contribution to micronutrient status. **The Working Group recommend for adults that individuals' consumption of red and processed meat should not rise; that higher consumers should consider a reduction; and as a consequence of this the population average will fall. Adults with intakes of red and processed meats greater than the current average, especially those in the upper reaches of the distribution of intakes where the scientific data are more robust, might benefit from, and should consider, a reduction in intake. It is not recommended that adults with intakes below the current average, should reduce their intakes. The wider nutritional implications of any reduction should be assessed**. As a guide to help identify where people's patterns of consumption lie in the distribution of intakes, the current average consumption of red and processed meats in the UK is around 90g/day cooked weight (8–10 portions per week), and consumers in the upper reaches of the distribution of intakes above 140g/day cooked weight (12–14 portions per week). This latter figure represents one standard deviation above the mean. 15% of consumers eat more than this amount. **These recommendations should be followed in the context of COMA's wider recommendations for a balanced diet rich in cereals, fruits and vegetables**. There is insufficient evidence to make recommendations on the

8

consumption of white meat or fish or on different cooking methods in relation to cancer risk (see 9.3.9).

S.3.4.5 Energy and obesity Overall, there is moderate to strong evidence that maintaining a healthy weight would reduce the risk of post-menopausal breast cancer and endometrial cancer and weak evidence that it would reduce the risk of colorectal cancer. There is no evidence that increasing obesity protects against cancers. Breast cancer is the most common cancer in women in the UK, accounting for about 25% of the cancers in women. England and Wales share one of the highest rates of breast cancer in the world. Endometrial cancer accounts for about 3% of cancers in women. **The Working Group therefore endorsed current advice to maintain a healthy body weight, in the BMI range of 20–25, and to prevent weight gain with age, through regular physical activity and eating appropriate amounts of food conforming to COMA dietary recommendations** (see 9.4).

S.3.4.6 Total fat Overall, there is weak evidence to conclude that higher total fat intakes in adult life result in higher risks of colorectal cancer, insufficient evidence to conclude that total fat intakes influence risk of prostate cancer, and moderate evidence to conclude that total fat intake in adult life does not influence the risk of breast cancer independently of BMI. **The Working Group made no specific recommendations on fat intake**. Following current dietary advice to reduce the proportion of energy from fat would not be expected to influence the risk of cancer directly, though it might reduce the likelihood of obesity (see 9.5).

S.3.4.7 Vitamins A, C, E and ß-carotene Overall, there is not enough evidence to conclude that vitamins A, C, E or β-carotene protect against the development of various cancers. Higher intakes of the antioxidant vitamins, β-carotene, vitamin C and vitamin E have been variously associated with lower risks of breast cancer, colorectal cancer, lung cancer, gastric cancer and cervical cancer in case-control and prospective studies. Most of the intervention trials that have been carried out so far with supplements of these vitamins have failed to confirm a hypothesised protective effect of these vitamins on cancer. If these vitamins exert a protective effect at an early stage of the carcinogenic process, for example by protecting against free-radical induced DNA damage, the relatively short-term trials reported so far would be unable to demonstrate a protective effect even if one existed. Alternatively, the observed associations may relate to a substance or mixture of substances in the diet for which intakes of these nutrients are acting as a marker (see 9.6).

S.3.4.8 The intervention studies also highlight the lack of information on the long term safety of sustained intakes of moderate to high doses of micronutrient supplements. In particular, the finding of an increased incidence of lung cancer in those taking β-carotene supplements in two intervention trials in people at high risk raises the possibility that a change in the usual balance of carotenoids in the diet (for instance by high dose purified supplements) might lead to potentially adverse perturbations in their absorption, metabolism or function. Such

9

findings caution against the widespread use of moderate to high dose micronutrient supplements, which cannot be assumed to be without adverse effects (see 9.6).

S.3.4.9   Non-starch polysaccharides (*dietary fibre*)   Overall, there is moderately consistent evidence that higher intakes of dietary fibre from a variety of food sources would reduce the risk of colorectal cancer and pancreatic cancer. The definition and analyses of dietary fibre is not clear in most studies, but non-starch polysaccharides (NSP) is the common factor. **The Working Group therefore recommends an increase in intake of non-starch polysaccharides from a variety of food sources.** The COMA Panel on Dietary Reference Values recommended an increase in average intake of NSP in the adult population from 12g/day to 18g/day and the Working Group endorses this recommendation (see 9.7).

S.3.4.10   Other nutrients (starch, sugars, folates, selenium, calcium, iron and zinc)   These nutrients have variously been proposed to be involved in the causation or prevention of some cancers. However, there is not enough evidence to reach conclusions for any specific links (see 9.8).

S.3.5   *Recommendations*   Authoritative commentators have estimated that dietary factors might explain about one-third of the variation in cancer incidence worldwide. The Working Group did not repeat the exercise and there is no reason to challenge this estimate. Though the evidence for specific links between particular cancers and dietary factors is of variable quality, the extent of the evidence considered in this report does not exclude causal associations. Nevertheless, uncertainties arise from inconsistencies in design and outcome of epidemiological studies; from imprecision in measurement of dietary exposures and from ascertainment of cancer incidence; and from absence of data concerning mechanisms operating in humans. In addition the data are limited almost exclusively to adults. For some relationships, for example colorectal, post-menopausal breast and endometrial cancers the evidence for causality, though short of absolute proof, is moderately strong and the balance of evidence is firmly in support of prudent recommendations in respect of them.

S.3.5.1 **The Working Group made its recommendations in the light of existing COMA recommendations. The following summaries are derived from and are cross-referenced to the paragraphs containing the Working Group's more detailed recommendations with any quantified guidance:**

- **to maintain a healthy body weight within the BMI range 20–25 and not to increase it during adult life (S.3.4.5);**

- **to increase intakes of a wide variety of fruits and vegetables (S.3.4.1 and S.3.4.2);**

- **to increase intakes of non-starch polysaccharides (dietary fibre) from a variety of food sources (S.3.4.9);**

- for adults, individuals' consumption of red and processed meat should not rise; higher consumers should consider a reduction; and as a consequence of this the population average will fall (S.3.4.4);

- these recommendations should be followed in the context of COMA's wider recommendations for a balanced diet rich in cereals, fruits and vegetables (S.3.4.4).

Adoption of dietary patterns conforming to these recommendations would be expected to reduce the burden resulting from some of the commonest cancers in the UK significantly.

In addition the Working Group recommended:

- the avoidance of β-carotene supplements as a means of protecting against cancer (S.3.4.8);

- the need to exercise caution in the use of high doses of purified supplements of other micronutrients as they cannot be assumed to be without risk (S.3.4.8).

S.3.5.2 Varying degrees of certainty surround these conclusions which reflect the current evidence. We have made recommendations where the evidence is clearly sufficient. Further data are already accumulating in this rapidly evolving field. It is therefore likely that firmer conclusions in at least some aspects of our review will be possible in a few years. **We therefore recommend that this topic be the subject of further review in the future.**

S.3.6 *Research*

The challenge for the research community is to close the gap between the 30% of cancer deaths thought to be attributable to diet, and the relatively few more or less firm links established by this review.

S.3.6.1 More research should focus on the links between diet and nutritional factors and risk of cancer. Better markers of dietary exposure, of nutritional status and of risk of cancer should be identified (see 10.2.1).

S.3.6.2 Dietary studies which aim to elucidate the "reciprocal relationship" between meat consumption and fruit and vegetable consumption should be encouraged (see 10.2.2). This would require more precise definitions of meat and of fruits and vegetables.

S.3.6.3 Appropriate collection and storage of biological samples should be considered in prospective studies (see 10.2.3).

S.3.6.4 The mechanisms of interaction between nutritional factors and genetic predisposition should be studied (see 10.2.5).

11

S.3.6.5 Dietary factors (including preparation and cooking methods) and individual nutrients which might be important in influencing risk of cancer, their interactions and their metabolic handling should be better specified (see 10.2.6).

S.3.6.6 Research should be done on the possibility that factors operating at specific periods in the life cycle might be critical for determining later risk of cancers, in particular the nutritional influences on, and health consequences of, the timing of menarche (see 10.2.7).

S.3.6.7 The relationship between physical activity and risk of cancer should be studied (see 10.2.8).

S.3.6.8 The potential benefits and costs of the recommendations in this Report should be quantified (see 10.2.9).

1. Introduction

1.1 Background

1.1.1 The Committee on Medical Aspects of Food and Nutrition Policy (COMA) has not previously considered in detail the link between diet and cancer, though in 1991, in the Report on Dietary Reference Values[1], COMA considered the possible role of dietary fat in carcinogenesis. The White Paper, "The Health of the Nation" noted that there was mounting, although as yet inconclusive, evidence that diet and obesity might influence the risk of various cancers[3]. The European Code Against Cancer, first published in 1987 and revised in 1995, advises that certain cancers might be avoided and general health improved if a healthier lifestyle were adopted, including an increase in vegetable and fruit consumption, frequent consumption of high fibre cereals, avoidance of overweight and limited intake of fatty foods. These and related public statements have received wide media attention, and there is a perceived wisdom that there is now a causal link established between particular aspects of diet and the development of some cancers. In the light of these developments and of increasing public awareness of the possible benefits of dietary changes as well as the growing interest in the role of possible "protective" components of plant foods, in 1993 COMA convened a Working Group to examine the evidence relating aspects of diet to specific cancers. Though mindful that research into the cause of cancers was a particularly fast moving field, COMA felt that an authoritative review of the world literature in the context of the UK was timely.

1.2 Terms of Reference of the Working Group

"To advise on the relationship between nutrition and the development of cancer and to make recommendations."

1.3 Meetings of the Working Group

1.3.1 The Working Group met for the first time on 19 July 1993 and on eleven subsequent occasions. A Press Release, published on 21 June 1993, invited submissions of evidence from individuals and organisations engaged in research in this area. This invitation was also published in the professional press. The Working Group is grateful to those who responded. The names of those who submitted evidence are listed earlier. In addition, the Nutritional Epidemiology Group of the Nutrition Society was invited to conduct a critical and objective review of published epidemiological studies of diet and cancer. A scoring system was developed to enable the overall quality of the papers to be ranked in an objective manner (see Annex 1). This epidemiological review excluded animal data and studies which only explored mechanisms. Nevertheless, limited data on animal experiments have been addressed where they were considered relevant to the nutritional impact on human cancers (see section 1.5.4 and Chapter 7). Members of the Working Group prepared working papers which formed the

13

basis of the final Report. The Working Group developed its own terminology to describe the epimiological evidence, the extent and strength of evidence for mechanism and the overall evidence for a link between diet and cancer at specific sites (see Annex 2).

1.4 Perspectives of the Working Group

1.4.1 *Burden of cancers* Cancer is a major cause of ill health and death in virtually every country in the world. Although there are 81 different categories of cancer listed in the ICD codes, affecting almost every organ and tissue in the body, approximately two thirds of the UK cancer burden is attributable to about 15 cancer sites. The most common cancers in UK men are lung cancer, prostate cancer and colorectal cancer which between them account for about 40% of the total cancer burden in men. The most common cancers in UK women are breast cancer, colorectal cancer and lung cancer which account for about 45% of the total cancer burden in women. There are large differences in the effectiveness of treatments for different cancers by the time they are diagnosed so that the most important cancer sites for mortality are not necessarily the most common cancers. The terms of reference of the Working Group were to look at the relationship between nutrition and the development of cancer; this Report therefore focuses wherever possible on cancer incidence data.

1.4.2 *Avoidability of cancers* There are four types of evidence which suggest that the development of cancer is related to environment or lifestyle factors, and might therefore be prevented by changes in them[4]. These include alcohol and tobacco use, exposure to chemical hazards, to sunlight and ionizing radiation, or to air and water pollutants, reproductive and sexual behaviour, viral infections, and diet.

(i) Variation between and within settled communities Age adjusted cancer incidence rates vary widely from country to country with up to 300-fold difference in cancer incidence for some cancers. Although this might partly be explained by genetic differences in populations, other types of evidence show that environmental factors are also important. Equally, different population groups within stable communities may show substantial variation in patterns of disease, such as vegetarians. Such groups may differ in a number of lifestyle or environmental factors from their peers.

(ii) Variation with migration Studies in migrants show that susceptibility towards cancer is not fixed and that migrant populations begin to take on the cancer rates of the host population within one or two generations.

(iii) Variation with time There are changes in cancer incidence within populations within less than one generation, which cannot be explained by inherited genetic changes in the population, implying an environmental or lifestyle cause of the change.

(iv) Specific known causes Various agents have been identified as causes of particular cancers and their elimination results in the reduction of cancer incidence. For example, 2-naphthylamine, has been shown to be a human bladder carcinogen.

14

1.4.3   Estimates of the contribution made by diet to variations in cancer incidence in the USA were made by Doll and Peto in 1981. They estimated, by comparing the incidence of each cancer with the lowest reliable incidence recorded
elsewhere, that about 75-80% of cancer cases in the US in people under 65
might be avoidable. They then estimated, based mostly on data from international comparisons of diet and cancer, that about 35% of cancer deaths in the
US might be attributable to variations in diet and were therefore preventable by
changes in dietary patterns. However, they commented that this was an imprecise
estimate and the correct figure could conceivably range from about 10% to
about 70%. This was compared to estimates of 30% attributable to smoking,
about 3% to alcohol, less than 1% to food additives, about 4% to occupation,
about 7% to reproductive behaviour and a possible 10% to infections[4]. In 1992
Riboli[5] estimated the proportions of specific cancers attributable to "*known, preventable risk factors*" and to "*suspected risk factors*". The proportions attributable to *known, preventable risk factors* ranged from 10% (for overweight after
menopause for breast cancer) to 85% (for tobacco and alcohol for cancer of the
larynx). That attributable *to suspected risk factors* ranged from 10% (for low
consumption of fruit and vegetables for cancers of the oral cavity and pharynx)
to 50 - 60% (for a combination of low consumption of fruit and vegetables, high
consumption of salt and salted foods and *Helicobacter pylori* infection for gastric
cancer). In 1995 Willett[6] estimated that about 32% of all cancers might be avoidable by changes in diet. These and similar analysis forms an important background to the Working Group's considerations. However, the Working Group did
not consider it appropriate or feasible to attempt to repeat such an exercise. The
Working Group were concerned to identify links between particular aspects of
diet and specific cancers in order to provide a sound basis for public health policy. It was not COMA's intention to address the issue of estimating the total contribution of dietary variation to variation in cancer risk, which requires a quite
different set of data and expertise. Nevertheless, the relatively few more or less
secure relationships identified by this review do not argue against the validity of
this estimate. Rather the difference between the two highlights the need for
research on the causal pathways which might help to bridge the gap. Diet
remains likely to be a key factor influencing the risk of cancer.

1.4.4   *Diet and nutrition*   The foods and drink which comprise the human diet
are made up of innumerable chemical constituents. Some, such as water, are
major components, but others occur in smaller amounts. Some, which may occur
only in microgram quantities in a usual daily intake, are essential nutrients, such
as vitamins or minerals. Others, while not essential, contribute to the nutritional
value of the diet, for example the carotenoids, some of which act as precursors
of retinol. Many dietary constituents, whether essential nutrients or not, may
have more than one metabolic role. Vitamin C contributes to the body's antioxidant defences in addition to its vitamin roles. Still other substances may have no
essential nutrient function, though sharing metabolically important (eg antioxidant) properties, such as polyphenols (see 7.6.4). We have considered all these
substances, essential or not, to be relevant to our remit. There are in addition a
number of substances in foods which are classified as additives or contaminants,
which may be natural or synthetic. We have not considered these to be part of

15

our remit. The relation between alcohol and cancer has been the subject of a thorough review by the Committee on Carcinogenicity[7], and we have not addressed this further.

1.4.5 *Scope of the Report* We have reviewed all the data directly relevant to the possible link between diet and the development of cancer in humans. In view of the already existing large body of literature addressing the issue of diet and cancer, we have not sought to identify new links between particular foods or food constituents and cancers, but to consider only the evidence relating to those links already hypothesized. Our consideration of the evidence was coloured by two general principles. Firstly, our interpretation of the data has focused on their relevance to the UK. Studies conducted in countries with very different diets and culture have the advantage of a wider range of exposures, but they may differ in a number of respects which might make it inappropriate to generalize their results. The degree to which studies can be generalised to be relevant to the UK depends on a number of factors, including the country of study, the usual dietary patterns in that country compared to the UK, the particular dietary component observed and the pattern of cancer incidence. There may also be differences inherent in the population, such as genetic or other constitutional predispositions. Some studies will, therefore, be more relevant than others. Studies of supplementation with particular nutrients in populations with much lower intakes than in the UK, or observations of "fruit and vegetable" consumption from countries whose fruits and vegetables are different from those eaten in the UK, might lead to inappropriate conclusions if applied indiscriminately. Though they make a valuable contribution to unravelling potential links between diet and cancer, such studies might have only limited relevance to the situation in the UK. Furthermore, our deliberations were confined to the major cancers which affect people in the United Kingdom (Chapter 2). Secondly, we have maintained a focus on evidence as it relates to humans. There is a wealth of data derived from animal experiments, often using extreme experimental conditions, which have provided insights into the processes involved in carcinogenesis. However such data are often not directly relevant to usual human exposures.

1.4.6 The term cancer embraces all malignant neoplastic disease, whatever its tissue of origin. Cancers arising from the epithelial tissues are called carcinomas, and those from the connective tissues are called sarcomas. Cancers of the haemopoietic system include leukemias and lymphomas.

1.4.7 We have found the evidence in humans to derive principally, though not only, from epidemiological data, and as such, to relate primarily to food consumption patterns. While some analyses have addressed calculated nutrient intakes, interpretation of this is beset by confounding, due to inherent interrelationships between particular nutrients, for instance because they coexist in similar foods (such as vitamin C and carotenes in vegetables). Equally, particular dietary patterns may also show inherent relationships between different foods - for instance meat free diets tend to be higher in vegetables. Consequently we have been cautious in extrapolating causality from observed associations in the absence of reasonable evidence for a mechanistic link which might occur in

16

humans. The principles on which we have based our judgements are detailed in Section 1.5. We have made recommendations on the overall balance of evidence. As for many public health recommendations this has not required absolute proof of causality

1.4.8 Similarly, the few intervention studies which have been conducted have, understandably, been in high risk groups for only relatively short periods of time in comparison with the natural history of cancer development. Consequently we have been careful not to overinterpret any apparently negative findings from such studies. On the other hand, positive findings from these trials, either for harm or benefit, are more helpful.

1.4.9 The Working Group found that there was not enough epidemiological evidence to report on a relationship between liver cancer and dietary factors, although they noted that in the UK, carcinoma of the liver is generally associated with alcoholic cirrhosis. Alcohol is outside the scope of this report and so liver cancer has not been included in Chapter 5.

1.5   Interpretation of Data

1.5.1   There are a number of generally recognised principles for evaluating whether an observed association between an exposure and disease is likely to be causal[8-10]. It should be noted that it is more difficult to conclude that there is evidence for a lack of causality than for a causal relationship. After critically evaluating large bodies of evidence, the International Agency for Research on Cancer (IARC) classifies agents or mixtures as 1) carcinogenic to humans, 2A) probably carcinogenic to humans, 2B) possibly carcinogenic to humans, 3) not classifiable, and 4) probably not carcinogenic to humans[10]. The same types of categories can, in principle, be used for agents or mixtures which are potentially protective against cancer.

1.5.2   The Working Group applied a number of principles for evaluating the evidence. These drew heavily on criteria developed by IARC[10], originally to evaluate data on pure chemicals. We found these principles extremely valuable in guiding our deliberations, but inevitably the data to which they were applied were often imperfect. Our conclusions therefore should be perceived as judgements based on a rigorous interrogation of the available data. By and large, the relative risks of cancers attributed to intakes of particular foods or food components were small in comparison to those found, for instance, in smoking or for some occupational carcinogens. Nevertheless, because diet appears to be related to some of the most common cancers, even a small change in relative risk might have large consequences in terms of public health. The significance of different degrees of confidence that any particular relationship might be causal is discussed in more detail in Chapter 4, but as for many lifestyle determinants of health in no case was a causal relationship established with certainty.

1.5.3   The main factors guiding our deliberations were:

(i)   *The type of epidemiological study* (the limitations of different types of study are discussed in section 4.1): evidence from all studies contributes to

17

the assessment but prospective studies carry more weight than case-control or ecological studies;

(ii) *Consistency of results between studies*, both of the same design and of different designs, and between those conducted in different circumstances, is more likely to indicate a causal relationship than when results are inconsistent;

(iii) *The quality of the studies reviewed*, with more value placed on those of better quality and design, in particular if the results of different studies are inconsistent (this includes avoidance of measurement error, selection or observer bias, and whether the possibility of confounding has been taken into account adequately);

(iv) *A general tendency for the results of all studies to be in the same direction*, irrespective of whether individual studies are significant, is more likely to indicate a causal relationship, albeit one with a small relative risk, than when the relative risks are more or less equally distributed around unity. The possibility of bias arising due to a preference for only publishing studies with significant findings or which are in the "expected" direction was also considered;

(v) *The size of the relative risk* : a large relative risk is more likely to indicate a causal relationship than a small relative risk, although a small relative risk does not necessarily indicate a lack of a relationship nor a large relative risk confirm one;

(vi) *A graded response* is considered to be a strong indication of causality, although a lack of a graded response does not necessarily indicate a lack of a causal relationship as there may be a threshold effect;

(vii) *Evidence of an effect from randomised controlled trials* is particularly strong evidence for a causal relationship. However the lack of a demonstrated effect does not necessarily indicate a lack of a causal relationship as studies might not have the statistical power to demonstrate an effect even if one existed, or might not have gone on long enough to demonstrate an effect (due to the duration either of the intervention or of the follow-up), or might have been conducted at an inappropriate stage of the natural history of the disease.

(viii) *The exposure should precede the effect*. Evidence against such a temporal sequence argues against a causal relationship.

(ix) *Evidence for a plausible mechanism* is an important contributor to establishing a causal pathway. Often plausible mechanisms have been proposed, but evidence for (or against) their occurrence in humans is lacking. We have placed more value on such hypotheses when there is direct evidence that they may apply in humans.

1.5.4 Evidence from animal studies on the potential carcinogenic effects of dietary constituents needs to be carefully considered with respect to its relevance to humans, but may provide additional information of value, in considering causality and possible mechanisms for effects. The extrapolation to human carci-nogenesis of evidence that a substance is potentially anti-carcinogenic against chemically induced tumours in animal models requires even greater care. Evidence of plausible mechanisms of action, particularly when it is considered likely that the mechanism occurs in humans, is especially relevant if it involves the causal pathway to carcinogenesis[10]. Because of the problems of extrapolation of such findings to free-living humans, the extensive data relating to chemically induced tumours in standard animal models has not been part of our review, though we have referred to data where relevant.

1.5.5   A conclusion that a causal relationship does not exist can only be made once there are several studies of sufficient quality to exclude the possibility with reasonable certainty that bias, confounding or misclassification could explain the lack of an apparent relationship. In addition, no individual study should show any tendency for the relative risk to increase with increasing or decreasing levels of exposure. Moreover, as the latent period for the development of most human cancers is generally more than 20 years, studies in which the latent period is sub-stantially less than 30 years cannot provide evidence for lack of carcinogeni-city[10]. Prospective studies of diet and cancer generally assume that the measure of diet obtained at the beginning of the study represents the habitual diet before and during the study. This may not be warranted. Nevertheless, there are as yet few prospective studies of diet and cancer longer than 10 years.

1.5.6   Furthermore, the difficulties in obtaining accurate measures of habitual dietary intake mean that actual risk can be substantially underestimated. This makes it necessary to study large numbers of people before a modest change in relative risk becomes statistically significant. Very large epidemiological studies are required to observe statistically significant relative risks less than 2.0, even for relatively common cancers such as breast cancer. Less common cancers would require even larger studies. Such studies would have to be continued for many years to accumulate sufficient numbers of cases. Most epidemiological studies of diet and cancer reported so far are too small to have the power to detect small changes in relative risk. Non-significant relative risks of less than 1.5 found in studies without adequate statistical power may well be false nega-tives and cannot be taken to imply a lack of association. Furthermore, diets com-prise a large number of different components many of which may show correlations and this may be a further source of uncertainty surrounding attri-bution of effects to individual components with which they are correlated (see Chapter 8). This is a particular factor in relation to meat and vegetables but may occur with many other foods.

1.5.7   In fact, for most cancers the evidence is sufficient to establish neither a causal association, nor a lack of association. In these circumstances judgements have had to be applied to the variously inadequate evidence. It is not possible to present an algorithm for this more subjective element of our analysis, but the preceding paragraphs present the principles on which it was based.

1.6 Form of the Report

1.6.1 The estimates by Doll and Peto[4], despite the weakness of the evidence on which they were based, demonstrate the potential of diet to influence the risk of cancer in the population. Since 1981, there has been an enormous amount of research investigating the nature and strength of possible links between diet and cancer. The Working Group reviewed evidence from observational and experimental epidemiological studies. Though not reviewed systematically, studies in cell systems and in whole animals were considered in relation to potential mechanisms of action in humans. Each type of study has its weaknesses: observational epidemiology is usually open to many different possible explanations, despite best efforts to take account of as many factors as possible; whereas the relevance of animal models to human cancer is often not clear. Numerous factors were weighed when evaluating the quality of the evidence and the conclusions which could be drawn from the whole body of evidence. These are set out in Section 1.5 and Chapter 9 of the Report respectively. The data were not always consistent in approach, categorisation or results and in most, if not all cases the conclusions represent a judgement based on incomplete evidence. The public health implications of any dietary changes were considered in the light of the importance of each cancer and where possible, recommendations made.

1.6.2 Any dietary recommendations arising out of this review of diet and cancer need to be made in the light of the wider links between diet and health or disease. Therefore, in addition to considering the strength of a relationship between a constituent of the diet and a particular cancer, it is also necessary to take into account whether any recommendation might, if followed, have effects on health, particularly adverse effects, other than in relation to cancer. Recommendations to the general population which reduced risk of some cancers, but also had adverse effects would be unhelpful, though more targeted recommendations to particular at risk groups might be possible in some circumstances. Though we have not considered in detail the evidence underlying COMA's existing recommendations, we have made our recommendations in the light of them. The considerations surrounding the development of public health recommendations in this context are similar to those in relation to cardiovascular disease. COMA's Report on Nutritional Aspects of Cardiovascular Disease[2] contains a more detailed discussion of such general issues as the value of population and individual strategies and the nature of individual and population risks.

1.6.3 Multiple risk factors for cancer make independent contributions to relative risk, although they might also interact with each other. Factors other than diet are also important, and in some cases overwhelming eg. smoking and lung cancer. The concentration on diet in this report should not, therefore, be taken to imply that factors primarily outside the specific remit of this Group (e.g. smoking) are not of fundamental importance. In this report we have touched on those factors which inter-relate substantially with diet, while other important but less related factors may have received less attention or been omitted. The Working Group's recommendations are intended to complement those which address other environmental factors but which require a different public health focus, and in no way substitute for them.

1.6.4 Our Report first reviews the data on cancer incidence or mortality in the UK for those cancers whose development has been proposed to be influenced by diet (Chapter 2), and then describes the national diet, with a particular focus on those foods or nutrients thought to be involved in the development of or protection from cancer (Chapter 3). Chapter 4 presents the nutritional epidemiological context for our analysis of the data and Chapter 5 evidence for a dietary influence on the development of cancers at various sites. Chapter 6 addresses the links between energy balance, obesity and other anthropometric measures, and cancers. Chapter 7 summarises the mechanisms underlying the development of cancers as they might operate in humans, both at the cellular level, and at the level of whole organs, in relation to nutritional factors. Chapter 8 discusses the evidence for an effect of other metabolically active components of fruit and vegetables on the development of cancers. Chapter 9 synthesises for each cancer site the evidence for a dietary or nutritional link, draws conclusions and balances the implications of these conclusions against many other factors in relation to their possible impact on public health, in order to make recommendations. Chapter 10 summarises the key recommendations for research which we feel would advance our understanding of the impact of diet and nutrition on the development of cancer, the better to promote the nation's health.

2. Cancer in the United Kingdom

2.1 Introduction

2.1.1 This chapter outlines the salient features of the distribution of incidence and mortality from malignant disease in the United Kingdom, drawing attention to regional and other differences and to changes over time. The cancers included are those which are discussed elsewhere in the Report ie. breast, lung, colon, rectum, prostate, bladder, stomach (gastric), cervix, ovary, endometrium, pancreas, oesophagus, melanoma, mouth and pharynx (oro-pharyngeal) and larynx and testis.

2.2 Sources of Information on Cancer

2.2.1 *Definitions*

2.2.1.1 Cancer incidence varies markedly with age. The incidence and mortality rates presented have therefore, been age-standardised to the world standard population proposed by Segi[11] and modified by Doll *et al* [4] to allow for differences in the age structure of the populations being compared. The rates presented in text and tables are average annual rates per 100 000 population (the words 'average annual per 100 000' usually being omitted).

2.2.1.2 In the description which follows, the United Kingdom (UK) comprises England, Wales, Northern Ireland and Scotland; Great Britain (GB) refers to the three countries of England, Wales and Scotland.

2.2.2 *Cancer Incidence*

2.2.2.1 Incidence (the number of newly diagnosed cases of cancer in a particular period in a defined population) is the preferred measure for understanding the aetiology of cancer. Incidence figures, ie. cancer registrations, for eight of the 14 registries in England & Wales and for all five Scottish registries were published for 1983-1987 in the *Cancer Incidence in Five Continents* monograph[12]. Further information for the 14 registries in England & Wales in 1989 is provided by the Office for National Statistics (ONS) previously the Office of Population Censuses and Surveys[13] and by Sharp *et al*[14] for the 15 Scottish Health Boards covering the period 1981–1990 and Scottish Health Statistics[15] for 1993 data. Reliable incidence data are not yet available for Northern Ireland.

2.2.2.2 Cancer incidence (average annual incidence for 1983–87) is provided for Japan (Osaka) and the United States (Surveillance, Epidemiology and End Results Program (SEER) representing 9 States) simply as an international comparison with figures for England & Wales and Scotland[12].

2.2.2.3 Publication of cancer registration statistics in England and Wales tends to be delayed by the need for the data to be collated and validated by the individual cancer registries, and because some registries' submissions to ONS (previously OPCS) are later than others. Detailed cancer registration data for 1989 were published by OPCS (now ONS) in 1994; provisional registrations for 1990 were published in 1995[31].

2.2.2.4 The relative frequency of cancer at selected sites expressed as a percentage of registrations of all malignant neoplasms in 1989 is shown for England, Scotland and Wales in Table 2.1 and Figures 2.1a and 2.1b. Malignant neoplasms are those coded 140-208 (excluding 173—non-melanoma neoplasm of skin) in the 9th revision of the International Classification of Disease[16]. Benign tumours and *in situ* cancers are excluded. The malignant neoplasms discussed in this Report represent nearly 70% of all cancers in England & Wales and nearly 80% in Scotland. The geographical distribution of the cancers discussed in this Report is presented in Table 2.2.

Figure 2.1a   Percentage of registrations of malignant neoplasms (male) for selected sites for 1989

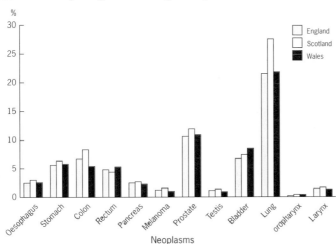

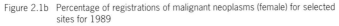

Figure 2.1b   Percentage of registrations of malignant neoplasms (female) for selected sites for 1989

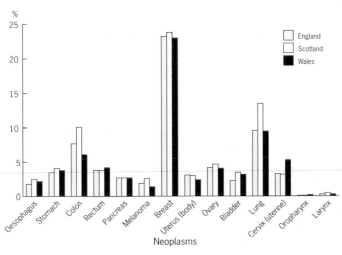

Table 2.1   Percentage of Registrations of malignant neoplasms* for England, Wales and Scotland for selected sites for 1989

	England				Scotland				Wales			
	M		F		M		F		M		F	
All Malignant Neoplasms*	109,147		111,298		11,012		11,469		8,413		8,371	
	n	%	n	%	n	%	n	%	n	%	n	%
Oesophagus	2,735	2.5	2,043	1.8	329	3.0	283	2.5	222	2.6	181	2.2
Stomach	6,118	5.6	3,893	3.5	697	6.3	465	4.1	490	5.8	318	3.8
Colon	7,345	6.7	8,594	7.7	917	8.3	1,168	10.1	457	5.4	508	6.1
Rectum	5,246	4.8	4,215	3.8	487	4.4	441	3.8	444	5.3	350	4.2
Pancreas	2,734	2.5	3,045	2.7	297	2.7	308	2.7	196	2.3	223	2.7
Melanoma	1,272	1.2	2,129	1.9	179	1.6	297	2.6	82	1.0	120	1.4
Breast (F)	–	–	25,837	23.2	–	–	2,727	23.8	–	–	1,931	23
Uterus (body)	–	–	3,494	3.1	–	–	342	3.0	–	–	199	2.4
Ovary	–	–	4,758	4.2	–	–	536	4.7	–	–	342	4.1
Prostate	11,596	10.6	–	–	1,312	11.9	–	–	922	10.9	–	–
Testis	1,178	1.1	–	–	148	1.3	–	–	76	0.9	–	–
Bladder	7,293	6.7	2,521	2.3	823	7.4	398	3.5	716	8.5	272	3.2
Lung	23,444	21.5	10,740	9.6	3,024	27.5	1,555	13.5	1,832	21.8	793	9.5
Cervix (uterine)	–	–	3,705	3.3	–	–	376	3.2	–	–	443	5.3
Oropharynx	200	0.2	103	0.1	41	0.4	15	0.1	33	0.4	13	0.2
Larynx	1,493	1.4	347	0.3	191	1.7	58	0.5	117	1.3	25	0.3
TOTAL for above sites	65.4		67.9		77.5		78.7		67.3		69.2	

Sources:
England and Wales   *Cancer Registration Statistics for England and Wales* in 1989[13]
Scotland   *Cancer Registration Statistics Scotland* 1981–1990[14]
* ICD 9 codes 140 to 208, excluding 173

24

Table 2.2 Age standardized incidence rates

	Oesophagus		Stomach		Colon		Rectum		Pancreas		Lung		Melanoma	
	M	F	M	F	M	F	M	F	M	F	M	F	M	F
Scottish Registries[a]														
North	9.4	4.7	17.0	7.5	24.2	22.2	12.4	8.2	7.4	6.5	65.4	18.3	6.0	6.5
North East	9.0	4.0	17.4	7.8	22.1	20.0	16.9	8.6	8.2	5.3	69.9	24.5	3.6	6.3
East	8.5	4.9	18.7	9.3	25.0	19.9	13.1	9.1	7.0	5.8	72.2	26.9	4.5	7.3
South East	6.2	3.5	21.0	9.4	21.6	19.0	14.1	8.6	8.6	6.1	85.7	29.3	5.0	7.5
West	9.3	4.5	19.0	9.7	21.1	17.7	12.6	7.7	8.5	5.7	97.2	33.6	4.2	6.9
English Registries[b]														
Northern	8.4	3.9	17.7	7.3	19.5	14.4	15.1	7.2	6.6	4.8	79.0	32.5	2.8	4.3
Yorkshire	7.8	3.3	17.3	7.4	20.1	14.9	15.0	9.1	7.0	5.3	67.0	25.0	4.1	7.1
Trent	6.6	3.0	14.9	6.3	17.6	14.8	15.1	7.6	6.6	4.2	57.5	18.8	3.6	6.0
East Anglian	6.1	3.3	14.3	5.3	18.9	13.7	13.3	7.2	5.8	5.0	49.3	17.5	4.5	6.0
North West Thames	6.9	3.2	12.6	5.2	15.1	16.0	11.1	7.6	8.5	6.2	58.8	22.9	4.3	5.7
North East Thames	5.4	3.6	16.4	6.6	17.4	14.5	12.1	7.5	6.7	7.2	62.5	23.8	4.6	6.1
South East Thames	7.0	3.3	14.1	5.7	17.6	14.1	11.7	6.5	7.5	6.1	58.8	23.2	4.2	5.3
South West Thames	6.6	3.2	14.2	4.5	18.6	15.0	12.6	8.1	8.6	5.7	49.7	18.9	4.2	6.3
Wessex	9.3	3.9	14.0	4.4	22.1	19.1	12.9	8.8	6.2	4.9	55.7	19.6	5.6	10.1
Oxford	3.8	2.7	14.9	4.6	17.0	14.5	12.2	7.0	7.0	6.4	48.0	16.2	3.4	6.8
South Western	6.6	3.5	13.2	5.2	16.0	14.5	12.9	8.4	7.0	4.5	42.3	15.0	6.2	9.2
West Midlands	9.1	3.8	17.7	7.1	22.5	15.8	16.4	8.4	6.1	5.0	62.6	20.2	3.5	4.6
Mersey	8.7	5.1	18.9	8.4	21.4	17.9	16.9	8.7	8.7	5.4	77.5	32.1	3.5	4.7
North Western	8.8	4.3	17.4	7.4	19.2	14.2	15.3	7.8	7.3	5.7	75.5	27.7	3.8	6.1
SCOTLAND[a]	**8.5**	**4.2**	**19.2**	**9.3**	**21.8**	**18.6**	**13.4**	**8.1**	**8.3**	**5.8**	**88.1**	**30.5**	**4.4**	**7.0**
WALES[b]	**9.2**	**4.6**	**19.9**	**8.1**	**18.8**	**13.3**	**18.7**	**10.7**	**8.1**	**6.0**	**76.6**	**25.9**	**4.2**	**5.2**
ENGLAND AND WALES[b]	**7.4**	**3.6**	**15.9**	**6.3**	**18.9**	**15.1**	**14.2**	**8.0**	**7.1**	**5.5**	**61.6**	**22.6**	**4.1**	**6.2**
JAPAN[a,c]	**8.4**	**1.8**	**73.6**	**32.7**	**14.8**	**10.1**	**11.6**	**6.3**	**8.9**	**5.0**	**41.5**	**11.7**	**0.2**	**0.2**
USA[a,d]	**4.0**	**1.3**	**8.0**	**3.5**	**31.1**	**23.6**	**15.4**	**9.6**	**8.2**	**6.0**	**64.3**	**29.9**	**10.8**	**8.8**

Table 2.2 continued

	Breast	Uterus (body)	Ovary	Prostate	Testis	Bladder		Cervix	Oropharynx		Larynx		All Sites	
	F	F	F	M	M	M	F	F	M	F	M	F	M	F
Scottish Registries[a]														
North	71.8	9.9	13.1	26.8	4.4	14.3	3.8	15.1	0.6	–	5.5	0.7	321.4	271.4
North East	59.5	8.6	14.6	31.5	5.3	18.9	6.7	13.7	0.8	0.3	4.0	0.5	333.8	269.6
East	66.6	8.6	12.1	26.3	5.3	21.9	6.2	11.3	0.5	0.5	5.1	1.3	327.9	275.4
South East	67.8	9.7	14.0	30.3	5.1	25.2	7.0	15.2	0.7	0.2	4.9	1.3	352.4	285.9
West	59.8	6.3	11.7	26.1	4.8	22.0	7.3	12.4	0.8	0.2	6.2	1.2	340.5	256.2
English Registries[b]														
Northern	62.5	7.2	10.8	23.3	3.5	20.2	6.9	11.8	1.1	0.5	6.4	1.4	302.4	243.0
Yorkshire	65.3	8.1	11.7	27.5	4.2	18.1	5.0	15.0	0.7	0.1	4.3	0.6	308.5	256.9
Trent	58.6	7.9	11.4	24.6	3.5	17.5	5.2	10.7	0.6	0.2	4.1	1.0	274.5	228.7
E Anglia	70.8	10.2	12.2	30.0	5.3	14.8	3.5	9.6	0.5	0.4	3.4	0.7	282.0	237.4
NW Thames	68.6	9.4	13.8	25.4	4.4	19.3	5.4	7.4	0.4	0.4	5.0	0.6	279.3	241.9
NE Thames	69.5	8.9	11.9	25.5	4.4	17.6	4.5	8.8	0.1	0.3	2.8	0.8	286.0	243.6
SE Thames	66.0	8.8	13.6	26.1	4.9	18.3	5.2	10.9	0.7	0.2	3.2	0.6	278.0	235.4
SW Thames	68.4	8.0	11.8	27.1	5.7	17.1	5.9	9.5	0.4	0.3	3.0	0.6	275.1	239.2
Wessex	80.3	9.1	14.2	34.6	6.2	23.7	7.8	14.5	0.6	0.2	4.4	0.6	296.7	273.9
Oxford	63.4	8.8	10.9	23.9	4.3	17.0	4.4	6.6	0.3	0.1	2.9	0.5	255.5	223.2
S Western	70.0	8.7	10.9	27.7	3.9	17.3	4.9	11.3	0.1	0.1	3.4	0.5	275.3	250.1
W Midlands	72.0	9.1	13.4	26.6	4.2	19.9	6.2	12.5	1.1	0.1	5.0	0.9	305.4	259.9
Mersey	72.2	9.8	11.7	27.5	6.6	22.8	8.5	16.4	1.1	0.2	5.6	1.1	345.6	289.2
N Western	63.8	6.0	11.3	24.6	4.2	20.6	6.9	12.4	0.9	0.6	5.7	1.0	308.2	251.9
SCOTLAND[a]	**62.6**	**7.7**	**12.6**	**27.8**	**5.0**	**22.1**	**7.0**	**13.2**	**0.7**	**0.2**	**5.5**	**1.2**	**340.7**	**266.8**
WALES[b]	**76.8**	**7.6**	**14.0**	**35.0**	**4.8**	**30.8**	**8.2**	**21.0**	**1.6**	**0.4**	**5.2**	**0.8**	**360.9**	**295.3**
ENGLAND AND WALES[b]	**68.2**	**8.4**	**12.3**	**27.2**	**4.5**	**19.6**	**5.9**	**11.8**	**0.7**	**0.3**	**4.3**	**0.8**	**295.1**	**250.7**
JAPAN[a,c]	**21.9**	**2.7**	**5.5**	**6.6**	**1.4**	**8.2**	**2.0**	**13.2**	**0.5**	**0.1**	**4.0**	**0.3**	**265.4**	**155.2**
USA[a,d]	**89.2**	**19.2**	**12.5**	**61.8**	**4.9**	**23.9**	**5.9**	**7.3**	**1.7**	**0.7**	**6.8**	**1.4**	**325.8**	**276.3**

Sources:
[a] Cancer Incidence in Five Continents Volume VI [12]
[b] Cancer Statistics for England and Wales in 1989 [13]
[c] Osaka Registry
[d] Surveillance, Epidemiology and End Results (SEER) Program (White population)

Table 2.3 Mortality rates for selected cancers and for all cancers for the period 1983-1987[a,b] by sex

	Oesophagus		Stomach		Colon		Rectum		Pancreas		Breast	Uterus (body)	Ovary	Prostate	Bladder		Lung		All Sites	
	M	F	M	F	M	F	M	F	M	F	F	F	F	M	M	F	M	F	M	F
Scotland	8.9	4.0	14.3	7.3	13.4	11.2	8.1	5.0	7.6	5.5	27.8	7.8	8.1	13.0	7.4	2.4	78.5	26.3	200.6	136.3
Northern Ireland[b]	5.6	2.9	14.8	6.3	15.6	12.5	7.5	3.7	6.9	5.4	26.2	6.1	7.6	13.7	5.2	1.5	56.4	15.4	174.2	119.3
Wales[b]	6.6	3.0	17.8	7.3	13.6	10.2	9.0	4.5	7.6	5.2	29.5	5.9	8.6	14.2	6.9	1.9	59.7	16.9	183.0	125.8
England and Wales	6.7	3.0	14.8	6.0	12.5	10.4	8.2	4.5	7.7	5.1	29.2	7.7	8.7	14.8	7.5	2.2	64.2	19.3	184.0	126.3
US (White)	3.7	0.9	5.0	2.2	15.1	10.8	2.9	1.7	7.6	5.5	22.4	5.0	3.2	3.3	4.1	1.2	55.3	21.5	158.9	108.2
Japan	6.9	1.1	40.8	19.0	7.8	5.9	6.2	3.4	8.0	4.5	5.8	5.2	6.5	14.2	2.3	0.7	27.7	7.7	149.8	79.9

Source:
[a] *Cancer Mortality and Mobidity Statistics*[17]
[b] Kilpatrick, Personal communication

27

2.2.3   Cancer Mortality

Cancer mortality, the number of deaths attributed to cancer in a defined population, is published annually for England & Wales by ONS (previously OPCS), for Scotland by the Registrar General (Scotland) and for Northern Ireland by the Registrar General. Mortality data for the UK over the period 1983 to 87 have been extracted from Tominaga *et al*[17] and are shown in Table 2.3. Data for Wales in 1987 were provided by the Welsh Cancer Registry. Figures 2.2a and 2.2b show a between country comparison of age standardized incidence rates in three main cancer sites for men and women in Scotland, Wales, England and Wales, Japan and the USA. Mortality tends to reflect the underlying incidence, but is influenced by the varying success of treatment and by the natural history of cancer at different sites in the body.

Figure 2.2a   A between country comparison of age standardized incidence rates for selected cancers (male)

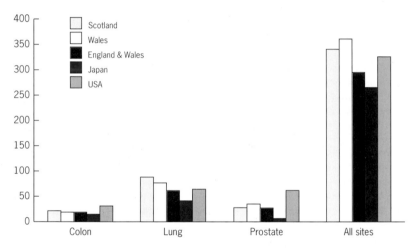

Figure 2.2b   A between country comparison of age standardized incidence rates for selected cancers (female)

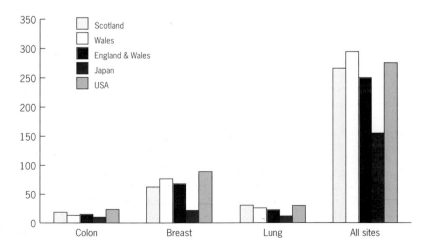

2.2.4 Data Comparability

The data presented cover slightly different time periods. This had been dictated by a variety of reasons, ranging from a conscious decision to present aggregated five year figures (1983 to 1987) for Scotland to provide sufficient numbers to obtain a robust estimate of incidence, to the quotation of time trend data published by Coleman et al[18] which covered slightly different periods for incidence (1973 to 1987) and mortality (1975 to 1988). Despite these differences and variation in registry and death certification practice within the UK and the other countries cited, valid broad comparisons can nonetheless be made.

2.2.5 Rates of Change (trends)

2.2.5.1 Trends in cancer mortality are difficult to interpret, being influenced by change both in incidence and in survival over time. Trends in incidence are a preferred indicator of change, being unaffected by changes in treatment and survival, although increasingly influenced by improved diagnostic techniques and screening programmes for breast and cervical cancer. However, cancer mortality data are available over a longer time span.

2.2.5.2 Changes in the age-standardised mortality rates between 1953 and 1987 for the countries in the UK have been published by Tominaga et al[17]. A selection of these trends is illustrated for selected cancers (Table 2.4 and Figures 2.3a and 2.3b). Coleman et al[18] provide international trend data expressed as the mean percentage change per 5 year period for 1973 to 1987 (incidence) and 1975 to 1988 (mortality) for the age-span 30–74 years. The publication provides data for Scotland and two English regions—West Midlands and South Thames.

2.2.5.3 Trends over time for some of the cancers considered in this Report vary considerably, and are discussed for each cancer site reviewed.

2.2.6 Differences in registration efficiency.

2.2.6.1 The quality of cancer registration in GB is known to vary. In general, Scottish data are held to be more reliable when compared by conventional indices of reliability ie. the proportion diagnosed histologically and the proportion of registrations based on a death certificate only. These indices were published for Scotland and for seven of the regional registries in England & Wales in Parkin et al[12]. Data quality for these seven registries was similar to that for Scotland but data for the other seven registries included in the tables in this paper, are considered to be less complete. Incidence rates and trends might also be influenced by policies of the different Cancer Registries.

2.2.6.2 While there are known to be variations in the completeness of registration within England and Scotland, the major differences in incidence observed are likely to be true. Supporting evidence includes the higher levels of the cancers associated with lower social class, such as oesophagus, stomach and lung in the North and Mersey and the lower levels of these sites recorded in more prosperous areas such as Wessex and East Anglia. Conversely, the cancers associated with prosperity such as breast and body of the uterus are of higher incidence in these latter registries.

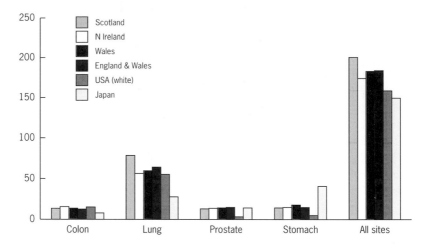

Figure 2.3a A between country comparison of mortality rates for selected cancers for the period 1983-87 (male)

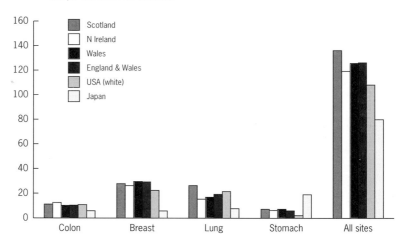

Figure 2.3b A between country comparison of mortality rates for selected cancers for the period 1983-87 (female)

2.2.6.3   The incidence data for Wales may be slightly inflated due to the methods of data collection used, based for the most part on Hospital Activity Analysis and the Patient Episode Database for Wales, which make it difficult to identify duplicate entries and metastatic disease[19].

2.3   Cancer in the UK

2.3.1   Cancer is a major cause of morbidity and mortality in the UK. About one in three people will develop cancer at some time during their life and cancer accounts for about one in four of all deaths. Approximately 300 000 cases of cancer are registered each year in GB and cancer is responsible for some 160 000 deaths.

Table 2.4 Time trends in the incidence (1973–1987) (from one Registry in each country) and mortality (1975–1988) (National data) from selected cancers by sex and selected country (age group 30–74)-estimated mean percentage change per 5 year period

Site	England + Wales[a]				Scotland				Ireland[b]				USA[c]				Japan[d]			
	Incidence		Mortality		Incidence		Mortality		Incidence		Mortality		Incidence		Mortality		Incidence		Mortality	
	M	F	M	F	M	F	M	F	M	F	M	F	M	F	M	F	M	F	M	F
Oesophagus	0.1	10.1	15.1	2.9	12.6	5.3	13.2	7.0	–	–	4.3	−1.5	17.1	−1.0	2.7	0.8	−2.1	−7.5	−0.9	−14.1
Stomach	−2.7	−8.7	−15.8	−19.0	−4.0	−5.6	−14.4	−14.8	–	–	−18.1	−29.8	−7.2	−3.6	−9.9	−12.8	−3.2	−7.6	−17.3	−21.5
Large Bowel	6.7	0.7	−1.9	−5.1	3.7	−0.4	−3.6	−8.5	–	–	−2.1	−9.2	7.7	0.7	−3.8	−8.2	28	22.6	10.7	3.9
Pancreas	−3.4	1.2	−5.2	1.8	−4.2	5.0	−9.4	0.6	–	–	−1.0	−11.1	−5.7	8.0	−6.0	0.9	20.4	13.8	9.5	4.8
Melanoma	41.4	54.2	14.2	12.5	54.0	52.0	22.5	5.5	–	–	38.6	16.6	30.3	20.1	9.2	2.6	9.2	21.1	5.2	4.1
Breast	–	5.6	–	2.6	–	5.0	–	2.1	–	–	–	1.7	–	13.8	–	1.3	–	29.9	–	8.8
Uterus (body)	–	1.8	–	−10.0	–	4.8	–	−8.6	–	–	–	−21.1	–	−23.5	–	−28.2	–	35.2	–	20.0
Cervix	–	3.0	–	−6.4	–	2.7	–	−7.1	–	–	–	−1.4	–	−18.5	–	−15.9	–	−13.5	–	−12.8
Prostate	14.1	–	13.4	–	19.3	–	13.5	–	–	–	0.0	–	25.1	–	2.3	–	3.8	–	10.1	–
Testis	10.3	–	−32.4	–	15.0	–	−32.6	–	–	–	−21.1	–	−16.9	–	−32.1	–	37.2	–	−18.3	–
Bladder	2.4	7.1	−4.6	−0.9	12.9	15.5	−4.5	−3.0	–	–	−0.9	−5.8	8.6	4.4	−14.7	−11.5	23.8	9.5	−9.0	−17.7
Lung	−7.1	17.5	−10.1	14	−2.4	26.2	−7.8	20.6	–	–	0.5	10.6	1.0	27.8	1.8	27.7	13.8	10.8	9.8	6.9

a Incidence data from West Midlands registry
b Incidence data unavailable
c Incidence data from Seattle registry
d Incidence data from Osaka registry
Source: Trends in Cancer Incidence and Mortality (Coleman et al 1993)[18]

Table 2.5 Deaths from common malignant neoplasms by age and sex for 1994 (provisional), England and Wales

Causes of death		All ages	Under 15	15–24	25–34	35–44	45–54	55–64	65–74	75–84	85 and over
						Age					
All causes, all ages	**M**	**266,368**	**3,360**	**2,189**	**3,792**	**5,620**	**12,802**	**31,195**	**76,124**	**88,143**	**43,143**
	F	**285,087**	**2,475**	**832**	**1,715**	**3,611**	**8,640**	**18,985**	**53,845**	**94,086**	**100,898**
Malignant neoplasms	M	72,835	192	207	453	1,222	4,333	11,564	25,441	22,181	7,242
	F	66,877	118	130	516	1,801	4,941	9,441	19,299	19,721	10,910
Malignant neoplasm of stomach	M	4,636	–	4	8	52	217	699	1,703	1,499	454
	F	2,951	–	1	10	44	100	254	719	1,092	731
Malignant neoplasm of colon	M	5,107	–	2	7	67	300	834	1,738	1,566	593
	F	5,781	–	2	12	56	254	648	1,548	1,865	1,396
Malignant neoplasm of pancreas	M	2,778	–	–	4	48	218	494	953	818	243
	F	3,027	–	2	1	34	131	377	900	1,021	561
Malignant neoplasm of trachea, bronchus and lung	M	21,114	–	1	20	184	1,153	3,516	8,496	6,260	1,484
	F	11,009	1	–	10	130	652	1,682	4,410	3,149	975
Malignant neoplasm of female breast	F	12,830	–	1	155	698	1,703	2,274	3,146	2,998	1,855
Malignant neoplasm of ovary	F	3,858	–	7	33	117	433	825	1,233	895	315
Malignant neoplasm of prostate	M	8,686	–	–	1	3	64	558	2,498	3,803	1,759
Malignant neoplasm of bladder	M	3,140	–	–	1	13	94	337	1,053	1,149	493
	F	1,625	–	–	1	4	28	123	417	617	434

Source: OPCS, 1995[31]

2.3.2 Cancer is largely a disease of the elderly, the peak in the age distribution occurring in men and women aged 65 to 79. Only about 6% of cancers in men and 9% in women occur at ages below 45. The frequency distribution by age group for the incidence of all malignant neoplasms registered in 1989 in England & Wales is shown in Figure 2.4[13].

Figure 2.4   Incidence of all malignant neoplasms: Frequency distribution by age-group, 1989

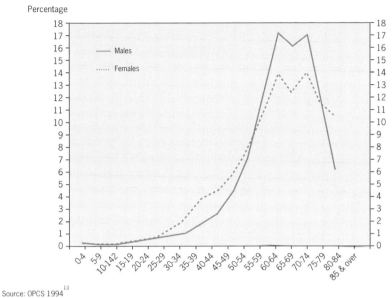

Source: OPCS 1994[13]

2.3.3 The age distribution of deaths from cancer shows a similar pattern to incidence, with the largest number of deaths occurring in those aged 65 to 84 (see Figure 2.5 for deaths from all malignant neoplasms). Table 2.5 shows the number of deaths for malignant neoplasms at different sites by age and sex. For all sites the peak occurs in those aged 65 to 84 years.

Figure 2.5   Deaths from malignant neoplasms by age and sex for 1994, England and Wales

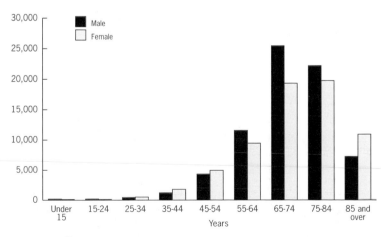

Source: OPCS 1995[15]

33

2.3.4   There are considerable differences in the incidence of cancer within the UK, with much higher rates overall in Wales and Scotland than in England & Wales (Table 2.2). Indeed if the contribution of Wales to the combined England & Wales figures were removed the disparity would be even greater. Rates in both sexes in Wales (male: 360.9; female: 295.3) and Scotland (male: 340.7; female: 266.8) are higher than in England & Wales combined (male: 295.1; female: 250.7). Much of the excess in women in Wales is due to breast cancer. Such variation is unlikely to be due to chance. While there may be differences in genetic susceptibility, it is likely that most of the variation is linked to the environment, using that word in the broad sense of all that impinges on the human organism.

2.3.5   Within England, there are also differences. For example, the rates in males in Mersey (345.6) are 26% greater than those in Oxford (255.5) and the rates in females for the same areas are 22% higher in Mersey. Again, such variations are unlikely to be due to chance. In Scotland, the regions are more uniform. There is only an 8% difference in male incidence and 10% for females between the highest and the lowest regions. Only the Mersey registry in England, however, has a higher rate of incidence for cancer in men than anywhere in Scotland. Over 70% of the English registries record a lower incidence in women than does Scotland.

2.4   Cancer at Specific Sites

2.4.1   *Breast*

2.4.1.1   Breast cancer is a very common cancer affecting women world-wide. The populations currently at highest risk are in Europe and North America where the risk is 5 times higher than in Asia. Even within western Europe, there is a 2-fold difference between the highest (Geneva) and lowest (Spain) incidence rates. Changes in the epidemiology of breast cancer are occurring in response to breast cancer screening programmes.

2.4.1.2   In 1989, 28 000 incident cases of breast cancer were registered in England & Wales and nearly 3000 in Scotland, representing 23% of the cancers in women. At regional level, recorded rates of incidence are generally higher in the Midlands and south of England, falling towards the north (Table 2.2). The highest rate, 80.3 was recorded in Wessex. Broadly speaking, the same picture is seen in Scotland with the highest rates in the southern half of the country. The exception to this is the Highland area, which records similar rates to those in the central and southern areas of Scotland. The standardised registration ratios (SRRs) for breast cancer by Health Authority in England from 1986 to 1990 are shown in Figure 2.6.

2.4.1.3   The UK mortality rate for breast cancer varies only minimally between the constituent countries and is the highest in Western Europe (Table 2.3). England & Wales have the highest mortality from breast cancer in the world.

2.4.1.4   Time trend analysis shows that breast cancer incidence continued to increase in England & Wales and in Scotland by about 1% a year over the period 1973 to 1987 (Table 2.4). There are signs that the rate of increase in incidence has begun to flatten in some populations including Ireland and Scotland. Trends

Figure 2.6   Standardised registration ratios (SRRs) for female breast cancer by Health
              Authority in England (April 1996 boundaries), 1986 to 1990.

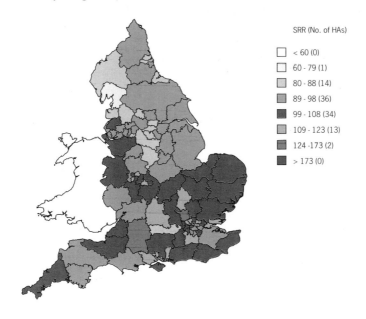

SRR (No. of HAs)

☐ < 60 (0)
☐ 60 - 79 (1)
▨ 80 - 88 (14)
▨ 89 - 98 (36)
▨ 99 - 108 (34)
▨ 109 - 123 (13)
▨ 124 -173 (2)
■ > 173 (0)

Source: Department of Health 1996[354]

Figure 2.7   Time trends in mortality from female breast cancer over the period 1953-1957 to
              1983-1987 for selected countries. Rates in Germany, France and Italy are lower than
              elsewhere. Most countries show a slight rise but rates appear to have stabilised in
              Scotland, Eire and in Northern Ireland.

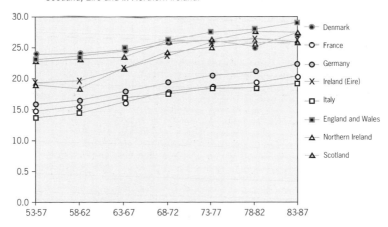

Source: Tominaga et al, 1994[17]

in mortality rates are increasing in several European countries; the increase in
UK mortality rates is about 0.5% a year (see Fig 2.7).

35

Figure 2.8   Standardised registration ratios (SRRs) for lung cancer by Health Authority in England
(April 1996 boundaries), 1986 to 1990.

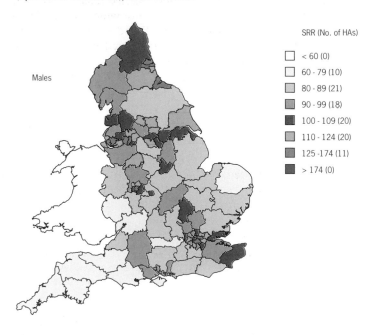

Males

SRR (No. of HAs)

☐ < 60 (0)
☐ 60 - 79 (10)
◻ 80 - 89 (21)
▨ 90 - 99 (18)
▨ 100 - 109 (20)
▨ 110 - 124 (20)
▨ 125 - 174 (11)
■ > 174 (0)

Source: Department of Health 1996[354]

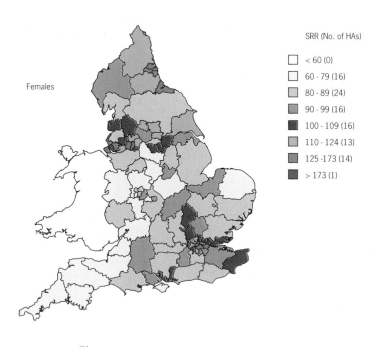

Females

SRR (No. of HAs)

☐ < 60 (0)
☐ 60 - 79 (16)
◻ 80 - 89 (24)
▨ 90 - 99 (16)
▨ 100 - 109 (16)
▨ 110 - 124 (13)
▨ 125 - 173 (14)
■ > 173 (1)

Source: Department of Health 1996[354]

36

2.4.2   *Lung*

2.4.2.1   Lung cancer, more accurately cancer of the trachea, bronchus and lung, is the most common cancer in the world, but with wide geographical variation. It is the most frequent cancer among men in GB and is second only to breast cancer in women. In 1989, 34 000 cases were registered in England, 2600 in Wales and 4500 in Scotland. In England & Wales, the disease accounts for 22% of all cancers in men and 10% in women. In Scotland, 28% of cancers in men and 14% in women are lung cancer (Table 2.1).

2.4.2.2   Within GB there are very substantial differences in incidence (Table 2.2, Fig 2.8). Scottish rates (highest in the West: males, 97.2; females, 33.6) are much higher than in Wales and England. In England the highest rates occur in the Northern (males, 79.0; females, 32.5), Mersey (males, 77.5; females, 32.1) and North Western (males, 75.5; females, 27.7) registries where they are virtually double those in the South-West registry (males, 42.3; females, 15.0), differences which are highly statistically significant. Throughout GB, incidence in males is at least twice as high as that in females and in some areas–North of Scotland, West Midlands and Trent–the rate is three times more. Figure 2.8 shows the standardised registration ratios (SRRs) for malignant neoplasm of the lung for males and females by Health Authroity in England (1986 to 1990).

2.4.2.3   Male mortality rates (Table 2.3) within Scotland, Northern Ireland, England and Wales are approximately 40% higher than elsewhere in Europe. Scottish women have the highest mortality rates (26.3) and are closely followed by the other countries in the UK. Lung cancer has consistently resisted all current methods of treatment and has a very high mortality, with only around 6% of patients surviving five years. Therefore incidence and mortality trends have followed similar patterns.

Figure 2.9a   Time trends in mortality from lung cancer (males) over the period 1953-1957 to 1983-1987 for selected countries. The fourfold international differences in male mortality are now 2-fold. Mortality rates have fallen in Scotland and in England and Wales but continue to rise in most other countries.

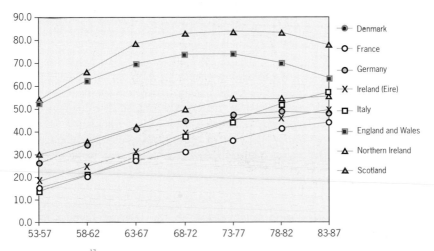

Source: Tominaga et al, 1994[17]

Figure 2.9b   Time trends in mortality from lung cancer (females) over the period 1953-1957 to
1983-1987 for selected countries. There is a universal rise most marked in the UK
and Denmark.

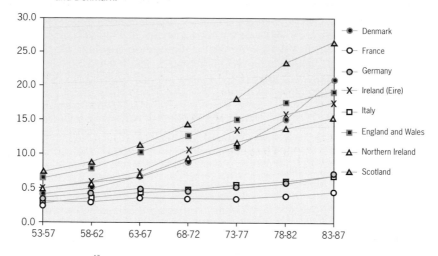

Source: Tominaga et al, 1994[17]

2.4.2.4   Male lung cancer incidence in the UK is declining by over 1% annually, as are the mortality rates, undoubtedly the result of a decline in tobacco
smoking habits (Table 2.4, Fig 2.9a). In Scotland, the most rapid rate of decline,
3% a year over the period 1973 to 1978, was in men aged 30–44. In women,
incidence continues to rise throughout GB (Fig 2.9b) by over 3% per annum in
England & Wales and 5% in Scotland. Mortality rates in women also continue to
rise at a rate of 3% in England and 4% in Scotland.

2.4.3   Colon and Rectum

2.4.3.1   Many registries report these two sites together because of the difficulties of identifying the exact origin of tumours around the rectosigmoid junc-
tion. Some 17 000 cases of colon cancer were registered in England & Wales in
1989 and 2000 in Scotland contributing 7% and 9% of all cancers respectively.
Rectal cancer accounted for about 4% of cancers in England, Scotland and
Wales with just over 11 000 cases being reported (Table 2.1).

2.4.3.2   The incidence rates for colon cancer in men and women are generally
fairly close. This is in contrast to rectal cancer, for which incidence in females is
just over half of that experienced by males (Table 2.2). The incidence of colon
cancer is highest in Scotland, whereas rectal cancer incidence is highest in
Wales, in both males and females. These differences probably reflect differences
in site assignment, since the total incidence for colon and rectum combined in
Wales (males 37.5, females 24.0) is very similar to that in Scotland (males 36.6,
females 28.1).

2.4.3.3   Mortality rates from colon cancer in the UK are highest in Northern
Ireland and higher in men than in women (Table 2.3). Mortality rates have
improved generally throughout the UK, most notable amongst Scottish women.
Mortality rates from rectal cancer are similar in all parts of the UK.

2.4.3.4   Slight increases in the incidence of colorectal cancer have occurred in the UK over the period 1973 to 1987, more marked in men (Table 2.4). A decline in mortality rates has occurred over a similar period, particularly in Scottish women.

2.4.4   *Prostate*

2.4.4.1   Prostatic cancer is the second most common cancer of men in GB. 12 500 cases were registered in England & Wales in 1989 and 1300 in Scotland, representing about 11% of the cancer burden. In England there is some evidence of a north/south divide in incidence (Table 2.2), with the lowest rate found in the Northern registry (23.3) and the highest in Wessex (34.6). Men in Scotland experience similar levels of incidence to those elsewhere in GB, although rates in the North East (31.5) and South East registries (30.3) are around 15% higher than elsewhere in Scotland.

2.4.4.2   Incidence is increasing rapidly in most populations. Time trend analysis between 1973 and 1987 suggests that the incidence of prostate cancer has continued to increase in the UK by between 3 and 4% annually, the higher rate relating to Scotland (Table 2.4). This increase may be due partly to earlier and improved means of detection and diagnosis. The removal of tissue for prostatic hyperplasia has resulted in the detection of increasing numbers of small, non-invasive carcinomas, many of which will probably not progress.

2.4.4.3   Mortality rates are uniform throughout the UK, although increasing in incidence, at a rate of around 3% each year. There is little variation throughout Europe with increases generally less than 1%.

2.4.5   *Bladder*

2.4.5.1   Cancer of the bladder accounts for around 6 to 8% of cancers in men and 3% in women in GB. In 1989, 10 000 cases were registered in England, 1200 in Scotland and 1000 in Wales. The registration of bladder cancers is probably not uniform between registries. The so-called benign papilloma of the bladder, a diagnosis which is increasingly rarely made, may or may not be included with the overtly malignant lesions.

2.4.5.2   There are quite substantial variations in incidence throughout GB, the levels in men in Wales (30.8) being 50% greater than in Scotland or England. In Scotland the highest levels are found in the South-East (25.2); in England, in Wessex (23.7) and Mersey (22.8). The lowest rate (14.8) is in East Anglia. Rates in women are usually about one third those in men, with parallel geographical distribution.

2.4.5.3   The incidence of bladder cancer has been rising slowly in most of Western Europe. In England and Scotland the rise has been greater in women than in men. In general mortality is about one-third incidence and has been falling by about 1% a year over the period 1975 to 1988, except in women in England & Wales. This suggests improving survival and possibly earlier detection.

Figure 2.10 Standardised registration ratios (SRRs) for stomach cancer by Health Authority in England (April 1996 boundaries), 1986 to 1990.

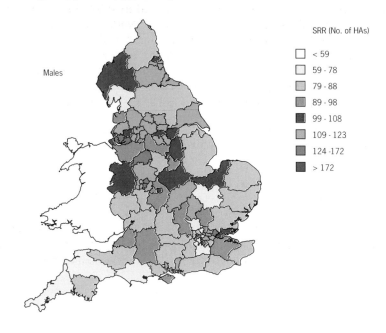

Males

SRR (No. of HAs)

- [ ] < 59
- [ ] 59 - 78
- [ ] 79 - 88
- [ ] 89 - 98
- [ ] 99 - 108
- [ ] 109 - 123
- [ ] 124 -172
- [ ] > 172

Source: Department of Health 1996[354]

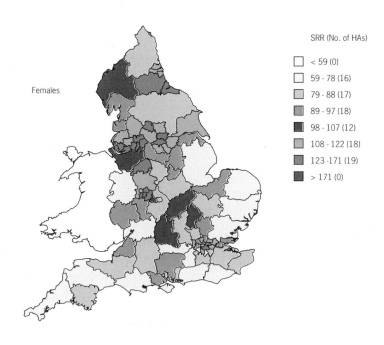

Females

SRR (No. of HAs)

- [ ] < 59 (0)
- [ ] 59 - 78 (16)
- [ ] 79 - 88 (17)
- [ ] 89 - 97 (18)
- [ ] 98 - 107 (12)
- [ ] 108 - 122 (18)
- [ ] 123 -171 (19)
- [ ] > 171 (0)

Source: Department of Health 1996[354]

2.4.6 *Stomach (Gastric)*

2.4.6.1   Gastric cancer in GB accounts for some 6% of cancers in men and 2% in women. Twelve thousand cases were registered in 1989 (Table 2.1). Incidence is higher in Scotland, Wales and the registries of North and North-West England (Table 2.2). The lowest incidence rates are found within South West Thames (14.2), South East Thames (14.1) and the South Western (13.2) registries, all of which are one third lower than that of South East of Scotland (21.0), with the highest incidence. Although the rate for gastric cancer among the female population is less than half that of males, it is similarly distributed (Fig 2.10).

2.4.6.2   For both men and women, the mortality rates for gastric cancer are similar in the countries of the UK and do not reflect the geographical variations in incidence.

2.4.6.3   The frequency of gastric cancer in both men and women is showing a world wide long-term decline (Figs 2.11a and 2.11b). Falls in the incidence and mortality from gastric cancer are observed all over the UK. However, the rate of decline, about 3% a year, is greater in South Thames than in either the West Midlands or Scotland. Mortality is falling at a faster rate in England & Wales than in Scotland.

2.4.7 *Cervix*

2.4.7.1   Cancer of the cervix is the second most common cancer of women worldwide, but fifth in England, fourth in Scotland and second in Wales. It is the most common cancer in GB among women aged 20–35. Approximately 4000 cases were registered in England & Wales in 1989 and 400 in Scotland, accounting for between 3 and 5% of the total cancer burden.

Figure 2.11a   Time trends in mortality from stomach cancer (males) over the period 1953-1957 to 1983-1987 for selected countries. There have been substantial falls over the 30 years. The higher rates in Germany and Italy are apparent, as is the clustering of rates in the UK. Danish and French rates are currently the lowest.

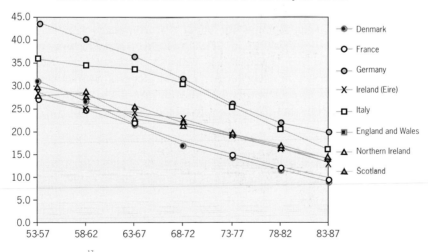

Source: Tominaga et al, 1994[17]

Figure 2.11b Time trends in mortality from stomach cancer (female) over the period 1953-1957 to 1983-1987 for selected countries. There have been substantial falls over the 30 years. The higher rates in Germany and Italy are apparent, as is the clustering of rates in the UK. Danish and French rates are currently the lowest.

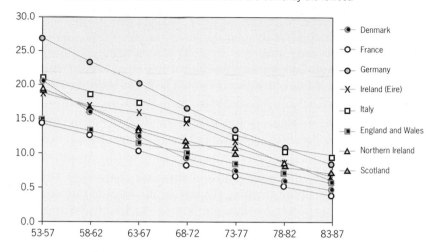

Source: Tominaga et al, 1994 [17]

2.4.7.2   The incidence of cervical cancer is some 50% higher in Wales than in England and Scotland and incidence is higher in the north of England than the South (Table 2.2).

2.4.7.3   In most developed countries with a national cervical cancer screening programme, the incidence and mortality has fallen. This has not been the case in GB where the overall trend in incidence from 1973 to 1987 was for an increase of 0.5% per year over the whole age range examined (30–74), and of about 5% per year in the younger age group (30–44).

2.4.8   *Ovary*

2.4.8.1   Ovarian cancer accounts for about 4% of cancers in women in GB, with 5600 cases being registered in 1989. Incidence rates are highest in Wales (14.0), slightly higher than in England & Wales or Scotland (12.6). Regions with higher rates of incidence in either breast, body of uterus or ovarian cancer (Table 2.2) not infrequently also exhibit higher rates at one of the other sites. Regions with lower rates follow suit, North East Scotland excepted, with low breast and high ovarian cancer rates.

2.4.8.2   Mortality from ovarian cancer is similar throughout the UK. Survival is relatively poor (25–35% at 5 years) but is improving due to earlier diagnosis and improved chemotherapy.

2.4.8.3   Time trends for GB indicate a continued increase in incidence of 2% a year. However, mortality trends suggest a marginal reduction for both England & Wales and to a lesser extent Scotland.

2.4.9 Endometrium (Body of uterus)

2.4.9.1   Cancer of the body of the uterus (also known as endometrial cancer) contributes 3% of cancers in women in GB with 3700 cases being registered in 1989 for England & Wales and 340 for Scotland. The incidence shows some regional variation (Table 2.2). Particularly low rates, in GB terms, are experienced within the North-Western registry of England (6.0), where incidence is nearly half that of East Anglia (10.2). The West of Scotland has a rate of 6.3, lower than the GB average.

2.4.9.2   The 5 year survival from cancer of the uterine body is high and the disease is not, therefore, a major cause of mortality. Mortality rates for the UK are generally lower than in Europe.

2.4.9.3   Time trends for 1973 to 1987 show that the incidence of this cancer has only marginally increased in England & Wales, while increasing by 1% a year in Scotland. Mortality trends show that the rate is decreasing throughout the UK by about 2% per annum (Table 2.4).

2.4.10 Pancreas

2.4.10.1   The 7000 cases of pancreatic cancer reported in GB in 1989 accounted for about 2.5% of all malignancies. Incidence rates for pancreatic cancer are generally greater in males than females and rates are fairly uniform throughout GB. Mortality rates are similar to incidence rates, reflecting the poor prognosis for this disease.

2.4.10.2   The trend over time for both incidence and mortality rates in GB is in line with the European average with a small reduction in males and a slight increase in females.

2.4.11 Oesophagus

2.4.11.1   Cancer of the oesophagus accounts for about 3% of cancers in men and 2% in women. Approximately 5000 cases of oesophageal cancer were registered in England & Wales in 1989 and 600 in Scotland (Table 2.1). Incidence rates were about twice as high in men than in women in the three countries. Incidence in both sexes is somewhat higher in Scotland and Wales than in England & Wales. There is moderate variation in incidence within Scotland and England & Wales (Table 2.2), the highest rate in England & Wales occurring in the Wessex (9.3) and the lowest in the Oxford registries (3.8).

2.4.11.2   Mortality rates reflect the incidence rates, being higher in men than in women and higher in Scotland than England. Mortality rates for both men and women are lowest in Northern Ireland (Table 2.3).

2.4.11.3   The incidence of oesophageal cancer in GB continues to increase. The trend over the period 1973 to 1987 was an increase of 2–3% a year amongst males, and of about 1% a year in females. An increase in mortality from oesophageal cancer has occurred in Scotland and England & Wales (Table 2.4). The recent increase in both sexes of the frequency of adenocarcinoma of the lower third of the oesophagus remains unexplained.

2.4.12 *Malignant Melanoma of Skin*

2.4.12.1 Skin cancers are among the commonest cancers. Non-melanoma skin cancer is more prevalent than malignant melanoma of the skin, which has been linked to dietary factors, whereas the former has not. Only malignant melanoma is considered in this report. About 4000 cases of melanoma were registered in GB in 1989, contributing approximately 1.5% to all cancers. The disease is usually commoner in females. There is considerable variation in incidence within GB. In general, risk is somewhat greater in regions close to the sea such as northern Scotland, Wessex and south-west England.

2.4.12.2 Rapid increases in the incidence of malignant melanoma have been reported over the last 20 to 30 years in many Caucasian populations, greater than the rate of increase of any other cancer. Rates of increase of 10% per year occurred in Scotland and England & Wales over the period 1973 to 1987 (Table 2.4). There has been a parallel increase in mortality rates of 3 to 5% a year (higher in men).

2.4.13 *Larynx*

2.4.13.1 Laryngeal cancer is uncommon in men and extremely rare in women. In 1989, registrations in men in England, Scotland and Wales accounted for less than 2% of cancers (Table 2.1). As with cancers of the oropharynx, risk is associated with alcohol and tobacco usage and changing trends in incidence reflect changes in usage. The incidence of laryngeal cancer in England is falling while that in Scotland may be increasing.

2.4.14 *Oropharynx*

2.4.14.1 Cancers of the oropharynx are rare in GB, less than 400 cases being registered in 1989. Incidence in women is about half that in men (Table 2.1). Mortality follows incidence in males; the recent trend in Europe has been a rise in mortality, but not in the UK.

2.4.15 *Testis*

2.4.15.1 Testicular cancer accounts for 1% of all cancers in men, about 1400 cases being registered in 1989 in GB. Incidence rates are slightly higher in Scotland and Wales than in England & Wales. The highest incidence rates for testicular cancer are in Mersey (6.6) and Wessex (6.2) and the lowest in the Northern (3.5), Trent (3.5) and South Western (3.9) registries (Table 2.2). The age incidence curve for testicular cancer has two peaks, one in the twenties, and one later in life possibly reflecting the relative frequency of the main histological types, teratomas having an earlier peak frequency than the more common seminomas.

2.4.15.2 Incidence is increasing almost everywhere in Europe, and around 2% per year in England and 3% in Scotland (Table 2.4). Mortality has fallen dramatically in most European countries by around 4 to 6% annually over the period 1975 to 1988. This fall is attributed to the success of chemotherapy with cisplatin, with 5 year survival rates now reaching 85%.

44

2.5 Cancer and socioeconomic variations

2.5.1 There are wide differences in the levels of cancer between socio-economic groups. Scrutiny of the data in Table 2.2 shows for example, a higher incidence of lung cancer in the less affluent areas of the north of England and south of Scotland, and higher incidences of breast and uterine cancer in the affluent south of England.

2.5.2 ONS (previously OPCS) undertook a social class analysis of the 1984 cancer registrations in England and Wales[20]. Social class groups were derived from the cross-classification of occupation and status. Cancer incidence, calculated as proportional registration ratios (PRR), for different social classes for selected cancers are shown in Table 2.6. The PRR is the ratio of the proportion of registrations from each cancer in a social class group to the proportion of registrations in the general population, expressed as a percentage. If the observed number of registrations is greater or less than expected, the PRR will be greater or less than 100.

Table 2.6 Proportional Registration Ratios[a] (PRR) for males and females aged 15–74 by site and social class, 1984[b]

Site		Social class by occupation					
		I Professional	II Intermediate	III N Skilled non-manual	III N Skilled manual	IV Partly Skilled	V Unskilled
Oesophagus	M	90	106	104	117	108	120
	F	–	132	86	94	134	147
Stomach	M	78	103	94	127	116	127
	F	[127]	104	103	169	142	184
Colon	M	122	114	105	87	85	82
	F	[146]	99	105	94	101	95
Rectum	M	81	91	102	92	98	88
	F	[89]	109	94	87	81	113
Pancreas	M	131	138	106	115	119	122
	F	[61]	146	87	149	117	141
Melanoma	M	150	108	115	57	67	34
	F	[97]	111	95	67	58	51
Breast		121	109	109	89	80	78
Uterus		[155]	83	97	68	74	100
Cervix		[55]	72	83	90	117	146
Prostate		140	101	103	75	73	65
Testis		124	114	134	83	91	85
Bladder	M	112	85	95	82	83	75
	F	[56]	74	121	122	97	81
Lung	M	77	96	106	129	135	139
	F	[72]	104	113	168	160	146
ALL SITES	M	101	100	101	101	101	101
	F	99	102	101	101	99	101

[a] PRR of all registrations for each social class
[b] Source: OPCS 1988[21]
[ ] small numbers (< 20)

45

2.5.3 Overall, there is no difference in the total cancer burden by social class. Social class gradients are seen for some cancers–gastric and lung (men and women), and cervix, where the PRR is higher in the lower social classes. Higher incidence in higher social classes is seen for colon cancer (men), melanoma (men and women), breast and prostate cancers.

2.5.4 Carstairs and Morris[21] examined both incidence and mortality from cancer in Scotland in the light of a "deprivation index" derived from data collected by the Census and made available for Post Code Sectors. There were substantial differences in incidence for many forms of cancer (Table 2.7), some being more common in more affluent, and others in less affluent, groups. Overall, the occurrence of the cancers they examined was more frequent in those classified as deprived.

Table 2.7   Standardised Registration Ratios for selected cancers by deprivation category, Scotland 1979–1982

	Deprivation Category		
	Affluent 1	Median 1	Deprived 7
Oesophagus	[78]	92	148
Stomach	79	103	138
Colon	104	99	96
Rectum	100	98	109
Melanoma	[164]	101	[54]
Breast (F)	114	100	89
Cervix Uteri	[67]	94	166
Bladder	92	100	120
Lung	69	100	183
All Sites	95	100	122

Figures are not available for Testis
Adapted from Carstairs and Morris (1991)[21]
[ ] small numbers

2.6   Trends over time

2.6.1   The changes in the pattern of cancer incidence and mortality that have occurred during this century provide clues to possible aetiologies of different cancers, with certain caveats. Adoption of new habits such as smoking tend to occur in a birth cohort manner. Similarly, when such habits are abandoned, it is the young who fail to take them up. For example, the decline in gastric cancer in Japan could be observed in younger men in 1960 at a time when overall rates were still rising[22].

2.6.2   The rest of this Report is concerned with describing and attempting to interpret the effects of different dietary components (see section 1.4.4) on the incidence of cancers at different sites. Whatever hypotheses are advanced, they must be consistent with the observed patterns and changes in patterns of cancer occurrence to be plausible, although this might be difficult to interpret due to the multifactorial nature of most cancers.

46

3. The British Diet

3.1 Sources of information

3.1.1   Information can be obtained from four sources: the National Food Survey (NFS),[23] conducted by the Ministry of Agriculture, Fisheries and Food (MAFF); the Dietary and Nutritional Survey of British Adults (British Adults Survey)[24] and the National Diet and Nutrition Survey: children aged 1½ to 4½ years[25], conducted for MAFF and DH; the 1983 survey on the diets of British Schoolchildren[26]; and the Total Diet Study conducted by MAFF[27]. Further information is available from other surveys, but Government surveys are uniquely designed to be broadly representative of the population, and therefore have been used to supply the information presented here.

3.1.2   *The National Food Survey*   The NFS is a continuous survey of the amounts and cost of foods obtained by private households in Britain and of their nutrient content. About 8000 households per year participate in this nationally representative survey which has been conducted since 1940. The householder keeps a seven day record of the description, quantity, and cost of all food entering the home for human consumption. Information on confectionery, alcoholic and soft drinks purchased for consumption inside and outside the home and meals purchased outside the home has also been collected since January 1992. However, the values quoted here generally exclude contributions from these sources in order to provide consistency for dietary trends. The NFS provides information on long-term trends in national food and nutrient intakes and variations in intake by groups of the population (e.g. by regional and socio-economic characteristics). It cannot, however, provide information about the nutrient intake of individuals within the population.

3.1.3   *The National Diet and Nutrition Surveys (NDNS)*   Following the success of the British Adults Survey an NDNS programme has been set up, which is intended to cover all age groups beyond infancy (children aged 1½–4½ years, young people aged 4–18 years, adults aged 16–64 years and adults aged 65 years and over) in a rolling programme over about a decade. Each survey will combine dietary assessments, obtained from weighed intakes, with anthropometry and measures of nutritional status and other relevant physiological variables. The British Adults Survey carried out over 1 year in 1986 to 1987 provides detailed nutrient and food intake data for approximately 2200 individuals aged 16-64 years and provides valuable data on the detailed composition of the diets of individuals throughout Britain[24]. The results of the survey of pre-school children (conducted in 1992/93), were published in 1995[25].

3.1.4   *British Schoolchildren*   A previous study on the diets of British Schoolchildren was carried out in 1983[26], with 2300 children aged 10–11 and

Table 3.1 Average Daily Intakes of selected nutrients by children

AGE (years)	1½–4½*		10/11**		14/15**	
	% energy		% energy		% energy	
Total energy Kcal	1140		1955		2181	
Fat g	45.7	36	83.1	38	96.2	38
Saturated fatty acids g	20.6	16.2	—	—	—	—
Mono-unsaturated fatty acids g	14.2	11.1	—	—	—	—
Polyunsaturated fatty acids g	5.9	4.6	—	—	—	—
Carbohydrate g	155	51	258	50.2	282	49.3
NME sugars g	57	18.7	—	—	—	—
Non-starch polysaccharides g	6.1	—	—	—	—	—
Vit C mg	46.8	—	49	—	48.6	—
Vit E mg	4.3	—	—	—	—	—
Carotenes ug	872	—	1460	—	1550	—
Iron mg	5.5	—	9.3	—	10.8	—
Calcium mg	637	—	768	—	809	—

*   Source: National Diet and Nutrition Survey Children 1½–4¼ years, Gregory *et al* 1995[24]
** Source: Diets of British Schoolchildren, 1989[26]

14–15 years successfully completing the study. Nutrient and food intake data were collected using a seven day dietary record with the height and weight of each child also being recorded. The study over-sampled in some areas in order to increase the number of children from less advantaged families involved in the survey. The data provided are limited and only available for certain nutrients.

3.1.5   *Total Diet Study*   MAFF's Total Diet Study (TDS), which has been carried out annually since the early 1960s, is a market-basket type survey[28]. Foods representing the average UK diet (based on the National Food Survey) are purchased from a variety of retail outlets in 24 towns each year, selected to be representative of the UK, prepared and combined into 20 groups of similar foods for analysis. It is used to provide, as far as possible, an estimate of the average intake of any nutrient or non-nutrient of current interest. Recent analyses of the TDS have included selenium and individual fatty acids.

3.2   Trends in the British Diet 1950–1995

3.2.1   The broad pattern of changes in the British diet over the last 50 years can be seen from the results of the National Food Survey, shown in Figures 3.1 and 3.2. There was a decline in the proportion of food energy derived from carbohydrate and a corresponding increase in the proportion of energy derived from fat in the years following the Second World War but the balance of energy from carbohydrate, fat and protein has remained comparatively steady over the last 20 years (Figure 3.1). There have, however, been substantial changes in the types and quantities of foods consumed over this period (Figure 3.2).

3.2.2   *Milk*   During the Second World War, successful efforts were made to increase milk consumption, after which milk intake remained relatively stable at about 390ml/day until the mid 1970s. Whole milk consumption fell to about 340ml/day in 1980 and to 116ml/day in 1995. Skimmed milks, which were hardly consumed in 1980, rose to a consumption level of 158ml/day in 1995.

Figure 3.1   Trends in the proportion of energy from fat, protein and carbohydrates

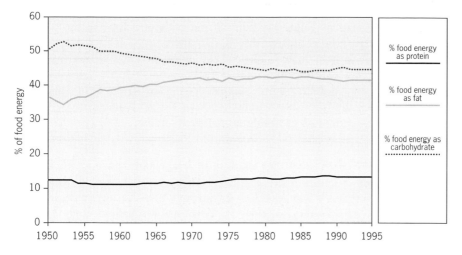

Source: National Food Survey 1950-1995

Figure 3.2   Trends in consumption of major food groups

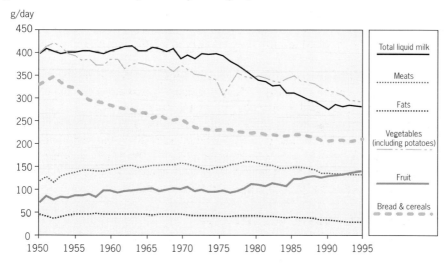

Source: National Food Survey 1950-1995

This trend seems to be continuing and currently 58% of the milk consumed in the house is skimmed (mainly semi-skimmed) milks.

3.2.3   *Fats and oils*   Total consumption of fats and oils remained steady at around 50g/day from the mid 1950s to the early 1970s, but consumption has now dropped to around 31g/day in 1995. The relative importance of individual foods within the fats group has changed, with an increased consumption of low and reduced fat spreads, and vegetable oils in place of butter, margarines and lard. Butter consumption decreased from about 24g/day in the late 1950s, to 16g/ day in 1980, to about 5g/day in 1995.

3.2.4 *Meats* The data for meat consumption are from both the NFS and the British Adults Survey[24]. The classifications in these two surveys are different, the NFS refers to meat as purchased (i.e. raw and with wastage) and those in the NDNS are for meats as eaten (i.e. cooked and without waste) so the data from these surveys cannot be compared directly. In addition the NFS is for the whole population whereas the British Adults Survey is for men and women aged 16 to 64 years only. The NFS does not include foods purchased and eaten out of the home whereas the British Adults Survey does. Data from both surveys are shown here since the NFS shows trends and the British Adults Survey provides estimates of the distribution of absolute intakes in adults.

3.2.4.1 The NFS shows that consumption of beef, lamb and pork rose sharply in the mid 1950s, but since then there has been a steady decline in consumption of red meats, particularly lamb, and a considerable increase in poultry consumption (see Figure 3.3). Poultry (34g/day in 1995) has reached an equivalent level of consumption of beef, lamb and pork combined (35g/day in 1995). The consumption of bacon and ham followed a similar rise in consumption during the 1950s with a steady decline since 1970 to reach a level of consumption in 1995 similar to beef (beef 17g/person/day; bacon and ham 16g/person/day). The mean household consumption of red meat (beef, lamb and pork), averaged over the

Figure 3.3   Trends in consumption of meats

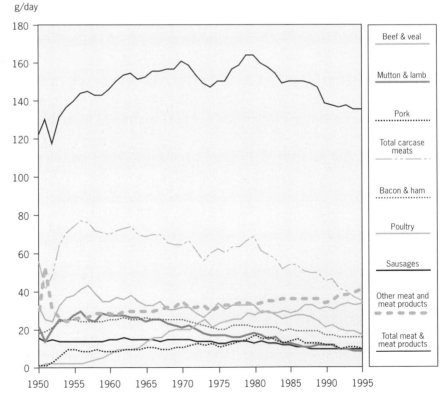

Source: National Food Survey 1950-1995

years 1993 to 1995, is 38g/day and that of bacon and ham is 16g/day. Meat products, with the exception of sausages, have shown a steady rise since the 1950s (see Figure 3.3). Among meat products, the most important change has been the increasing popularity of convenience products.

3.2.4.2   The vast majority (98%) of the British Adults Survey participants ate meat on 1 or more days of the survey week, while 1.6% ate no meat at all, of whom 0.7% consumed fish but no meat. These data cannot distinguish between those who never eat meat or fish from those who consume it occasionally (ie less than once a week). On average men (16 to 64 years) ate meat and meat products ten times and women (16 to 64 years) eight times during the 7-day recording period. The average consumption of red and processed meat (beef, lamb and pork, including that in meat products) was 92g/day for consumers only. One standard deviation above the mean consumption was 144g/day, representing the 85th percentile. Extreme consumers (97.5th percentile) averaged 214g/day. The average consumption of all meat (including poultry and poultry products) was 112g/day for consumers only. Extreme consumers (at the 97.5th percentile) ate 236g/day. There was a good correlation between the frequency of consumption and the amount consumed during the 7-day recording period (Males, Spearman's Correlation Coefficient 0.63; Females, Spearman's Correlation Coefficient 0.67).

3.2.5   *Fish*   Total fish consumption has fallen on average from about 27g/day in 1950 to 21g/day in 1995, of which about 6g was oily fish. Fish consumption is highly skewed and in the British Adults Survey consumers of oily fish had intakes of about 19g/day.

3.2.6   *Bread and other cereal products*   In 1950 bread consumption was 234g/day, falling to 154g/day by 1970 and to 108g/day in 1995. In terms of the contribution of bread to total energy intake, it has declined from 15% in 1970 to 13% in 1995. The consumption of National Wheatmeal Bread, introduced during the Second World War, declined rapidly after white bread was reintroduced in 1955. Although consumption of wholemeal bread increased from 1978 until 1986, this has not reversed the long term decline of bread consumption in the home. Other cereal products (e.g. breakfast cereals, rice, pasta, cakes and pastries) represented 19% of the total energy intake, a rise of 5% since 1970.

3.2.7   *Potatoes*   Total potato consumption has declined by 49% since 1950 from 277g/day to 142g/day, of which 115g/day is fresh potato. The percentage contribution from fresh potatoes to the total energy intake in the household diet has reduced slightly from 5% in 1970 to less than 4% in 1995.

3.2.8   *Vegetables other than potatoes*   Over the past few decades the range of vegetables purchased by British consumers has increased markedly. Total vegetable consumption has risen since 1950 (120g/day), to a high of 174g/day in 1986, but recently has gradually fallen to about 152g/day in 1995. Fresh vegetables still form most of the market (65% of total purchased), followed by canned (21%), frozen (9%) and other processed vegetables (Figure 3.4). Some vegetables will not be included in these figures, as they are 'hidden' in other

51

Figure 3.4   Trends in consumption of vegetables (excluding potatoes) and fruit

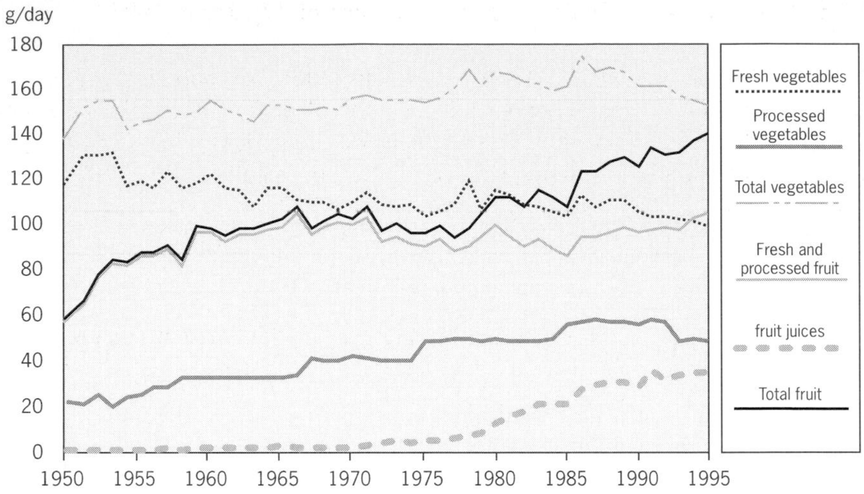

g/day

Legend:
- Fresh vegetables
- Processed vegetables
- Total vegetables
- Fresh and processed fruit
- fruit juices
- Total fruit

Source: National Food Survey 1950-1995

foods and classified elsewhere, e.g. ready meals that contain vegetables but also contain meat or fish will be classified as meat or fish products.

3.2.8.1   The British Adults Survey was used to obtain estimates of the average frequency of consumption by the adult population per week. Men and women ate vegetables excluding potatoes eight times per week, ie, eight servings during the 7-day recording period. There was a good correlation between the frequency of consumption and the amount consumed during the 7-day recording period (Males, Spearman's Correlation Coefficient 0.70; Females, Spearman's Correlation Coefficient 0.75).

3.2.8.2   *Fresh green vegetables*   Consumption of fresh green vegetables has declined from 56g/day in 1950 to 32g/day in 1995. Consumption of brassicas and peas and beans have fallen to a third of the 1950 levels, whereas consumption of leafy salads has doubled from 4 to 8g/day.

3.2.8.3   *Other fresh vegetables*   Consumption of these vegetables has increased slightly from 62g/day in 1950 to 67g/day in 1995. Consumption of carrots has increased to 16g/day, but that of other root vegetables and tomatoes (now 7 and 14g/day respectively) has fallen by a third over the same period. Consumption of alliums has remained fairly constant and is now 13g/day. Consumption of other fresh vegetables, including red/green peppers, celery, cucumbers, mushrooms and courgettes has reached 18g/day.

3.2.8.4   *Processed vegetables*   Canned vegetable consumption (excluding potatoes) increased to a peak of 33g/day in 1970 and has stayed fairly constant with 1995 intakes of 32g/day. Canned tomato consumption has doubled from 3 to 7g/

52

day between 1970 and 1994 and bean (including baked bean) consumption has fallen from a peak of 19g/day in 1987 to a value of 17g/day in 1995.

3.2.8.5 *Frozen vegetables* These have substituted not only for canned vegetables, but also for fresh vegetables in the case of peas and beans. Consumption of frozen vegetables and products has increased from 7g/day in 1970 to 14g/day in 1995. Consumption of frozen peas has increased slightly since 1970 to 5g/day. There has been a large increase in the consumption of other frozen vegetables and products throughout the 1970s and 1980s from 4g/day in 1970 to 9g/day in 1995.

3.2.8.6 Consumption of vegetable products other than frozen (including vegetable salads, vegetable ready meals, vegetarian products, vegetable pies etc.) has also grown extensively, from less than 1g/day in 1970 to 5g/day in 1995.

3.2.9 *Fruit* Total consumption of fruit has almost doubled since 1950 from 73g/day to 142g/day in 1995. The consumption of fresh fruit increased by about one third between 1950 and 1970, (from 58g/day to 78g/day) and has now risen to 96g/day in 1995. This equates to a rise in the percentage contribution of all fruit to total energy intake from 2% in 1970 to 4% in 1995. The figure of 4% in 1995 breaks down into 2% from fresh fruit and over 1% from fruit juice. Consumption of canned fruit also increased during the 1950s and 1960s from 7g/day in 1950 to a high of 20g/day in 1966 and has subsequently fallen to 6g/day. The largest change has been in the consumption of fruit juice, which has increased dramatically and at 35ml/day now accounts for nearly 25% of total fruit and fruit products consumed. Fresh fruit accounts for 67% of the market, canned fruit 5% of the market and dried and frozen 2% of the total market.

3.2.9.1 As with vegetables, the British Adults Survey was used to obtain estimates of the frequency of consumption by the adult population per week. Men ate five servings and women ate seven servings of fruit (including fruit juice) per week. There was a very strong association between the frequency of consumption and the amount consumed during the 7-day recording period (Males, Spearman's Correlation Coefficient 0.95; Females, Spearman's Correlation Coefficient 0.95).

3.2.9.2 *Citrus fruits* The consumption of oranges rose between 1952 and 1970 from 11g/day to 15g/day and has since fallen to 10g/day in 1995. This fall is partly offset by the increased consumption of fruit juice and other citrus fruits.

3.2.9.3 *Other fresh fruit* The most popular fresh fruits are apples followed by bananas. Banana consumption was only 5g/day in 1950, had risen to 12g/day by 1970 and was 25g/day in 1995 (108% increase since 1970). Apple consumption, on the other hand, has decreased by around 23% to 26g/day in 1995.

3.2.10 *Beverages* Tea consumption (measured as dry weight) has shown a sharp decrease from a level of 11g/day in the early 1960's to its current level of 6g/day. Coffee consumption tripled between 1950 and 1973, reaching a level of over 2g/day, but has since remained fairly constant. Consumption of other beverages, such as cocoa and other branded food drinks, was 1g/day in 1995.

3.2.11 *Soya and Related Products* The NFS shows that there has been a significant increase in the consumption of novel protein foods, including "soya mince" and textured vegetable protein from 1976 to 1995. However absolute intakes of novel protein foods are still low, averaging less than 1g/day. This total cannot be attributed to soya protein alone, as this NFS category also includes novel protein foods that are not based on soya, e.g. textured mycoprotein.

3.3 Nutrient intakes

3.3.1. *Fats and fatty acids* Although there has been a steady reduction in the amount of fat in the diet during the last twenty years, there has been virtually no change in the average contribution made by fat to energy derived from food (Figure 3.5). This is because the amount of carbohydrate and the amount of energy in the diet has also decreased. The latest NFS data show that fat provides about 40% of food energy. However, there have been important changes in the types of fat and fatty acids consumed. Figure 3.6 shows the trends since 1955 in consumption of the main food groups contributing to total fat intake. The intake of saturated fatty acids has declined since 1980 from 19% of food energy to just below 16% in 1995. During this time there has been a corresponding increase in polyunsaturated fatty acids from 5% to 7% of food energy. Energy intake from monounsaturated fatty acids and trans fatty acids have remained fairly constant at approximately 15% and 2% of food energy respectively.

3.3.1.1 From the British Adults Survey, the average daily intake of fat was 102g (2.5–97.5 per centile: 50–156g) for men and 74g (2.5–97.5 per centile: 31–125g) for women, both corresponding to about 40% (2.5-97.5 per centile: 29-

Figure 3.5   Trends in proportion of food energy from fat and fatty acids

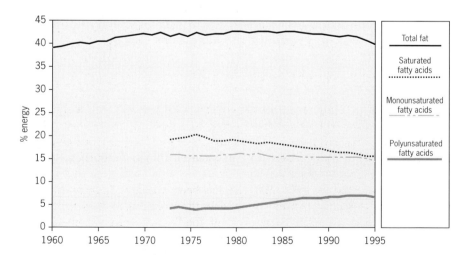

Source: National Food Survey 1950-1995

Figure 3.6   Trends in contribution made by food groups to fat intake

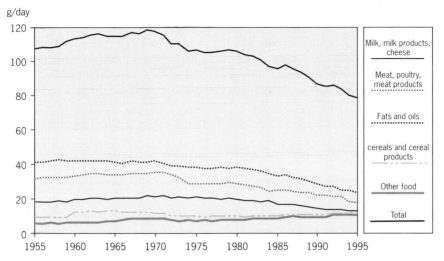

g/day

Source: National Food Survey 1955-1995

50%) of food energy. Women obtained a slightly higher proportion of total (and food) energy from saturated fatty acids than men. The main sources of fat in the diet are meat and meat products, cereal products (particularly biscuits, buns, cakes & pastries, puddings and ice cream), fat spreads, milk and fried vegetables (including chips and roast potatoes). The main sources of saturated fatty acids are similar, except that fried vegetables do not make such a significant contribution.

3.3.1.2   Intake of n-6 polyunsaturates was higher for men (mean 13.8g/day, 2.5–97.5 per centile: 5.1–29g/day, 5.1% total energy) than for women (9.6g/day, 2.5–97.5 per centile: 3.1–21.3g/day, 5.1% total energy). Dietary sources of n-6 polyunsaturates are vegetables (including roast and chipped potatoes), cereal products, fat spreads and meat and meat products. Population average intakes of longer chain n-3 polyunsaturates (e.g. EPA and DHA from oily fish) were about 0.1g/day for men and women. However, this result is skewed as a significant proportion of the population has a negligible intake of oily fish. Intakes in consumers of oily fish were higher at 0.3g/day for men and 0.2g/day for women. The average P/S ratio was higher for men than women (0.40 vs. 0.38).

3.3.1.3   Trans fatty acid intake in the average adult is approximately 5g/day (2.5–97.5 per centile: 1.0–11.3 g/day), which equates to about 2% of total food energy. Dietary sources of trans fatty acids are margarines, and shortenings in cakes, biscuits and pastry products, and milk and meat from ruminants.

3.3.2.   *Carbohydrates*   Since 1950, there has been a decline both in the absolute amount of carbohydrate in the diet and in the contribution it makes to food energy (Figure 3.1). In 1950 about 52% of food energy came from carbohydrates, mostly starch. Since that time, there has been a long term decline in the consumption of bread and potatoes and the amount of starch in the diet has fallen. Energy from carbohydrate contributed about 46% food energy in 1995, with 27% of food energy coming from starch and 11% from non-milk extrinsic sugars. From the British Adults Survey, men had an average carbohydrate intake of 272g/day (2.5–97.5 per centile: 131–435g/day) which is equal to 41.6% total energy, compared with 193g/day (2.5–97.5 per centile: 83–314g/day, 43% total energy) for women. The main sources of carbohydrate are cereal products (in particular bread and breakfast cereals) and potatoes.

3.3.3. *Non-starch polysaccharide (NSP)* Intakes have been calculated from NFS data since 1985. There has been a slight decrease in NSP intakes since 1986 from 13g/day in 1986 to just under 12g/day in 1995. About 45% of NSP is provided by cereal products such as bread and 51% by fruit and vegetables.

3.3.4. *Vitamin C* Absolute intakes of vitamin C have remained relatively constant since the 1950s. Though energy intakes have fallen considerably over this period, the concentration of vitamin C in the diet has increased (from 20mg/1000kcal in the 1950s to 29mg/1000kcal in 1995). From the British Adults Survey, no significant difference in intakes of vitamin C between men and women were found, although women had higher intakes from supplements than men. Average intakes from all sources were 75mg/day (2.5–97.5 per centile: 19–227mg/day) in men and 73mg/day (2.5–97.5 per centile: 14–209mg/day) in women. There were no age related differences for men in intakes of vitamin C from all sources, but women aged 16–24 years had intakes markedly lower than the overall average for women (mean 62mg/day, 2.5–97.5 per centile: 12–189mg/day). Approximately 80% of dietary vitamin C is provided by fruits and vegetables, and until the mid 1980s potatoes were the main source. Since that time, fruit juices have become the main source due to increased consumption.

3.3.5 *Vitamin E* Vitamin E has only been calculated from NFS data recently. A special analysis in 1979 estimated intake at 8.3mg/day. Tea was estimated to provide approximately 25% of total intake, but it has since been suggested that this is not bioavailable. Intake in 1995 was 9.5 mg/day; this excludes any contribution from tea. The NFS also noted an increase in the consumption of fats and oils rich in polyunsaturated fatty acids, which contributes to vitamin E intake. Oils and fats are currently the source of 48% of vitamin E, compared to 26% in 1979. From the British Adults Survey, vitamin E intakes from all sources, including supplements, were higher in men than in women (mean 11.7mg/day vs. 8.6mg/day, 2.5–97.5 per centile: 3.7–23.4mg/day vs. 2.6–20.4mg/day) and supplements were an equally important source in men as in women. Other significant sources of vitamin E are vegetables including fried potatoes (22%) and cereal products (21%).

3.3.6 *Retinol* Retinol levels have been recorded separately by the NFS since 1969. Levels peaked in the late 1970s and early 1980s at 1030µg/day, and have since reduced by approximately 28% to 740µg/day. The British Adults Survey found that retinol intakes were higher for men than for women, with mean daily levels of 1280µg and 1130µg respectively (2.5–97.5 per centiles: 190–6670µg vs. 135–5780µg). Approximately 58% of this total comes from liver and liver products, with a further 14% from milk and milk products, and 13% from fat spreads.

3.3.7 *Carotenes* The NFS has separately calculated intakes of β-carotene since 1969, when the diet contained 2110 µg/day. Intakes have since fallen to 1640µg/day in 1995. From the British Adults Survey, intakes are slightly higher in men than in women (mean 2410µg vs. 2130µg, 2.5-97.5 per centile: 250–7560µg vs 200–6520µg). Carotene intake is lower in the 16-24 year old age group (mean 1890µg for men vs. 1580µg for women, 2.5–97.5 per centile: 170–6490µg vs 170–5670µg). The principle source of β-carotene in the diet is carrots.

3.3.8. *Folate* Folate intakes from the NFS have increased from an estimated 213µg/day in 1980 to the current level of 237µg/day. From the British Adults Survey, the mean daily folate intakes for men were significantly higher than for women (mean 312µg vs. 219µg, 2.5–97.5 per centile: 145–562µg vs. 95–385µg respectively). The main sources of folate in the diet are cereal products (21%), vegetables (16%) and beers (10%).

3.3.9 *Iron* According to NFS data, iron intakes have been gradually declining since 1963. This decline probably reflects the reduction in total energy intake because the contribution of iron in 1995, at 5.3mg/1000 kcal, was similar to that in 1965 (5.4mg/1000 kcal). From the British Adults Survey, mean iron intake for men was 14mg/day (2.5–97.5 per centile: 6.5–27.1mg/day) and for women, 12.3mg/day (2.5–97.5 per centile: 4.7–30.7mg/day). Cereal products contributed 42% of dietary iron intake with meat and meat products contributing a further 23%.

3.3.10 *Calcium* From NFS data, calcium intakes have shown a similar pattern to iron intakes with levels gradually declining from the 1960s to the present day. This pattern followed a similar increase and decline in milk consumption over the same period of time. However, the concentration of calcium in the diet increased from 396 mg/1000 kcal in 1963 to 455 mg/1000 kcal in 1994. From the British Adults Survey mean calcium consumption for men was 940mg/day (2.5–97.5 per centile: 410–1607mg/day) and for women 730mg/day (2.5–97.5 per centile: 266–1317mg/day). Milk and milk products provide 48% of dietary calcium, and a further 25% comes from cereal products.

3.3.11 *Sodium and potassium* NFS data on sodium intakes are available from 1985 onwards. This excludes the contribution from table salt. During this period, intakes have decreased slightly to the current level of 2.5g/day. Potassium intakes have been reported since 1992 and are currently 2.5g/day. The British Adults Survey found that the average sodium excretion (best estimate of total sodium intake) was 173mmol/day in men and 132mmol/day in women. This is equivalent to 10.2g salt/day (3.9g sodium) in men and 7.8g salt/day (3.0g sodium) in women. Potassium intakes were 3.2g/day (82mmol/day) in men and 2.4g/day (62mmol/day) in women. The major dietary sources of sodium were bread (22%) and meat products (27%), particularly bacon & ham (11%). The major dietary sources of potassium were vegetables (28%) particularly potatoes (17%), meat & meat products (13%), milk & milk products (14%) and cereal products (14%).

3.3.12   *Selenium*   Neither the NFS nor the NDNS estimates intakes of selenium. From the British Total Diet Study, intake was estimated to be 60μg/day in the mid 1970s, 63μg/day in 1985 and 60μg/day in 1991[28]. Approximately half was derived from cereals and cereal products, 40% from meat and fish and 10% from milk and dairy products. Fruit and vegetables provided little or no selenium.

3.4   The diets of children

3.4.1   The National Diet and Nutrition Survey (NDNS) of Children aged 1½–4½ years was carried out between July 1992 and June 1993[25] and provides greater insight into food and nutrient intake by British pre-school children. Much of the following data are based on this report. Some data have also been taken from the survey on the Diets of British Schoolchildren which was carried out in 1983[26] and which contains less detailed information on nutrient intakes. Intakes of selected nutrients by children, obtained from the above two surveys of children, are presented in Table 3.1 (see p 48).

3.4.2   *Fat*   The average daily intake of total fat was 45.7g (2.5–97.5 per centile: 23.2–74.8g) for children aged 1½–4½ years. This corresponds to about 36% of food energy (2.5–97.5 per centile: 25–46%). The mean total fat intake for 10-11 year olds was 83.1g/day (2.5–97.5 per centile: 47.7–118.5g/day), whilst for 14-15 year olds it was 96.2g/day (2.5–97.5 per centile: 49.2–143.2g/day). The contribution to food energy was 38% in both cases, with a 2.5–97.5 percentile range of 34.6–41.4% for 10–11 year olds and a 2.5–97.5 percentile range of 34.2–41.8% for 14–15 year olds.

3.4.2.1   The average daily intake of saturated fatty acids by the 1½–4½ year olds was 20.6g/day (2.5–97.5 per centile: 9.4–34.7g/day) which is equivalent to 16.2% (2.5–97.5 per centile: 10.0–23.5%) of food energy. Cis-monounsaturated fatty acids contributed an average of 11.1% of food energy (2.5–97.5 per centile: 7.4–15.0%), with daily consumption averaging 14.2g (2.5–97.5 per centile: 6.9–24.0g/day). Average daily intake of cis-polyunsaturated fatty acids by this age group was 5.9g/day (2.5–97.5 per centile: 2.3–11.7g/day) providing on average 4.6% of food energy (2.5–97.5 per centile: 2.3–8.2%).

3.4.3   *Carbohydrates including fibre*   The average daily carbohydrate intake by children aged 1½–4½ years was 155g (2.5–97.5 per centile: 88–243g), equivalent to 51% of food energy (2.5–67.5 per centile: 39–64%). Non-milk extrinsic (NME) sugars provided 18.7% of food energy (2.5–67.5 per centile: 5.8–35.6%). Intakes of non-starch polysaccharides for this age group had a 2.5–97.5 per centile range from 2.5–11.4g/day (mean 6.1g/day).

3.4.4   *Vitamins C, E and total carotenes*   For children aged 1½–4½ years, the majority of vitamin C (93%) was obtained from food sources, with a mean daily intake from food of 48.6mg (2.5–97.5 per centile: 9.5–154mg) compared with an

58

intake from food and dietary supplements combined of 51.8mg (2.5–97.5 per centile: 9.5–157mg). There was no significant difference in intake between age groups. Mean daily intakes by the 10–11 year olds and the 14–15 year olds had a 2.5–97.5 per centile range of 40.6–44.7mg/day, with intakes being highest amongst the older boys. Thirty-five per cent of the children aged 1½–4½ years had intakes of vitamin C below the RNI. The intake of vitamin E by the 1½–4½ year olds was almost all accounted for by food sources, with an average intake from food of 4.3mg (2.5–97.5 per centile: 1.7–9.0mg). Those in the youngest age group (1½–2½ year olds) had significantly lower intakes than children aged 2½–4½ years. The mean intake of total carotenes (β-carotene equivalents) for 1½–4½ year olds was 872mg/day (2.5–97.5 per centile: 155–3002mg/day) which was all obtained from food sources. Average intake of carotenes increased with age, and was highest for boys in the oldest age group (3½–4½ years). The main sources of vitamin C were soft drinks (14.7%), fruit juice (9.5%), potatoes (5.5%) and vegetables (3.4%). Just under a quarter (23%) of the total vitamin E intake was obtained from fat spreads, with vegetables, including potatoes and snacks, providing slightly more (26%). Over half, 56%, of total carotenes intake came from vegetables, including potatoes and savoury snacks, with cooked carrots being the single largest provider.

3.4.5   *Calcium and iron*   For the 1½–4½ year olds, mean daily calcium intake was 637mg (2.5–97.5 per centile: 246–1255mg) for the whole sample population with mean total iron intakes being 5.5mg (2.5–97.5 per centile: 2.6–10.4mg). The average daily contribution to total iron intakes from food was 5.4mg (2.5–97.5 per centile: 2.6–9.2mg); all calcium came from dietary sources. Eighty-four per cent of children under four years had a mean total iron intake which was below the RNI, with 57% of those over four years having an iron intake below the RNI for that age group. Mean intakes of calcium were in excess of the RNIs for children aged 1½–4½ years. Mean calcium intakes by schoolchildren had a 2.5–97.5 per centile range of 725–961mg/day, with mean iron intakes having a 2.5–97.5 per centile range of 8.6–11.9mg/day. Boys had higher intakes of both nutrients. The main source of calcium in the toddlers diet was milk and milk products, which provided 64% of the mean intake, with milk providing 51% alone. For the 1½–4½ year olds the contribution of milk to calcium intake decreased with age, whilst the contribution from cereals and cereal products increased. The main source of iron in the diets of the toddlers was iron fortified cereals and cereal products, providing about half (48%) of the total intake.

3.5   Variations in diet and nutrition according to social class, income group and region

3.5.1   *Carcase meats (beef, lamb and pork).* Figure 3.7 shows that the average consumption of these meats, excluding that in meat products, (averaged NFS data over years 1993–1995) is similar in all income groups. The consumption is highest in the West Midlands and lowest in Scotland (Figure 3.8).

3.5.2   *Fruit and vegetables, excluding potatoes.* The NFS data averaged over years 1993–1995 show a trend to lower consumption of fruit and vegetables from income group A to income Group D (Figure 3.9). The consumption of fruit

Figure 3.7   Consumption of total carcase meat (beef, lamb & pork excluding that in processed meats and meat products) by income group

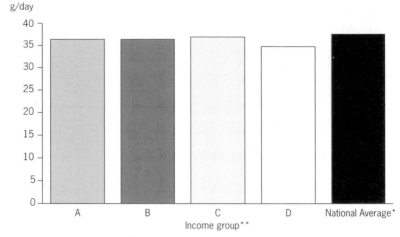

Source: National Food Survey, 1993-1995[23]

*Average of all groups including E1, E2 and OAP
**As described in the NFS Annual Reports

Figure 3.8   Consumption of total carcase meats (beef, lamb & pork excluding that in processed meats and meat products) by region

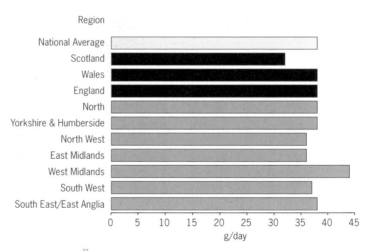

Source: National Food Survey, 1993-1995[23]

and vegetables is considerably lower in Scotland than in England and Wales and in the North and North West regions of England compared to the other regions (Figure 3.10).

3.5.3. *Fat and fatty acids*   The NFS indicates that there are no systematic differences in the proportion of energy derived from fat and saturated fatty acids in different regions or between different income groups of Great Britain. The British Adults Survey showed a similar pattern. However the P/S ratio was significantly lower in men and women in social classes IV and V compared to

60

Figure 3.9   Consumption of vegetables (excluding potatoes) and fruit by income group

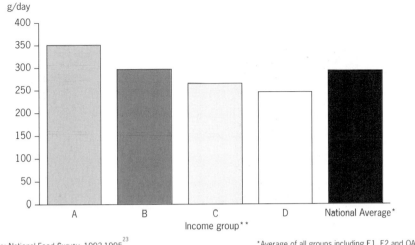

g/day

Source: National Food Survey, 1993-1995[23]   *Average of all groups including E1, E2 and OAP
                                                                        **As described in the NFS Annual Reports

Figure 3.10   Consumption of vegetables (excluding potatoes) and fruit by region

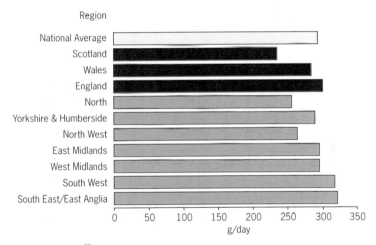

Source: National Food Survey, 1993-1995[23]

those in non-manual classes. The 1994 NFS data show that the difference in P/S
ratio between income groups is now small. Since about 1980, the decline in the
proportion of energy derived from saturated fatty acids has occurred in all
income groups and regions.

3.5.4   *Vitamins C and E, and β-carotene*   Figures 3.11–3.16 show the average
intakes of vitamins C, E and β-carotene by income group and region (averaged
NFS data over years 1993–1995). Both vitamin C and β-carotene intakes are
lower in income groups C and D compared with income groups A and B as
would be expected from the pattern of consumption of fruit and vegetables in
these income groups (see section 3.5.2). The British Adults Survey also showed

61

Figure 3.11   Vitamin C intake by income group

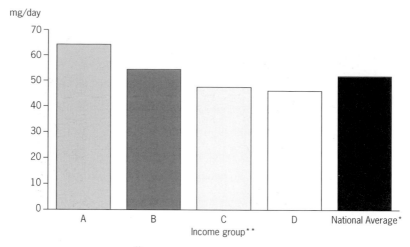

mg/day

Source: National Food Survey, 1993-1995[23]

*Average of all groups including E1, E2 and OAP
**As described in the NFS Annual Reports

Figure 3.12   Vitamin C intake by region

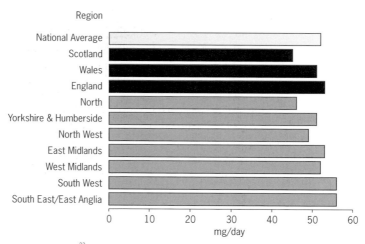

Source: National Food Survey, 1993-1995[23]

a strong effect of social class on intake of these nutrients, with lower intakes in social classes IV and V. Regional variations are less but tended towards a lower intake in the North. There were slightly lower intakes of vitamin C in the North West and in the West Midlands than in the South East. β-carotene intakes are lowest in the North West, West Midlands and Scotland. These differences in intakes were reflected in regional and social class differences in plasma levels of β-carotene and vitamin E measures in the British Adults Survey. Men in London and the South East and men in non-manual social classes had significantly higher levels of plasma carotene and vitamin E than men in the Northern region and

Figure 3.13 Vitamin E intake by income group

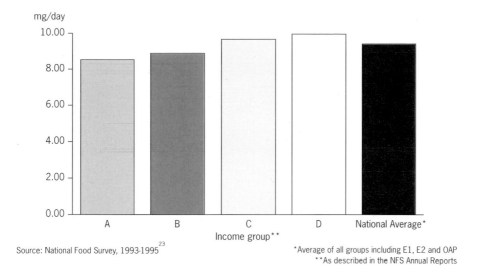

Source: National Food Survey, 1993-1995[23]

*Average of all groups including E1, E2 and OAP
**As described in the NFS Annual Reports

Figure 3.14 Vitamin E intake by region

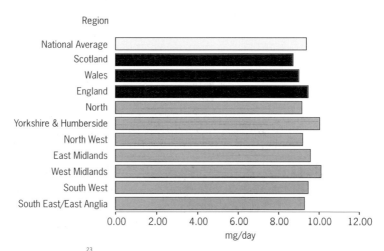

Source: National Food Survey, 1993-1995[23]

men in manual social classes. Women in London and the South East had significantly higher levels of plasma carotene than women living elsewhere but there were no differences in plasma vitamin E levels. A social class difference was also seen in women, with women in non-manual households having significantly higher levels of plasma carotene and vitamin E than women from manual households.

3.5.5. *Folate and Retinol* The British Adults Survey found that intakes of retinol and folate were lower in Scotland than in other parts of Britain for both men and women. For women, intakes of folate and retinol were lower in unemployed women and intakes decreased across the social classes, with those in social clas-

Figure 3.15   Beta-carotene intake by income group

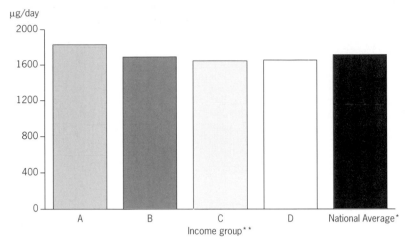

μg/day

Source: National Food Survey, 1993-1995[23]

*Average of all groups including E1, E2 and OAP
**As described in the NFS Annual Reports

Figure 3.16   Beta-carotene intake by region

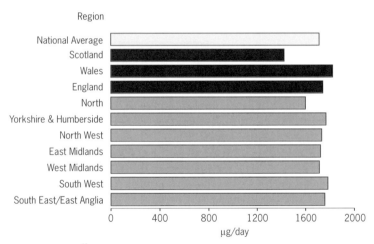

Source: National Food Survey, 1993-1995[23]

ses I and II having the highest intakes. There was very little variation in retinol and folate intake by men with region, employment status or social class.

3.5.6.   Tables 3.2a and 3.2b show intakes of starchy staples (including potatoes), vegetables (excluding potatoes), fruit, fish, meat and meat products recorded in the British Adults Survey by region. Only a few regional differences in the types of foods consumed emerged. Men and women from the North were less likely to eat pasta and rice and more likely to eat potatoes especially chips than those from the South East. Unlike men, fewer women in Scotland consumed whole-meal bread compared with women from other regions. Fewer vegetables and fruits were consumed in Scotland and the North and this was especially evident

Table 3.2a   Regional consumption of foods in women

Food Group	Mean consumption (grams/person/day)			
	Scotland	Northern	Midlands	London, SE
Staple starches				
Pasta	13	5	7	11
Rice	10	8	9	14
White bread	54	50	48	42
Wholemeal bread	16	23	28	43
Other Bread	13	15	12	14
Potato chips	35	38	31	24
Fried and roast potatoes	4	8	12	13
Other potato products	1	1	0	1
Other potatoes	51	54	59	57
Total staple starches	**197**	**202**	**206**	**219**
Carrots	1	1	2	2
Other salad vegetables	14	17	17	16
Raw tomatoes	10	14	16	21
Peas	9	15	14	12
Green beans	2	2	4	3
Baked beans	10	11	11	11
Leafy green vegetables	11	12	14	16
Cooked carrots	6	10	9	9
Fresh tomatoes	2	2	2	2
Other vegetables	33	35	34	44
Total vegetables	**98**	**119**	**123**	**136**
Fruit				
Apples and pears	20	21	34	31
Orange and other citrus	18	10	12	12
Bananas	10	7	12	11
Canned fruit in juice	1	2	2	4
Canned fruit in syrup	6	3	3	3
Other fruit	21	18	20	26
Total fruit	**76**	**61**	**83**	**87**
Fish				
Fried white fish	11	11	9	9
Other white fish	6	8	6	6
Shellfish	2	2	1	2
Oily fish	5	7	4	6
Total fish	**24**	**28**	**20**	**23**
Meat and meat products				
Bacon and ham	13	14	10	12
Beef and veal	36	29	28	31
Lamb	2	7	7	9
Pork	6	8	7	9
Coated chicken	1	2	1	2
Chicken and turkey	19	18	20	20
Liver	3	5	4	3
Burger and kebabs	6	5	5	6
Sausages	9	7	8	8
Meat Pie etc	11	16	14	11
Other meat products	18	10	11	11
Total meat and meat products	**124**	**121**	**115**	**122**

Source: Dietary and Nutritional Survey of British Adults—Further Analysis[933]

Table 3.2b   Regional consumption of foods in men

Food Group	Mean consumption (grams/person/day)			
	Scotland	Northern	Midlands	London, SE
Staple starches				
Pasta	14	8	7	12
Rice	17	17	16	21
White bread	84	87	86	79
Wholemeal bread	27	40	41	29
Other Bread	14	13	14	14
Potato chips	60	66	51	42
Fried and roast potatoes	11	14	21	22
Other potato products	1	1	0	0
Other potatoes	75	80	93	76
Total staple starches	**303**	**326**	**329**	**295**
Vegetables				
Carrots	1	1	1	1
Other salad vegetables	14	14	18	18
Raw tomatoes	14	12	17	16
Peas	10	20	21	17
Green beans	2	2	5	5
Baked beans	16	19	21	16
Leafy green vegetables	9	15	18	20
Cooked carrots	5	13	13	11
Fresh tomatoes	2	2	3	4
Other vegetables	37	39	45	49
Total vegetables	**110**	**137**	**162**	**157**
Fruit				
Apples and pears	24	24	29	31
Orange and other citrus	13	9	8	8
Bananas	9	9	9	7
Canned fruit in juice	1	2	2	2
Canned fruit in syrup	4	3	5	5
Other fruit	10	12	16	19
Total fruit	**61**	**59**	**69**	**72**
Fish				
Fried white fish	17	17	12	14
Other white fish	5	6	6	7
Shellfish	1	3	1	3
Oily fish	7	9	6	9
Total fish	**30**	**35**	**25**	**33**
Meat and meat products				
Bacon and ham	18	21	20	19
Beef and veal	45	46	41	45
Lamb	4	9	13	11
Pork	9	12	12	12
Coated chicken	3	2	1	4
Chicken and turkey	27	24	27	27
Liver	3	4	4	5
Burger and kebabs	10	9	6	11
Sausages	13	13	14	15
Meat Pie etc	26	32	24	22
Other meat products	19	19	17	15
Total meat and meat products	**177**	**191**	**179**	**186**

Source: Dietary and Nutritional Survey of British Adults—Further Analysis[933]

amongst men. More meat pies and other meat products were consumed by both men and women in Scotland and the North than in the Midlands and the South, and women but not men in Scoland ate more beef than women elsewhere.

3.5.7   Men and women in the higher social classes were more likely to eat fruit and fruit juice, vegetables especially salad vegetables, oily fish and shellfish, pasta, rice and wholemeal bread. More men and women in the lower social classes consumed potato chips or fried potatoes than in the higher social classes.

4. Epidemiology of Diet and Cancers

4.1 Types of epidemiological studies

4.1.1 *Introduction*

4.1.1.1 Epidemiology is the study of the distribution and determinants of disease, such as cancer, in and between populations. By describing the characteristics of populations or population subgroups it can identify factors which are associated with a higher or lower risk of disease, some of which may be causally connected. Although such evidence about causation is often circumstantial and incomplete it may allow the generation of hypotheses that can be tested by other means. It may also identify some factors whose influence on disease may not, for a variety of reasons, be easily or at all tested by other means. While epidemiological studies may produce associations from which causal inferences can be drawn, establishing causal links is much more difficult.

4.1.1.2 The strength of causal inference that can be drawn from epidemiological studies differs with different types of study design. Broadly, epidemiological studies can be divided into observational or experimental designs (either individual or population based). The distinction between observational and experimental studies is that in the latter the researcher determines the exposure, whereas in the former the researcher observes but does not determine exposure. Experimental studies assessing the effectiveness of interventions in a more realistic setting are called intervention studies. Individual-based observational studies may be further divided into cross-sectional, case-control, or cohort studies; individual-based experimental studies can be clinical or field trials. Observational studies in populations are known as ecological studies and population-based experimental studies are called community trials. The key principles of each type of study are described below in sections 4.1.2 to 4.1.6. When drawing causal inferences the most powerful studies are experimental studies, followed by individual based observational studies, particularly cohort studies. The review presented here mostly draws on case-control and cohort studies. For cancer, the experimental studies are fewer and are difficult to interpret as they often cannot involve all stages of cancer development; or outcomes may be restricted to a marker of cancer, rather than the cancer itself; or they may not have been continued for sufficiently long for an effect to be evident.

4.1.1.3 The findings from epidemiological studies need to be interpreted after considering the effects of chance, bias, and confounding. The interpretation of the findings of a study is usually guided by the levels of statistical significance of the results obtained. However, simply relying on the p-value, or whether the confidence interval included or excluded 1.0, may be misleading. The role chance played in obtaining the result needs to be considered. A study that makes many comparisons is likely, by chance alone, to find some statistically significant results; a study that does not show any statistically significant results may be flawed either in terms of the number of subjects included or the accuracy and relevance of the measure of diet used or may reflect a lack of association. The results should be interpreted on the basis of biological plausibility as well as statistical significance. The results may also be influenced by bias. Bias is a systematic effect that may influence the results of the study (and the publication of the results) either to increase or decrease the apparent effect; bias in the selection of subjects for inclusion in the study is one of the most important sources of bias but there may also be a bias in the way information is obtained from different subjects in the study (see 4.1.4). The effect reported in the study may have been due to an unmeasured confounding factor. Thus a correlation between alcohol consumption and lung cancer merely reflects the fact that heavy drinkers often tend to be heavy smokers as well. Even after adjusting for known confounders, it is always possible that residual confounding is still present. Without consideration of all of these factors when interpreting the study, misleading conclusions may be drawn. In the systematic reviews presented a scoring system has been used to judge the scientific quality of the study (see section 5.1.3 and Annex 1 for more details). Problems of interpreting dietary studies are explored further in section 4.2

4.1.2 *Ecological studies.* Ecological studies relate the rates of disease in different populations to characteristics of the same populations, such as diet. For example, the classic study of Armstrong & Doll[29] showed strong correlations between intakes of fat and of meat and incidence of cancer at several sites, including breast, colon and prostate (see Figure 4.1 for relationship between meat consumption and risk of developing colon cancer). Temporal changes in

Figure 4.1   The Relationship between meat consumption and colorectal cancer in various countries adapted from Armstrong & Doll (1975)[29]

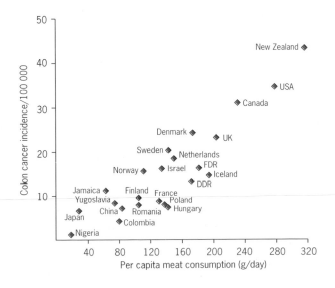

consumption of foods and nutrients have been related to changes in incidence of various cancers between 10 and 20 years later[30]. The main limitation of these studies is that there are many factors distinguishing different populations, many of which may not be known, which can act as confounders. Furthermore, the people with the disease and those exposed to the purported causative agent are not necessarily the same.

4.1.3 *Migrant studies.* As a type of ecological investigation, migrant studies have been used to disentangle the contribution of genetic and environmental factors to cancer causation by looking at the changes in disease incidence and mortality in people who move from one country to another. The groups that have been most extensively followed are the Japanese moving to the USA and immigrants to Australia. Over time the rates of cancer in the migrants approximate to those of the population of the host country. The substantial changes in risk seen within a generation in the migrants compared with their compatriots who remained at home has been interpreted as reflecting the influence of environment on cancer incidence. Dietary influences have been implicated for stomach, large bowel, breast and prostate cancers. While there may be an element of genetic predisposition for these cancers, this is clearly unlikely to differ over only a few generations, and so to account for changes in disease occurrence.

4.1.4 *Case-control studies.*

4.1.4.1 Case-control studies compare the dietary habits of people who have developed the disease under investigation (cases) with a group of people without the disease (controls). Case-control studies have the advantage that they can be carried out fairly quickly and are suited to the investigation of risk factors in rare diseases. They can also examine multiple risk factors simultaneously. They are, however, subject to two types of bias which may be particularly important in studies of diet and cancer: bias in the selection of patients and bias in the recall of past diet.

4.1.4.2 Two studies have examined the effects of recall and selection bias on estimates of cancer risk, by conducting a retrospective assessment of the diet of cases and controls who had previously been assessed in a prospective study. Comparing estimates of risk derived from a retrospective dietary assessment and from a contemporaneous dietary assessment in the same women, Giovannucci *et al*,[32] found higher risks based on the retrospective dietary assessment than with the contemporaneous dietary assessment. In the Canadian National Breast Cancer Screening Study, Friedenreich *et al*[33] reported that retrospective assessment of diet produced a slightly, but not statistically significant, higher risk than obtained from a contemporaneous dietary assessment in the same women. If bias of the size reported by Giovannucci does affect case-control studies, this might explain the discrepancy sometimes apparent between the results of cohort studies and case-control studies.

4.1.5 *Prospective cohort studies.*

4.1.5.1 Prospective cohort studies are not subject to the same potential biases as case-control studies and all aspects of diet and their interactions are potentially available for study. In a prospective study, a large population sample of presently healthy individuals is assessed for dietary and other lifestyle factors at baseline, and then followed for at least 5 years but usually 10 to 15 years or more until sufficient cases of cancer have arisen to evaluate risks. Such investigations are costly, and cohort studies of cancer have only been embarked upon relatively recently, as the accumulating evidence from case-control, migrant and ecologic studies has suggested that more detailed investigations are justified. However, latent periods between exposure and clinical cancer may be many years so that evidence accumulated even over 10 or 15 years may not cover the period of exposure. During the last ten years it has become increasingly clear that there are associations between the growth of the fetus and the development of some cancers in later adult life[34–36]. These observations are part of a wider body of ideas in which the metabolic capacity of an individual is influenced by fetal environment, which thereby sets, or programmes, metabolic behaviour for the remainder of that individuals life. The hypothesis proposes that the nutritional status and nutrient intake of the mother during pregnancy contribute directly to the susceptibility of the offspring to a wide range of potentially damaging exposures, for instance in food or in the environment, by modulating the individual's responses to them. Growth in childhood, maturation to adolescence and adult shape and size may all be influenced in part by this process. The cancers for which an association has been shown include ovary, prostate and breast[35–37]. If the development of cancer requires the accumulation of multiple hits, and cellular development during early life is one factor which acts in concert with other exposures at a later age, it may be necessary to consider the nutritional exposure of an individual over the whole lifespan.

4.1.5.2 Nested case-control studies   Dietary habits and other lifestyle factors are likely to change over the period of a prospective study, and the dietary intake of most individuals requires several repeated measures to be made in order to reduce inaccuracy in the assessments. Furthermore, if samples of blood and other biological specimens are obtained, they not only provide direct measures of nutritional status but can also be used as independent measures of diet or other risk factors. However, the need for repeat measures of diet and chemical analysis of biological material greatly adds to the expense if the information from all individuals is to be analysed. A recent approach has therefore been to store all baseline and follow up material such as dietary questionnaires and blood specimens, then to analyse the data several years later only from the cases in the cohort, and their matched controls. The specimens have to be stored at very low temperatures to minimise deterioration over the necessary long periods of time, but nested case-control studies potentially overcome some problems of measurement error encountered in the assessment of diet in cohort studies.

4.1.6 Intervention trials   Randomised intervention trials should remove the effects of bias and confounding completely if they are properly randomised. The randomised intervention trial tests the effect of a defined intervention in a specific population. They are good for demonstrating an effective intervention, although care should be taken in generalising the results to other populations not tested in the trial. However for practical reasons, randomised intervention trials are of limited use in testing some hypotheses, for instance those that require long term changes in behaviour. Demonstrating a protective effect of an intervention thought to act at an early stage in a disease, such as cancer, that develops over decades would require an intervention trial that also lasted over decades. Although intervention studies have the greatest scientific strength, their applicability is limited and their cost is great. They are often not feasible except in high risk groups from whom the applicability of findings to the general population may be debatable. Since there may be multifactorial nutritional causes and interactions between different dietary constituents in cancer, intervention with single, or even a few nutrients may be an inadequate test of a complex hypothesis.

4.1.7   *Estimates of risk*

4.1.7.1   The relative risk is used to express the strength of association between disease and a risk factor or measure of exposure such as diet. The relative risk is the ratio of the incidence of the disease in the exposed group, divided by the incidence of disease in the unexposed group. For retrospective studies, such as case-control studies, it is usually not possible to assess risk directly and it is estimated using the ratio of odds of disease (odds ratio). For most purposes there is little difference between these two measures of risk. The definition of exposed/ unexposed is usually arbitrary, as exposure is usually continuously variable, and depends on the way the researcher chooses to divide the distribution of the measure of exposure, such as diet. Where the distribution is continuous rather than a simple yes/no dichotomy, the researcher usually ranks subjects and then divides the distribution into groups such as thirds, fourths or fifths. Subjects are then allocated to these discrete groups: it is the custom to define the lowest level of exposure as the reference group (or "unexposed") and higher groups as the "exposed". If the relative risk or odds ratio is greater than one it indicates that the risk or odds of disease is greater when exposed (or at a higher level of consumption). If the risk or odds ratio is less than one it indicates that the risk is lower at higher levels of exposure. It may be misleading to compare directly risk estimates from different studies using different cut-offs (absolute and/or relative in terms of thirds, fourths and fifths) between lowest and highest levels of exposure. A further complication is that different studies use different levels of consumption, for example absolute or relative levels, as the reference category.

4.1.7.2   In order to assess how well the estimate of risk is likely to reflect the "true" effect, or that which would be obtained if the whole population had been measured rather than a sample, it is important to know how close the estimate derived from one sample might relate to the "truth" or underlying population effect. It is now common to express this as a confidence interval; this represents the range within which the risk that is being measured is likely to lie. It is commonly expressed as the 95% confidence interval; the higher the confidence level specified the wider the confidence interval. The width of this confidence interval will depend on the sample size; the larger the sample, the smaller the width of the interval. The convention is to say that if neither the upper nor the lower levels of the 95 per cent confidence interval encompasses one, then the difference in risk between levels of exposure is statistically significant. It is now possible to derive risk estimates and confidence intervals, adjusted for the effect of other factors. This allows an estimate of the effect of exposure on risk, independently accounting for these in a statistical sense. When comparing results across studies it is important to consider whether risk estimates have been adjusted, and whether the variables used in the analysis are comparable. Differences in results between studies may be related to the inclusion of different variables in the analysis rather than the underlying risk. An obvious example would be differences in risk estimates for lung cancer depending on whether or not smoking had been taken into account.

4.1.7.3   Any imprecision in measurements of exposure or outcome will tend to reduce the observed size of any actual association. The major source of such imprecision is the assessment of dietary exposure but there may also be imprecision in an ascertainment of cancer incidence.

4.1.7.4   Meta-analysis is a numerical summary, using statistical methods, of the results of a number of studies. It can be used to combine studies, which individually do not have sufficient power, to produce an analysis of greater power. Meta-analysis can also offer more precise estimates of the size of an effect than any individual study. However, the reliability of the estimated effect size depends on the quality of the analysis and the similarity of the combined studies. Meta-analyses of randomized controlled trials with standardised methodologies can give reliable estimates, but less confidence can be placed in combining the results of studies where methods of data collection and presentation might not be comparable. In addition, it is important to ensure that all relevant studies have been included, irrespective of their results, as a biased or incomplete review is potentially misleading.

4.1.8   *Public health implications*   From a public health point of view, the absolute effect the disease has on population mortality or morbidity is more important than the relative risk alone. More appropriate measures of this absolute effect are the *risk difference*, (sometimes called the attributable risk or excess risk or absolute risk) which is the difference in rates of occurrence between exposed or unexposed groups, or the *population attributable risk* which is a measure of the excess rate of disease in a total population which is attributable to an exposure[38]. From the latter it is possible to suggest the proportion by which the incidence rate of the population would change if the exposure was eliminated. The risk difference provides a measure of the absolute changes in the numbers of people affected by changes in the relative risk, given the underlying incidence rate of the cancer. At the same relative risk what determines the number of people in the population affected is the underlying incidence rate. For example, for a relative risk of 0.5, the incidence would decrease by 5 000 for a disease with an underlying incidence of 10 000 or by 500 for a disease with an underlying incidence of 1 000. From a public health perspective a small reduction in the relative risk of a common cancer can have more impact than a large reduction in the relative risk of a rare cancer.

4.2 The assessment of diet in case-control and cohort studies

4.2.1 Nutritional epidemiology provides the only direct approach to the assessment of risks from diet in human cancer, but there are particular problems associated with the measurement of diet. This is particularly so in case-control and large prospective studies held within single populations where there is little dietary variation between individuals but large measurement error associated with each assessment. In most epidemiological studies the requirement for measuring diet is to ensure that subjects are correctly placed in the distribution of food and nutrient intakes, so that when risk of cancer is assessed across thirds, fourths or fifths of the distribution, misclassification does not bias the outcome. The absolute intake of people at different ends of the distribution within studies is less likely to be as important as the ranking. If measurement error and resulting misclassification is not consistent across the range of intake, then there will be a biased estimate of effect. For example, energy intake is under-reported in obese subjects differently from the non-obese, and failure to allow for this may lead to bias. Adjusting nutrient intakes for energy is often done, but this will not correct for bias arising from differential measurement error.

4.2.2. *Dietary assessment in case-control studies* To assess dietary exposure, habitual consumption several years before cancer diagnosis is usually attempted for each individual. In case-control studies, investigators need to ask for details of past dietary habits during the course of an interview or questionnaire. However, reports of past dietary consumption are more closely related to present consumption, and the discrepancy is greater the longer the period of recall attempted[39]. This introduces reporting bias, see 4.1.4.1.

4.2.3 *Dietary assessment in prospective studies* More reliance is placed on findings from prospective studies, where a contemporaneous measure of habitual exposure is usually attempted. Methods that have been used to measure diet in prospective studies are described below (4.2.4–4.2.6). However, estimates of food intake may not directly reflect the actual exposure to any active constituent at the site of action. Methodological errors, as well as differences in absorption and metabolism of active constituents, and interactions with other dietary components, reduce the precision of the estimate of exposure.

4.2.4 *Food frequency questionnaires* To assess consumption of foods, the majority of prospective studies have used short lists of food, food frequency questionnaires (FFQ), in which participants estimate how often they have eaten certain foods over the recent past. These FFQ are designed to assess long term habits, over months or years, and comprise a list of foods most informative about the nutrients or foods of interest. The length of this list generally does not exceed 150 items. Various methods to assess portion sizes may be used, for example fitting average portion weights derived from other data to the respondents' chosen food and frequency selections[40]. To assess the frequency of food consumption, accompanying the food list is a multiple response grid in which respondents attempt to estimate how often selected foods are eaten. Up to ten categories ranging from never or once a month or less, to six times per day is a usual format. Because responses are standardised, FFQ can be analysed in

74

comparatively short periods of time so that large numbers of individuals can be investigated relatively inexpensively. Generally, only one response to a FFQ has been obtained from each individual during study follow up of several years in published results from existing cohorts.

4.2.5 *Other methods* Another method for obtaining information is the diet history, which is usually conducted by trained interviewers who obtain more detailed information on usual foods consumed, portion sizes, recipes and frequency of food consumption over the recent past. This method is less commonly used in cohort studies owing to the necessity for face-to-face interviews and consequent costs. The 24 hour recall method, using dietary information obtained by interview or by written record, has also been used in cohort studies, but is not a frequent method of choice. In this the actual foods consumed are described, together with information on portion weights. This method is also more costly due to the variety of foods consumed (at least 5000 different food items are available in most westernised food supplies), all of which require estimation of portion size and individual computer coding. Finally, participants may be asked to keep daily written records of the description and amount of food kept at the time of consumption. Provided records are kept for a sufficient length of time, this method is the most likely to represent what participants really do eat, and is generally used to assess the accuracy of other methods such as FFQ[41].

4.2.6 *Measurement error in dietary assessments* It is important to be able to distinguish between technical errors of measurement and true variability. People do not eat the same foods every day, and any method of dietary assessment must take this variability into account. This variability within individuals is different from that between individuals. Both within and between person variability are usually assumed to be randomly distributed, and affect the precision of the estimate of the population intake. Random errors reduce the power of studies to detect relationships between exposure and outcome, but do not bias the estimate of effect (risk ratio). On the other hand, systematic errors, eg through non-random over or under-estimation of diet (see 4.2.1), will bias the estimate of risk. Such systematic errors should be avoided as far as possible, and potential for such an effect in studies where they might have occurred should be considered. In addition confounding – failure to allow for the effects of other factors which are not randomly associated with diet – can introduce bias.

4.2.7 *Food tables* Many hypotheses concerning diet and cancer relate to the content of foods, such as nutrients, contaminants such as aflatoxins, heterocyclic amines, or to non-nutritive food constituents. An estimate of the content of these items of each food eaten is also required in order to obtain intake, unless biomarkers are available (see 4.2.13). Tables of food composition, with information about average content of the most commonly consumed foods, are generally available for most nutrients, but less comprehensively for food contaminants and non-nutritive constituents. Where food tables are used, the published levels are averages, and individual intakes may deviate substantially from the average due to preparation, cooking and storage practices, and because foods vary in their composition naturally depending on soil, season, and variety. There have also been technical problems in the chemical method of analysis for many nutrients and constituents, for example carotenoids and folates. Different countries also use different systems of analysis, so that average results may not always be comparable between countries, for example carbohydrate, NSP.

4.2.8 *Other sources of error* In the assessment of food consumption, people do not consume the same food from day to day and substantial error at individual level is introduced when diet is assessed from a single day's dietary investigation. However if the analysis is at group level then a single day's dietary investigation is a fairly good reflection of the group average and the error will be smaller. Participants using the FFQ may have difficulty in choosing the correct category of how often food is consumed, so that under or over estimation occurs. Restriction of the choice of food into a comparatively short list of around 150 foods or less, means that error associated with estimation of amounts of single items is more likely to be biased than when the full variety of foods is analysed, for example in a 24 h recall or record of food consumption. Restriction also makes methods inflexible and unable to cope with a variety of dietary hypotheses likely to emerge over the course of a prospective study lasting several years.

4.2.9 *Underreporting* Many FFQ are not designed to assess total dietary intake, and only information relating to the food or nutrient of interest at the time of the study is obtained. For example, in one prospective study the FFQ covered only 80 food items, and accounted for only 83% of mean total energy intake[42]. The term "underreporting" applies generally to underestimates of food intake, and has implications particularly for energy intake. This problem has been demonstrated by comparing dietary estimates with biomarkers of intake (see 4.2.13), and has been documented in all forms of dietary assessment including 24 hour recall[43,44], weighed records[45–47], diet history[48,49] and FFQ[50], although in general it is more likely with 24 hour recall than with diet history or records[51]. Overweight and obese individuals are particularly likely to underreport, though not all food items are affected equally[48,52]. Protein, sugars and fat tend to be underreported, but not carotenes, vitamin C, NSP or vegetables[50]. The adjustment of intakes of macronutrients for energy has been used to attempt to mitigate this source of bias, but it did not improve correlations between estimates of protein intake and 24 hour urinary excretion of nitrogen (a biomarker of protein intake)[53]. The extent to which it affects estimates of fat and carbohydrate intakes is not known, as no useful biomarkers for these exist.

4.2.10 *Dietary interactions and energy adjustment* Diets consist of a complex mixture of foods and beverages. The many different constituents likely to be important in influencing cancer risk may act independently or have additive effects. Some constituents are present in the same foods, and intakes therefore tend to be correlated, for example vitamin C, carotenoids, NSP, folate, and glucosinolates are all found in vegetables (see Chapter 8). This adds to the difficulty of distinguishing between causal and spurious associations in the statistical analysis of epidemiological studies. Attribution of risk or benefit to one aspect of diet without consideration of the potential interaction with other aspects of dict may be misleading. For example, Ursin et al[54] have recently shown in the US National Health and Nutrition Examination Survey (NHANES) that people who eat low fat diets also eat diets that are different in other ways which have also been suggested to be independently associated with cancer. They have suggested that risk for each aspect of diet should be considered after adjusting for the effects of other aspects of diet. Many studies have adopted the strategy of adjusting risk estimates for levels of energy intake, although the approach adopted has not been consistent across all studies[55,56]. Furthermore, the effect of energy adjustment depends on the correlation between the nutrient concerned and energy intake, and also on the correlation between the errors of measurement for these two quantities. The latter is heavily dependent on the dietary method used. Energy adjustment is inappropriate (and without effect) if there are zero correlations between energy intake and the nutrient concerned, for example in the case of carotene[53]. In addition dietary patterns may be associated with other non-dietary behaviours, for example smoking, which may have much greater effects on risk of cancer than any dietary component.

4.2.11 *Effects of measurement error on validity* In the absence of measurement error, there should be complete agreement between a chosen method and the 'true' habitual intake. However, methods of dietary assessment have different types of error structure, so that the magnitude of the error varies according to the method and may not always be predictable. To assess the validity of a measure assumes that there is a measure of truth available, which for dietary assessment is not the case; all that can be assessed is the accuracy of one measure compared with another measure (relative validity). In most epidemiological studies the main requirement is that the measure is able to rank subjects correctly. "Relative validation" studies are conducted prior to use of a particular method in some large prospective studies in order that the extent of measurement error can be determined and reduced if possible. Generally, methods are compared with results from records of food consumption, but some biomarkers (see 4.2.9) have been shown in metabolic studies to closely agree with habitual intake and can be used as an independent reference to assess the extent of measurement error associated with different methods. When validation studies are performed, most recent large cohort studies have found that the method used correlates significantly with the reference measure for some if not all nutrients. However, correlations between the reference and the estimate of intake are as low as 0.2 to 0.7, depending on the nutrient, method under study, and energy adjustment. Low correlations will mean that only about half or fewer individuals are placed in the same third or fifth of the distribution of intake as indicated by the reference method[40,50].

4.2.12 *Consequences of measurement error* It is generally concluded from validation studies that the measures used are adequate to detect differences between levels of dietary exposure, but the chance of detecting a small but biologically important difference in risk is reduced. Nevertheless, estimates of relative risks may be substantially reduced and low or non significant estimates cannot be taken to mean absence of an important effect of diet. Errors are assumed to be random, but this may not be the case. Confounding by other constituents, perhaps more easily measured (such as alcohol) may also occur. If errors are random, repeated observations lessen error substantially so that hypothetical estimates of relative risks could be substantially improved by repeated measures on each individual in cohort studies, using different methods if their errors are uncorrelated. Table 4.1 shows the hypothetical effect of repeat measures with uncorrelated errors on estimates of relative risks. The table also shows hypothetically the improvement in characterisation of relative risks which can be achieved by increasing the range of dietary exposure to which the cohort is exposed, as for example in an international, multicentre study.

Table 4.1   The estimated effect of measurement dilution error

Nutrient	'True' relative risk	Measured relative risks		
		One measure one centre	Two measures one centre	Two measures multicentre
Protein	10	2.5	3.9	5.3
Sugars	10	4.5	6.1	7.7
Starch	10	3.6	5.2	6.7
Energy	10	3.3	5.0	6.7
Fat % energy	10	3.4	5.2	7.0
Carotene	10	3.0	4.4	5.7
Vitamin C	10	2.4	4.3	6.2
Non-starch polysaccharides	10	4.5	6.1	7.7

Hypothetical estimates of 'true' relative risks of 10 for dietary exposures from a single dietary measurement on each individual in one single cohort, and two measurements with uncorrelated errors on each individual studied, either in a single cohort, or in a multicentre cohort.

4.2.13 *Biomarkers of dietary intake* Further improvement can be obtained if markers of habitual intake that can be measured in biological specimens are available. These have been used to assess the relative validity of different dietary methods, and to confirm that records of food consumption are more likely than other methods to rank subjects correctly when estimating habitual diet[50,57–60]. In cohort studies, the usefulness of biomarkers in characterising individual risk is illustrated in a follow up study of markers of aflatoxin exposure in relation to liver cancer. The range of aflatoxin contamination of foods is very great, so that use of food tables of average levels of contamination is unlikely to pick up individual exposure. Relative risks of cancer from aflatoxin consumption were only 0.9 and insignificant (confidence intervals 0.4–1.9) for individuals classified to have had high dietary exposure, as assessed by an interview of the frequency of consumption of 45 foods. However, aflatoxin exposure biomarkers in urine samples obtained from individuals in the cohort were able to detect substantial significant relative risks for liver cancer in the order of 6–10. Relative risks were 59.4 (CI 16.6–212.0) in individuals positive for urine biomarkers of both aflatoxin and hepatitis B[61].

4.2.14 *Conclusions* The effect of measurement error can be estimated and taken into account in well designed prospective studies. However, in much of

78

the existing epidemiological literature, where studies were instigated a number of years ago, relatively poor measures of dietary intake may account for conflicting results and erroneously low estimates of relative risk. Caution is therefore necessary in interpreting results from the existing body of literature. Measurement error can reduce estimates of relative risk substantially within single cohorts, but large multinational cohorts are one way of overcoming measurement error since the power from large numbers of participants with more varied dietary habits is greatly increased. Such large scale collaborative efforts that have been initiated recently include the European Prospective Investigation of Cancer (EPIC)[5] which has a cohort of 400 000 across nine countries of Europe. Accurate biomarkers may also be associated with less measurement error than some methods of dietary assessments. Estimates of risk from these newer prospective studies, and from those using biomarkers, are therefore likely to be substantially greater and more consistent than those hitherto reported.

5. Epidemiology of Diet in Relation to Specific Cancers

5.1 Review of epidemiology of diet and cancer

5.1.1 This chapter draws together the epidemiological literature linking diet with cancer. Chapter 3 details the British diet with which the findings in this chapter need to be considered and Chapter 4 sets out the important methodological issues related to epidemiological studies. The first section of this chapter (5.1) sets out the methodological approach to the epidemiological reviews; sections 5.2 to 5.16 present the epidemiological reviews of specific cancer sites.

5.1.2 The relationship between diet and cancer at different sites has been examined by reviewing case-control and cohort studies published in English between 1966 and August 1996. The review covered nine major sites: breast, lung, colorectum, prostate, bladder, gastric, cervix, pancreas and oesophagus. A review with commentary on individual studies and bibliography has been published[62]. More limited reviews were undertaken on ovarian, endometrial, skin melanoma, oropharyngeal, laryngeal and testicular cancers. The cancers are addressed in order of decreasing incidence in either sex. In the UK, carcinoma of the liver is generally associated with alcoholic cirrhosis. Alcohol is outside the scope of this report and so liver cancer has not been included in this chapter.

5.1.3 *Scoring system* A scoring system was developed to enable the overall quality of the papers to be ranked in a systematic manner (see Annex 1). Separate scoring systems were used for cohort and case-control studies because some markers of reliability (eg. control selection) apply to only one type of study and because the interpretation of results from cohort studies are *a priori* less prone to bias than those from case-control studies. The scoring focused on the study design, method of assessing dietary exposure, analysis and, for cohort studies, the definition of the cohort. The scoring was intended to reflect the amount and reliability of information on diet and cancer risk. The repeatability of the scoring system was assessed and found to be robust[63]. On the basis of the scores, studies were classified as low scoring (**L**) (score $\leq$ 45), intermediate (**I**) (46–64) or high scoring (**H**) ($\geq$ 65).

5.1.4 *Drawing conclusions* The Working Group drew its conclusions on the epidemiological evidence with a view to the criteria set out in section 1.5. It assessed the consistency of the body of evidence according to the statistical significance of the findings and their general direction, and categorised it as weakly, moderately or strongly consistent (see Annex 2 for the Working Group's Terminology used in the descriptions of evidence). In general, the evidence was classified as weakly consistent where half to two-thirds of the studies were in the same direction, as moderately consistent where two-thirds to three-quarters of the studies were in the same direction and as strongly consistent where more than three-quarters of the studies were in the same direction. However, absolute differences in intake are not apparent in the comparisons illustrated in Figures 5.1 to 5.46, and the range of intakes being considered from one study to another may be very different. The Working Group attempted to take this into account when drawing conclusions. The quality of the studies was also taken into account.

5.1.5   Figures 5.1 to 5.46 are included to illustrate the reported estimated relative risks or odds ratios and the 95% confidence intervals for highest versus lowest levels of consumption of dietary factors for specific cancers (see 4.1.7). However, some studies failed to report relative risk (RR) or odds ratio (OR) but did report whether there was a significant association; whilst these have been included in the text they cannot be included in the relevant figures. Where the 95% confidence intervals (95% CI) were not reported but the RR or OR were, the information for the RR or OR has been included on the figure without the 95% CI.

5.1.6   In drawing conclusions the Working Group were aware of the possibility of reciprocal relationships for instance between the consumption of meat and of fruit and vegetables, but the data available did not enable this effect to be separated out. In addition, the length of studies might influence the likelihood of a positive finding in that shorter studies would have greater potential of producing false negative results (see also 4.1.5).

5.2   Breast Cancer

5.2.1   *Introduction*

5.2.1.1   Breast cancer is the most common cancer in women in the UK, affecting over 30 000 women each year. England and Wales have the highest mortality rates from breast cancer in the world. Two highly penetrant susceptibility genes for breast cancer have been identified and account for up to 4 per cent of breast cancers and up to 10% of ovarian cancers. Among established risk factors are family history of the disease, early menarche and late age at menopause. Thus women with early menarche (aged 12 or younger) have an almost four-fold increased risk compared with women with late menarche (13 or older) and long duration of irregular cycles. Age at first birth is important; women with a first full-term pregnancy before the age of 20 have half the cancer risk of nulliparous women or of women delaying the first birth until age 30–35. Other established risk factors are low parity and post-menopausal oestrogen replacement therapy. Many of these risk factors point indirectly to hormonal involvement.

5.2.1.2   Breast cancer rates vary more than five-fold between countries, suggesting that there are environmental causes which could potentially be modified. International comparisons[64–66], comparisons within countries[64,67,68], and time trends within countries[69–72] are all consistent with a positive relationship between mortality from breast cancer and fat consumption, and negative relationships with cereals and pulses. Key *et al*[73] have, however, suggested that some of the observed secular trend in the UK is an artefact related to changes in coding for causes of death over time. When they took these changes into account Key *et al*[73] suggested the relationship with fat was weaker. Studies of Japanese migrants to the USA have suggested that rates move toward the US rates and away from rates of Japanese in Japan[72].

5.2.1.3   It has been hypothesised that breastfeeding reduces the risk of breast cancer. Several large studies since the 1960s have failed to find an association between breastfeeding and the risk of breast cancer for cancers which are diagnosed post-menopausally, but the results for pre-menopausal breast cancers are conflicting. The UK National Case-Control Study Group in a population case-control study of 755 matched pairs with breast cancer diagnosed before the 36th birthday found an increasing reduction of risk with each baby breastfed for a minimum of 3 months[67]. The prospective USA Nurses' Health Study found no overall protective effect of breastfeeding[74]. A large case-control study examined all women diagnosed with breast cancer over a 30 month period in 1990-92 in 3 centres in USA. All women were 54 years of age or less, and all were below 45 years in two of the centres. A protective effect of 10% attributable to breastfeeding applied to women who had breastfed for at least 2 weeks and was relatively unchanged by the number of children so fed[75]. Any effect on risk of pre-menopausal breast cancer from breastfeeding is likely to be mediated hormonally rather than due to any nutritional effect.

5.2.2   Meat and fish

5.2.2.1   Meat consumption has been positively associated with breast cancer in most case-control studies which have examined this (see figure 5.1). Of 20 case-control studies[76–95], 17 observed higher risks associated with higher total meat, red meat or processed meat consumption, although only 11 studies were statistically significant[84,86-95]. The relative risks ranged from 1.1 to 3.5 in the studies finding higher risks associated with higher consumption. One study in Greece[83] found no association and another in Japan[82] found a non-significantly lower risk associated with higher meat consumption. However, a retrospective nested case-

Figure 5.1   Estimated Odds Ratios (95% CI) for incidence of breast cancer for highest versus lowest consumption of meat in case-control studies

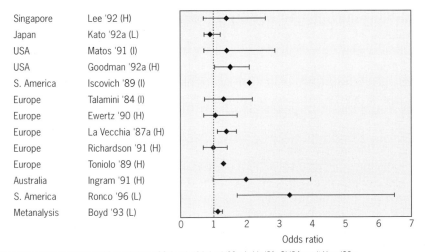

OR missing for Katsouyani '86; Hislop '86a; Holmberg '86; Landa '94; Levi '93a; Lubin '81; Qi '94; van't Veer '90a

control study, carried out as part of the Nurses' Health Study[32], found some evidence of recall bias in reporting red meat consumption in cases compared with controls, suggesting that this effect might be a result of bias rather than a true difference in intake.

5.2.2.2   Five out of 9 prospective studies have observed significantly higher relative risks associated with higher total meat or red meat consumption[42,96–99] (see Figure 5.2). The New York University Women's Health Study[96] and the study by Vatten et al[97] both found relative risks of the order of 1.8. The study by Hirayama found relative risks of 2.4 for daily meat consumption compared with diets that excluded meat. However there were only 14 cases in the daily meat eating group. A study in Norwegian women found a relative risk of 2.3 in those eating meat more than 5 times a week compared with those eating meat twice a week or less[42]. Three further prospective studies[100–102] have found non-significantly higher risks associated with total meat or red meat consumption with relative risks around 1.2 to 1.3. The Nurses' Health Study[103] found no relationship between meat consumption and risk of breast cancer. No study has found significantly lower risk of breast cancer with higher meat consumption. Overall therefore, 8 out of 9 prospective studies have found higher risk of breast cancer associated with higher total meat or red meat consumption. However, of the four higher scoring studies[42,97,101,103], two[101,103], failed to find significantly higher risks of breast cancer associated with meat consumption and of the four studies which found significantly higher relative risks, two[96,98] had low scores according to the criteria described in section 5.1.3 and Annex 1.

Figure 5.2   Relative risks (95% CI) for incidence of breast cancer for higher versus lower consumption of meat in cohort studies

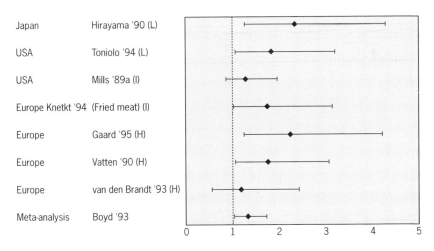

Japan	Hirayama '90 (L)	
USA	Toniolo '94 (L)	
USA	Mills '89a (I)	
Europe Knetkt '94	(Fried meat) (I)	
Europe	Gaard '95 (H)	
Europe	Vatten '90 (H)	
Europe	van den Brandt '93 (H)	
Meta-analysis	Boyd '93	

Studies without RR include: Nomura '78 (NS higher risk); Hunter '93 (no relationship)

5.2.2.3   The method of cooking meat in relation to risk of breast and other cancers has been investigated in some studies as a result of the hypothesis that mutagenic compounds induced by heating (cooking) meat are involved in processes leading to cancer (see 7.13.4.10). Knekt et al [99] found, in a cohort study in Finland, an elevated risk of breast cancer (energy adjusted RR 1.80 (CI 1.03—3.16)) and other female hormone-related cancers among women with high intakes of fried meat (such meats included all meats prepared by the pan-frying method but excluded oven-roasted meats). This finding is supported by case-control studies reporting significant associations between fried meat intake and breast cancer risk[78,87,94]. In the Finnish cohort[99], a separate analysis on the consumption of fried meat and other meats suggested that increased breast cancer risk was specifically associated with fried meat intake.

5.2.2.4 A meta-analysis of studies (13 case-control and 5 cohort studies) of dietary factors and breast cancer risk[104] produced a summary estimate of relative risk for highest versus lowest consumption of meat of 1.18 (95% CI 1.06-1.32). In cohort studies there appeared to be a graded effect with increasing number of servings per week. Figure 5.3 shows the relative risk according to the number of servings of meat per week in four of the cohort studies[42,96,97,102]. The relative risks for six or seven servings per week compared with no meat eating or one or two servings per week are estimated to be between 1.3 and 2.4.

Figure 5.3   Relative risks for incidence of breast cancer for the number of servings of meat per week in cohort studies

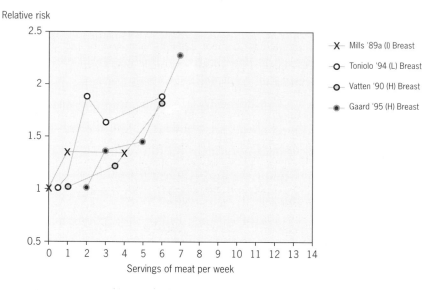

5.2.2.5   Conclusions   There is moderately consistent evidence that higher meat consumption, particularly red or fried/browned meat, is associated with a higher risk of breast cancer. The evidence is largely in the direction of higher risks with higher frequency of consumption (number of servings per week), which in British adults is strongly correlated with the amount consumed (see 3.2.4.2). Nevertheless half the higher scoring prospective studies have failed to find statistically significant relative risks. The relative risks for consumers of six or seven servings of meat, especially red meats, per week compared with one or two servings per week or less are estimated in the range of 1.3 to 2.4. There are insufficient data on poultry or fish consumption and the risk of breast cancer to draw conclusions.

5.2.3 Milk and dairy products

5.2.3.1 In a comparison of different countries, a higher intake of milk products was associated with increased breast cancer mortality[29]. Case-control and cohort studies in individuals have, however, proved less consistent. Knekt et al[105], during a 25 year follow-up period in a prospective study in Finland found a significant inverse relationship between milk intake and incidence of breast cancer, the age adjusted relative risk of breast cancer being 0.42 (95% CI 0.24–0.74) between the highest and lowest tertiles of milk consumption. One other prospective study[96] found a significant inverse relationship between milk and milk products and breast cancer incidence in New York City women but two other prospective studies[106,107] found no association. A fourth prospective study[42] in Norwegian women found the consumption of whole milk was associated with an elevated risk for those who consumed 5 or more glasses (0.75 litres) per day, while there was no significant higher risk among consumers of similar amounts of skimmed or semi-skimmed milk. Case-control studies have resulted in inconsistent findings, with more studies suggesting a positive association or no association than those suggesting an inverse association.

5.2.3.2 <u>Conclusions</u> There is inconsistent evidence that milk consumption is associated with risk of incidence or mortality of breast cancer.

5.2.4 Fat

5.2.4.1 An association between rates of breast cancer and fat consumption in different countries has long been described[4]. However, there are many possible reasons for such an association.

5.2.4.2 Some, but not all, case-control studies have tended to suggest a higher risk of breast cancer with higher dietary fat intake. Of 20 case-control studies of breast cancer which presented odds ratios for estimates of total fat intake, 12[77,79,81,86,93–95,108–112,155] suggested a higher risk of breast cancer associated

Figure 5.4   Odds Ratios (95% CI) for incidence of breast cancer for highest versus lowest consumption of total fat in case-control studies

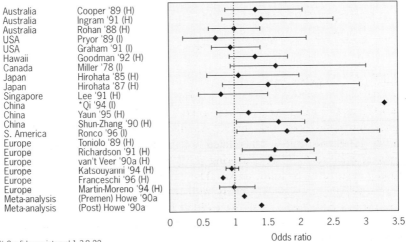

*Qi '94 95% Confidence interval 1.3-8.22

85

with higher total fat intake (see Figure 5.4). However, the confidence intervals of six of these studies included 1.0. The others found either no effect[113–118] or a significantly lower risk with higher fat intake[119]. A pooled analysis of 12 case-control studies which divided studies into those in post-menopausal women and those in pre-menopausal women found a significant effect of fat intake in post-menopausal women but not in pre-menopausal women [120]. For several of the study sites included in this summary Howe *et al*[120] recalculated fat intake before combining data. The risk of breast cancer associated with fat intake was reduced somewhat when three statistically heterogeneous studies were excluded from the analysis but it remained statistically significant. A meta-analysis of studies of dietary fat and breast cancer risk[104] found the summary of relative risk for the 16 case-control studies that examined fat as a nutrient was 1.21 (95% CI 1.10–1.34).

5.2.4.3   However, in contrast to the case-control studies, prospective studies of fat intake and subsequent risk of breast cancer in middle-aged women have not found an association between fat intake and subsequent risk of disease (see Figure 5.5). The relative risks are equally distributed around 1.0. Of nine prospective studies which have examined fat intake and subsequent risk of breast cancer, one found no association[121] and four[101,122–124] found relative risks of less than one, although the confidence intervals included 1.0 for three, and four[42,96,125,126] found relative risks greater than one but the confidence intervals included 1.0 in all four studies.

Figure 5.5   Relative risks (95% CI) for incidence of breast cancer for highest compared to lowest consumption of total fat in cohort studies

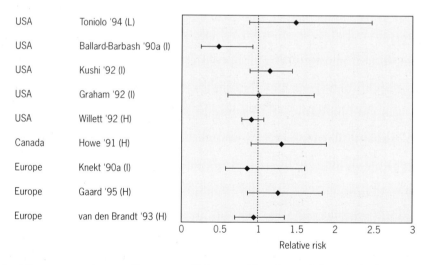

5.2.4.4   The prospective studies were all large with substantial statistical power to detect an effect; if an effect exists, it is likely, therefore, to be small. The Nurses' Health Study followed over 89 000 women for 8 years and found that the risk of breast cancer in women in the top fifth compared with that in women in the lowest fifth of fat intake was 0.9 (CI 0.77–1.07) after adjusting for energy intake[55]. In addition, no effect was seen when post-menopausal women were analysed separately. The Netherlands cohort study included over 62 000 women aged 55–69 (ie mostly post-menopausal). After 3 years, the risk of breast cancer in women in the highest quintile compared with women in the lowest quintile for fat intake was 0.95 (CI 0.68–1.34) after adjusting for energy intake[101]. The NHANES study followed 5 485 women for 2 years and found a significant inverse effect of fat intake on risk of breast cancer[124]; however this study used a 24 hour dietary recall method which may not adequately represent the habitual diet.

5.2.4.5 The four prospective studies which found non-significantly higher relative risks associated with higher fat intakes were the Canadian National Breast Screening Study[125], the Iowa Women's Health Study[126], the New York University Women's Health Study[96] and the Norwegian Women's Study[42]. A case-control study nested in the Canadian National Breast Screening Study with follow-up for about 5 years reported a relative risk of 1.3 (CI 0.9–1.9) between highest and lowest fourths of fat intake using a logistic regression method applied to cases and matched controls from within the cohort who had not developed breast cancer by the end of the follow-up period[125]. Most of the women who developed breast cancer were pre-menopausal at the start of the study. The Iowa Women's Health Study followed over 34 000 women for 3 years and assessed their diet using a food frequency questionnaire similar to that used in the Nurses' Health Study. This study found a relative risk of 1.15 (CI 0.88–1.50) for women in the highest quarter of fat intake compared with those with the lowest after adjusting for energy intakes[126]. The New York Women's Health Study followed over 14 000 women for 6 years and found a relative risk of 1.49 (CI 0.88–2.46) after adjusting for energy intake. The relative risks were similar when pre- and post-menopausal women were analysed separately. The Norwegian study which followed over 31 000 Norwegian women for an average of 10 years[42] found a relative risk of 1.23 (CI 0.86–1.76) in women in the highest quarter of fat intake compared with those in the lowest after adjusting for energy intake. A pooled analysis of seven prospective studies, involving over 335 000 women followed-up for up to 7 years, found no evidence of either a higher risk of breast cancer in women with the highest fat intakes compared with those with the lowest intakes or of a positive association between fat intake and risk of breast cancer[127]. And a meta-analysis of seven cohort studies of dietary fat and breast cancer[104] found a summary relative risk of 1.01 (CI 0.90–1.13). When this study extracted the relative risks comparing the highest to the lowest level of fat intake for both cohort and case-control studies (23 studies), the summary relative risk was 1.12 (CI 1.04–1.21).

5.2.4.6 All the prospective studies described above were in western populations with relatively high fat intakes. The lowest category of fat intakes in the Nurses' Health Study was 25% dietary energy and in other studies was around 30–35% dietary energy. There was no evidence in the pooled analysis that women with fat intakes less than 20% of energy had a lower risk of breast cancer, although this was based on only 84 cases[127]. This would imply a non-linear relationship which is not suggested by the international correlations which gave rise to the hypothesis[55]. Overall, therefore, the prospective studies to date do not support the hypothesis that higher total fat intakes in middle-aged women increase the risk of breast cancer. It is possible that the studies have not been long enough for an association to become apparent. It remains possible that dietary fat intake during childhood and adolescence may affect breast cancer risk several decades later[127].

5.2.4.7 Two studies have explored the discrepancy between the results from case-control studies and prospective studies by conducting nested case-control studies within a prospective cohort[32,33]. The retrospective case-control studies might have been biased by a more inaccurate recall of past diet in those with breast cancer than in the controls (recall bias) and by unrepresentative participation of cases and controls (selection bias). Conducting case-control studies in a population whose diets have previously been assessed prospectively enables the effect of bias on measurements of risk to be assessed. Giovanucci et al[32] assessed the effects of both selection bias and recall bias and found that although both cases and controls tended to overestimate fat intake retrospectively compared with prospectively, women with breast cancer tended to do this to a greater extent than women without breast cancer. There was also a tendency for self-selection in that among the controls but not the cases, the women who had a lower intake of fat and saturated fatty acids in the prospective assessment were more likely to respond to the retrospective questionnaire. The effect of these biases was to produce an apparent odds ratio greater than 1.0 in the retrospective study which was not seen in the prospective analysis (prospective: RR 0.9 and retrospective: OR 1.4). This study suggests that small biases in mean intakes can produce large biases in odds ratios between extreme fifths of intake leading to an overestimation of the risk in case-control studies. This effect might explain the difference between the results of the case-control studies and the prospective studies. However, the study by Friedenreich et al[33] found little evidence of significant recall bias. There was some suggestion that cases may have over-estimated consumption of high-fat foods compared with controls in that the retrospective assessment of diet produced slightly, though not statistically significant, higher estimates of risk compared with the results from the prospective assessment of diet in the same women.

5.2.4.8 Saturated fatty acids   Although a number of case-control studies have found higher intakes of saturated fatty acids in cases compared with controls[81,93,128,129] (see Figure 5.6), a recent European study[119] showed no association. The results from prospective studies for saturated fatty acids are similar to those for total fat and it is possible that the same problems with bias as were seen for total fat in Giovannucci's nested case-control study are also operating in these case-control studies[32]. Of nine prospective studies, one found a significantly higher risk with higher saturated fatty acid consumption which disappeared after adjusting for energy intakes[42], and five found non-significantly higher relative risks for women in the highest fifth of fat consumption compared with women in the lowest[96,101,121,125,126] (see Figure 5.7). The Nurses' Health Study[55] and the Finnish Health Study[122] found essentially no effect of saturated fatty acids although the Nurses' Health Study did find a significant inverse trend with saturated fatty acids in post-menopausal women. Nevertheless, the relative risk for women in the highest fifth of saturated fatty acid consumption compared

Figure 5.6   Odds Ratio (95% CI) for incidence of breast cancer for highest compared to lowest consumption of saturated fatty acids in case-controled studies

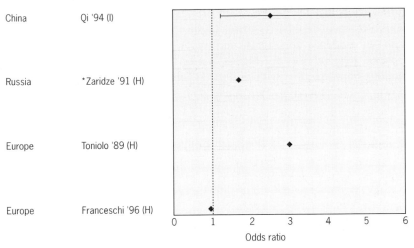

China   Qi '94 (I)

Russia   *Zaridze '91 (H)

Europe   Toniolo '89 (H)

Europe   Franceschi '96 (H)

Odds ratio

* Zaridze '91 95% Confidence interval 0.24 - 11.78; Gerber '89 no OR

Figure 5.7   Relative risks (95% CI) for incidence of breast cancer for highest compared to lowest consumption of saturated fatty acids in cohort studies

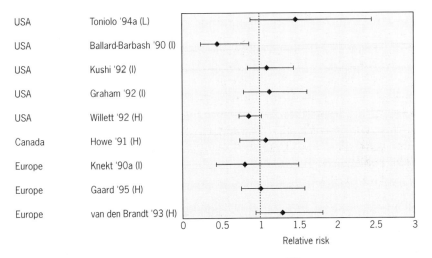

USA   Toniolo '94a (L)

USA   Ballard-Barbash '90 (I)

USA   Kushi '92 (I)

USA   Graham '92 (I)

USA   Willett '92 (H)

Canada   Howe '91 (H)

Europe   Knekt '90a (I)

Europe   Gaard '95 (H)

Europe   van den Brandt '93 (H)

Relative risk

with the lowest fifth was not significant. The NHANES[124] found a significantly lower risk of breast cancer with higher intakes of saturated fatty acids but the same reservations apply to this study as described previously. The pooled analysis of seven prospective studies found no evidence of an association between saturated fatty acid intake and risk of breast cancer[127].

5.2.4.9 Mono- and Polyunsaturated fatty acids   Two recent case-control studies[94,119] reported small inverse associations with consumption of both mono- and polyunsaturated fatty acids. Ronco et al [94] (intermediate scoring study) did not report odds ratios but Franceschi et al [119] (high scoring study) reported odds ratios for highest versus lowest quintile 0.81 and 0.70 respectively for mono- and polyunsaturated fatty acids. A cohort study in the Netherlands[101] does not

89

support a major role of mono- or polyunsaturated fatty acids in the aetiology of post-menopausal breast cancer since the following relative risks were reported: monounsaturated fatty acids, RR 0.75 (CI 0.50–1.12) and polyunsaturated fatty acids RR 0.95 (CI 0.64–1.40) for highest versus lowest quintile of consumption, with no evidence for significant trends. A second European cohort study[122] reported relative risks for highest versus lowest tertiles of 2.7 (CI 1.0–7.4) for monounsaturated fatty acids and 1.2 (CI 0.6–2.8) for polyunsaturated fatty acids. Howe *et al*[125] found a slightly elevated risk in a nested case-control study in a Canadian cohort of 1.2–1.3 in the highest quartile of monounsaturated fatty acids intake with marginally significant tests for trend. However, the RR estimates in the highest quartile were not significantly different from unity. Two US cohort studies[55,96] observed no effect of mono- or polyunsaturated fatty acids on risk of breast cancer. In a meta-analysis of case-control and cohort studies, Boyd *et al*[104] found summary RR for monounsaturated fatty acids of 1.09 (CI 0.99–1.21); for case-control studies alone RR 1.42 (CI 1.19–1.69) and cohort studies alone RR 0.95 (CI 0.84–1.08); and summary RR for polyunsaturated fatty acids consistently one or less than one but CIs did not exclude one in any analyses.

5.2.4.10 Conclusions Within the range of fat intakes found in Western populations, the evidence from case-control studies for an association between higher total and saturated fatty acids intakes and risk of breast cancer is weakly consistent. The evidence from prospective studies alone is moderately consistent that no such association exists. It remains possible that dietary fat intake during childhood and adolescence may affect breast cancer risk several decades later. The evidence for a lack of association between intakes of mono- and polyunsaturated fatty acids and the risk of breast cancer is moderately consistent.

5.2.5 *Fruits and vegetables*

5.2.5.1 Seven[86,88,91,128,130–132] out of the ten case-control studies identified have reported relative risks of developing breast cancer of less than one with

Figure 5.8   Odds Ratio (95% CI) for risk of incidence of breast cancer for highest compared with lowest consumption of fruits in case-control studies

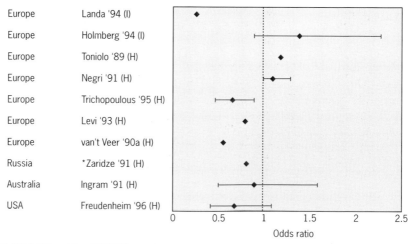

Europe	Landa '94 (I)
Europe	Holmberg '94 (I)
Europe	Toniolo '89 (H)
Europe	Negri '91 (H)
Europe	Trichopoulous '95 (H)
Europe	Levi '93 (H)
Europe	van't Veer '90a (H)
Russia	*Zaridze '91 (H)
Australia	Ingram '91 (H)
USA	Freudenheim '96 (H)

* Zaridze '91 95% Confidence interval 0.13-5.26

higher consumption of fruits (see Figure 5.8). The remaining three studies[81,85,133] reported a relative risk greater than 1. It is not clear from the data reported, how many of those studies reporting reduced risk of breast cancer with higher consumption of fruits are significant but several of the studies have 95% confidence intervals which include 1. Only two prospective studies[103,134] have been identified which reported fruit consumption separately. Rohan *et al*[134] found a relative risk of developing breast cancer with higher consumption of fruits of 0.81 (CI 0.57-1.14) and Hunter *et al*[134] reported no association with fruit consumption.

5.2.5.2   A number of case-control studies have reported decreased risk of breast cancer associated with higher consumption of total vegetables[34,76,85,88,93,128,131,132,135] but only four did not have confidence intervals which included 1 (see Figure 5.9). Two high scoring studies[86,89] showed an increased risk of breast cancer with higher intakes of total vegetables. Several case-control studies measured consumption of green and/or yellow vegetables and of these seven reported lower risk of breast cancer with higher consumption[76,82,84,87,91,133,136] (see Figure 5.9) and two[86,137] showed no association. Both the prospective American Nurses' Health Study[103] and the Canadian cohort study[134] found an inverse association with vegetable consumption and risk of breast cancer (RR 0.83 (CI 0.66–1.03) and RR 0.86 (CI 0.61–1.23) respectively).

5.2.5.3   Conclusions   The evidence from case-control studies is weakly consistent that higher intakes of fruits and moderately consistent that higher intakes of vegetables are associated with lower risk of breast cancer. There are few cohort studies on the effect of consumption of fruits and vegetables on the risk of breast

Figure 5.9   Odds Ratios (95% CI) for incidence of breast cancer for highest compared with lowest consumption of total and green vegetables in case-control studies

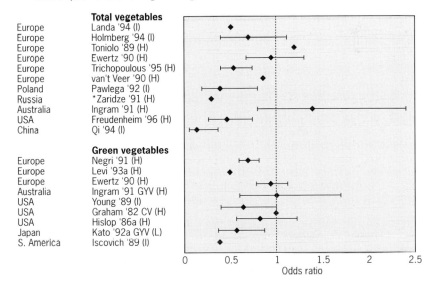

* Zaridze '91 95% Confidence interval 0.03-3.7; GYV green yellow vegetables; CV cruciferous vegetables

91

cancer. Such evidence as there is is weakly consistent that higher intakes of fruits are associated with a lower risk of breast cancer and moderately consistent that higher intakes of total and green/yellow vegetables are associated with lower risk.

5.2.6 Non-starch polysaccharides (Dietary fibre)

5.2.6.1   Assessment of dietary fibre intake in epidemiological studies has been difficult due to the lack of data on the fibre content of individual foods and the use of different methods of biochemical analyses to determine fibre content.

5.2.6.2   A meta-analysis of 12 case-control studies found a significantly lower risk (RR 0.85) of breast cancer associated with higher fibre (20g/day) intakes in postmenopausal women[120]. However, three out of four prospective studies have failed to find a relationship between fibre intake and future risk of breast cancer[55,121,126]. The fourth study[134] did find a significantly lower risk of breast cancer with higher intakes of dietary fibre (see Figure 5.10). Mechanisms by which dietary fibre or closely associated plant compounds may influence oestrogen metabolism are discussed in 7.13.2.8. The associations with green (and cruciferous) vegetables seen in some of the case-control studies may reflect components of vegetables other than fibre.

Figure 5.10   Relative risks (95% CI) for incidence of breast cancer for highest compared with lowest consumption of total fibre intake in cohort studies

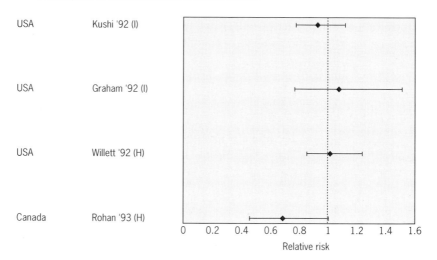

5.2.6.3   Conclusions   The evidence that higher intakes of fibre are associated with a lower risk of breast cancer is inconsistent.

5.2.7 Vitamin A, Retinol and Carotenoids

5.2.7.1   An inverse association has been observed between vitamin A intake (either total vitamin A, pre-formed retinol or carotenoids) and risk of breast cancer in several case-control studies[112,113,115,118,132,133,137–140] but not in others[76] (see Table 5.1). However, Marubini et al[138] found a small non-significant positive association between β-carotene intake and risk of breast cancer. A meta-analysis of 12 case-control studies found a lower risk of breast cancer with

92

higher vitamin A intakes in post-menopausal women after controlling for fat intake[120]. This analysis found that carotenoids appeared to have a stronger effect than pre-formed vitamin A.

Table 5.1 Estimated odds ratio (OR)* or relative risk (RR)* and 95% confidence interval (CI) for breast cancer for highest compared with lowest quantiles of intake of vitamin A, retinol and carotenoids in epidemiological studies

Study (Quality Score)	Location	Estimated OR or RR	CI
Case-control studies			
Freudenheim et al, 1996 (H)[136]	USA (Pre-menopausal)	0.46[d]	0.28–0.74
Graham et al, 1982 (H)[137]	USA	0.8[a]	p trend < 0.05
Lee et al, 1991 (H)[115]	Singapore (Pre-menopausal)	0.33[d]	0.16–0.69
Yuan et al, 1995 (H)[112]	China	0.9[b] 0.6[c]	0.6–1.2 0.4–0.9
Rohan et al, 1988 (H)[118]	Canada	0.83[a] 0.89[b] 0.85[d]	0.70–0.96 0.77–1.03 0.72–1.00
Ewertz & Gill, 1990 (H)[76]	N. Europe	1.2[d]	0.9–1.5
Negri et al, 1991 (H)[133]	S. Europe	0.73[a] 0.86[b] 0.74[d]	0.6–0.9 0.7–1.0 0.6–0.9
Graham et al, 1991 (I)[113]	USA	0.6[c]	0.4–0.8
Potischman et al, 1990 (I)[139]	USA	0.7[a] 0.8[e]	0.3–2.0 0.3–2.3
Katsouyanni et al, 1988 (I)[140]	S. Europe	0.46[a] 0.60[b] 0.56[d]	0.26–0.82 (90% 0.36–1.00 CI) 0.32–0.98
Marubini et al, 1988 (I)[138]	S. Europe	0.7[b] 1.2[d]	0.4–1.5 0.6–2.5
Cohort studies			
Hunter et al, 1993 (H)[103]	USA	0.84[a] 0.80[b] 0.89[c]	0.71–0.98 0.68–0.95 0.76–1.05
Graham et al, 1992 (I)[121]	USA	1.0[a] 0.9[b] 0.9[c]	0.7–1.3 0.7–1.3 0.6–1.3
Paganini-Hill et al, 1987 (I)[141]	USA	0.8[a] 0.8[b]	N/S trend N/S trend

* Odds ratio for case-control studies and relative risk for cohort studies
[a] Total vitamin A
[b] Preformed vitamin A
[c] Carotenoid vitamin A
[d] β-carotene
[e] Vitamin A from vegetable sources

5.2.7.2 A significant small inverse association between total vitamin A, retinol (including supplements) and carotenoid intakes and subsequent breast cancer incidence was found in the Nurses' Health Study[103] and an inverse association was found in a prospective study of retired people in California[141] but the latter was not statistically significant. A third prospective study[121] did not show a relationship (see Table 5.1). The association in the Nurses' Health Study remained after adjusting for known risk factors for breast cancer[103] during 8 years of follow-up. When the intakes of vitamin C and E were added, the inverse association of total vitamin A intake with the incidence of breast cancer was strengthened (RR 0.78 (CI 0.65–0.95)) in the highest quintile group as compared with those in the lowest. Overall the use of vitamin supplements was not significantly associated with breast cancer. Among women in the Nurses' Health Study with the lowest dietary intake of vitamin A, however, the use of vitamin A from supplements was significantly associated with a lower risk of breast cancer. This suggests that only women with a low intake of vitamin A from food may benefit from vitamin A supplements, and that vitamin A supplements are unlikely to influence the risk of breast cancer among women whose dietary intake of this vitamin is already adequate.

5.2.7.3 Two studies which measured blood concentrations of retinol and/or β-carotene[142,143] did not show a relationship with risk of breast cancer.

5.2.7.4 Conclusions There is weakly consistent evidence that higher intakes of vitamin A, either total, pre-formed retinol or carotenoids, are associated with a reduced risk of breast cancer. There is a suggestion that among women with the lowest dietary intakes of vitamin A, the use of supplements of vitamin A reduces the risk of breast cancer, but vitamin A supplements are unlikely to influence the risk of breast cancer among women whose dietary intake of vitamin A is high. There is insufficient evidence to draw conclusions on vitamin C and E and risk of breast cancer.

5.2.8 Phytoestrogens

5.2.8.1 Phytoestrogens (isoflavones and lignans) (see Chapter 8) have weak oestrogenic effects. The major source of phytoestrogens in the diet is soya products. Cross sectional studies have found that urinary phytoestrogen excretion is greater in Japanese women consuming a traditional diet (who have low rates of breast cancer) compared with women in Finland, the UK or the US (who have high rates of breast cancer)[144–152]. Urinary lignan excretion and faecal phytoestrogen excretion is higher in vegetarians, who have a lower risk of developing hormone dependent cancers[153], than those consuming an omnivorous diet[145,154]. Of three case-control studies of soya and breast cancer risk, one found a significant inverse association between breast cancer risk and soy protein intake in premenopausal Chinese Singaporean women[115]. A case-control study in China found no difference in soy protein intake between cases and controls, although the average levels of soy protein consumption was similar to that consumed by Singaporean women[112]. An earlier case-control study in Japan found no difference in soyabean consumption between cases and controls[155]. Two prospective studies have found inverse associations between miso soup, tofu and soya bean paste soup and risk of breast cancer in Japanese women[100,156].

5.2.8.2   Conclusions   There is insufficient evidence to draw conclusions on the effect of phytoestrogens on the risk of breast cancer.

5.2.9   Conclusions   *Breast Cancer and Diet*

There is moderately consistent evidence that higher meat consumption, particularly red and fried meat, is associated with a higher risk of breast cancer. The evidence for an association between higher total and saturated fat consumption and risk of breast cancer is inconsistent within the range of fat intakes found in Western populations but there is moderately consistent evidence for no association between intakes of mono- and polyunsaturated fats and risk of breast cancer. There is weakly consistent evidence that higher intakes of fruits and moderately consistent evidence that higher intakes of vegetables are associated with lower risk of breast cancer, but the evidence that higher intakes of fibre are associated with lower risk is inconsistent.

5.3   Lung Cancer

5.3.1   *Introduction*

5.3.1.1   Smoking is by far the most important cause of lung cancer. In Europe and North America it is estimated that about 90% of the cases of lung cancer in men and 70–80% in women are caused by smoking[157]. Among current cigarette smokers, the risk of lung cancer death increases substantially with the amount smoked[158], with RRs ranging from 15 for smokers of less than 20 per day to 48 for smokers of more than 30 per day. Past/occasional cigarette smokers have a RR of more than 6 compared with non-users of tobacco. Persons who smoke pipes or cigars have a RR of more than 4 for lung cancer death[158]. The potential for confounding by smoking is great in particular as it is difficult to characterise precisely exposure to tobacco smoke, whether by smoking or from environmental tobacco smoke. Other factors are also relevant. These include exposure to asbestos, arsenic and ionising radiation. Both incidence and mortality are inversely related to social class.

5.3.1.2   Smoking causes several histological types of lung cancer, notably squamous cell carcinoma, small cell carcinoma and adenocarcinoma. Many studies either do not report the distribution of histological types in the study population, or have failed to distinguish between the different histological types in analysing their relationships to diet. Consequently the published data do not allow the relationships between diet and the various types of lung cancer to be separately identified, and we have not attempted this in the following section.

5.3.1.3   A number of international studies[159–161] have reported positive associations between dietary fat (animal but not vegetable) intake and lung cancer, although others have not[162,163]. Schrauzer *et al*[164] suggested inverse associations with selenium. Chen *et al*[165] found a negative association between plasma ascorbate and mortality rates from lung cancer in China. Higher lung cancer rates in the north of Italy have been associated with higher consumption of animal foods and lower consumption of vegetables (including cereals) and fish[166,167].

5.3.2 *Fruits and vegetables*

5.3.2.1   The majority of case-control studies which have examined the relationship between vegetable consumption and lung cancer have found that higher consumption of vegetables is associated with lower risk of lung cancer[168–179] (see Figure 5.11), one study found no relationship[180] and one[181] found higher consumption associated with an increased risk. The estimated relative risks for total vegetable consumption when comparing highest with lowest intakes ranged from 0.14 to 1.1. Associations have been seen for dark green vegetables, yellow and light green vegetables, carrots, raw and salad vegetables. In general the estimated relative risk decreased with increasing numbers of servings of vegetables per week (see Figure 5.12).

Figure 5.11   Odds Ratios (95% CI) for incidence of lung cancer for highest versus lowest consumption of total vegetables in case-control studies

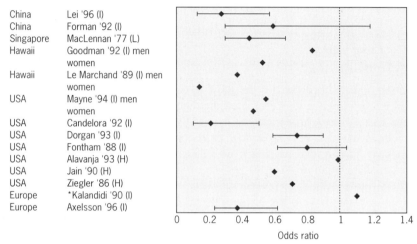

* Kalandidi '90 95% Confidence interval 0.4-2.7

Figure 5.12   Odds Ratio for incidence of lung cancer for numbers of servings per week of total vegetables in case-control studies

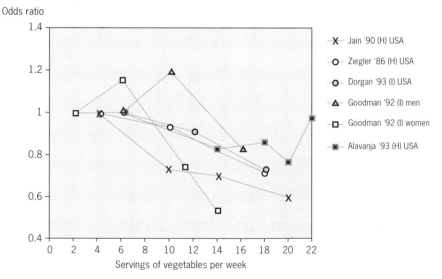

5.3.2.2 Two out of five prospective studies which measured vegetable consumption have found a lower risk of lung cancer associated with higher vegetable consumption[182,183] and two[158,184] found a higher risk with higher consumption although the confidence intervals include 1.0 (see Figure 5.13). The only high scoring study[185] found no effect of vegetable consumption in smokers and a reduced risk in non-smokers. A study in the Netherlands[186] found a lower risk of lung cancer associated with higher onion consumption but not with leek or garlic consumption. All studies attempted to adjust for smoking; however smoking has such a strong effect that it is difficult to account for it completely. The relative risk with increasing number of servings of vegetables per week was different in the two studies reporting this[158,182] (see Figure 5.14).

Figure 5.13 Relative risks (95% CI) for incidence of lung cancer for highest compared to lowest consumption of total vegetables in cohort studies

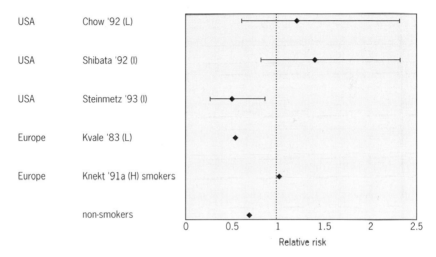

Figure 5.14 Relative Risks for incidence of lung cancer with number of servings per week of total vegetables in cohort studies

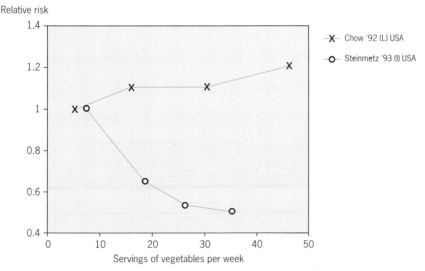

5.3.2.3   The majority of case-control studies show that higher fruit consumption is associated with lower risk of lung cancer[169–171,173,175,177,181,187,188] (see Figure 5.15). This effect was actually confined to low scoring studies and high scoring studies do not show this effect. A high scoring study in China[189] found a significantly higher risk of lung cancer with increased consumption of fruit as did a study by Goodman et al[173] for men but not for women. Five other studies (four of which were high scoring) found no significant association[172,174,179,180, 190]. The estimated relative risks for total fruit consumption when comparing highest with lowest intakes ranged from 0.33 to 1.5. The evidence for decreased relative risk with increasing numbers of servings of fruits per week is inconsistent in those studies for which the number of servings per week is available[170,173,174,179,180,187,189] (see Figure 5.16).

Figure 5.15   Odds Ratio (95% CI) for incidence of lung cancer for highest compared with lowest consumption of fruit in case-control studies

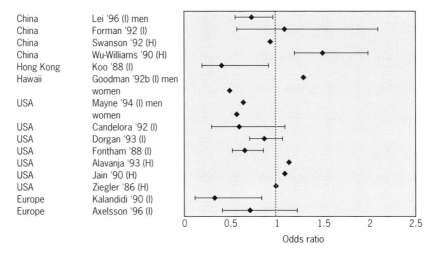

Figure 5.16   Odds Ratio for incidence of lung cancer with number of servings of fruit in case-control studies

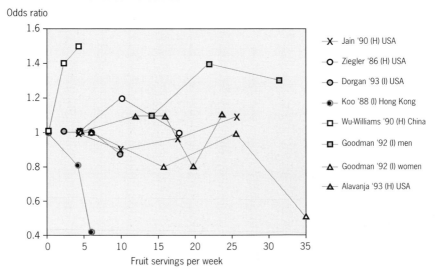

5.3.2.4 Higher consumption of fruits has been associated with a subsequently lower risk of lung cancer in the majority of prospective studies. Seven out of eight prospective studies have found a lower risk of lung cancer associated with higher fruit consumption[158,182,183,185,191–193], although three studies failed to find statistically significant relationships[158,182,183] (see Figure 5.17). Only one study[184] showed an increased relative risk of lung cancer for higher fruit consumption but this was not significant. For those studies recording the number of servings of fruits per week, there was a decreased risk with increasing number of servings (see Figure 5.18).

Figure 5.17 Relative risks (95% CI) for incidence of lung cancer for highest compared to lowest consumption of fruit in cohort studies

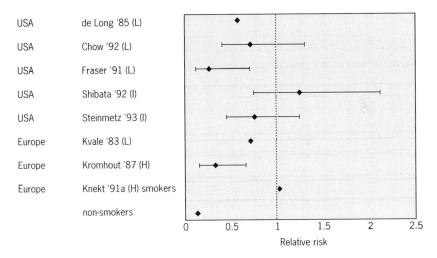

Figure 5.18 Relative risks for incidence of lung cancer with number of servings per week of fruit in cohort studies

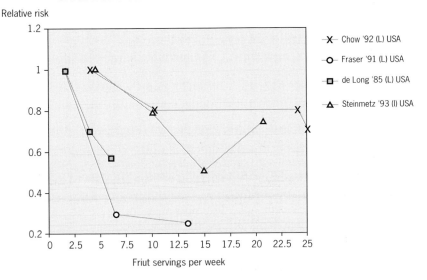

5.3.2.5 Conclusions There is moderately consistent evidence that higher consumption of fruits and weakly consistent evidence that higher consumption of vegetables are associated with a lower risk of lung cancer. It is likely that the effects of smoking have not been taken into account completely. The estimated relative risks for high consumption versus low consumption vary considerably between studies but are generally between 0.5 and 0.7.

5.3.3 Vitamin A, Retinol and β-carotene

5.3.3.1 The effect of β-carotene and/or vitamin A intake was examined in 18 case-control studies: in 14 of these an apparently protective effect of β-carotene and/or vitamin A was observed[169–171,176,177,194–202] (see Table 5.2). Alavanja et al[180] found no association between vitamin A and β-carotene intakes and risk of lung cancer and Goodman et al[173] found no association in men but a decreased risk with higher intakes of vitamin A and β-carotene intake in women. Seven studies[169,174,176,180,181,200,202] found an increased risk of lung cancer with higher intakes of retinol.

5.3.3.2 Of the nine prospective studies[122,141,158,182–184,193,203,204] identified which calculated an index of vitamin A and/or β-carotene intake, two high scoring studies found lower risk of lung cancer associated with higher intakes of β-carotene[185,193] but one in non-smokers only. Risk of lung cancer was inversely associated with vitamin A intake in one intermediate and two low scoring studies[183,203,205]. The study by Shibata et al[184] found a lower risk in women but not in men for higher intakes of β-carotene and three studies[141,158,182] found no association between intakes of vitamin A and/or β-carotene.

5.3.3.3 Six prospective studies which measured serum β-carotene concentrations found lower lung cancer risk associated with higher serum levels of β-carotene[142,206–210] (see Table 5.3). The risk of lung cancer in those with the lowest serum concentrations of β-carotene was generally about twice that of the risk in those with the highest concentrations. Serum retinol concentrations did not show the same association suggesting that β-carotene does not need to be converted into retinol to be active[206,207]. The study in Hawaiian men of Japanese ancestry found that the relationship between serum β-carotene and subsequent risk of lung cancer decreased from RR 3.4 to RR 2.2 after adjusting for smoking[208].

5.3.3.4 Smokers tend to have lower intakes of β-carotene, and also lower serum levels of β-carotene for the same intake[184]. In addition, the studies measuring serum levels of β-carotene found considerable degradation during storage even at $-70°C$, and samples subjected to repeated thawing showed even greater degradation. If cases were subjected to more frequent thawing than controls, then this could introduce a bias and give the appearance of a protective effect of β-carotene. It is also possible that β-carotene is acting as a marker for other dietary components or for a "healthier" lifestyle. Adjusting for potential confounders may not take account of other differences between people who consume large amounts of fruit and vegetables and those who consume only small amounts.

Table 5.2 Estimated odds ratio (OR)* or relative risks (RR)* and 95% confidence intervals (CI) for incidence of lung cancer for highest compared to lowest quantiles of intake for dietary vitamin A, retinol and β-carotene in epidemiological studies

Study (Quality Score)	Location	Estimated RR	CI
Case-control studies			
Alavanja et al, 1993 (H)[180]	USA (non-smokers)	0.98[a] 1.33[b] 1.00[c]	
Dartigues et al, 1990 (H)[195]	France	0.23[a] 0.24[c]	0.14–0.40 0.14–0.48
Samet et al, 1985 (H)[200]	USA	0.71[a] 1.11[b] 0.77[c]	0.53–1.00 0.77–1.43 0.56–1.11
Ziegler et al, 1984 (H)[202]	USA	1.11[a] 1.25[b] 0.77[c]	
Jain et al, 1990 (H)[174]	Canada	1.19[a] 1.21[b] 0.89[c]	1.02–1.44[b]
Byers et al, 1987 (I)[194]	USA	Men 0.67[a] 0.56[c] Women 0.83[a] 0.77[c]	p for trend 0.12 p for trend 0.001 p for trend 0.37 p for trend 0.32
Candelora et al, 1992 (I)[169]	USA (never smokers)	0.4[a] 1.2[b] 0.4[c]	0.2–0.8 0.6–2.4 0.2–0.8
Dorgan et al, 1993 (I)[170]	USA	0.79[c]	0.64–0.97
Fontham et al, 1988 (I)[171]	USA	0.89[b] 0.88[c]	0.72–1.12 0.70–1.11
Goodman et al, 1992b (I)[173]	USA	Men 0.9[a] 1.0[c] Women 0.71[a] 0.67[c]	
Gregor et al, 1980[197]	UK	All men 0.46[a†] Smokers 0.28[a†] All Women 1.88[a†] Smokers 2.28[a†]	p <0.05 p <0.05
Hinds et al, 1984 (I)[196]	Hawaii	Smokers 0.56[a]	0.26–1.00
Le Marchand et al, 1989 (I)[176]	Hawaii	Men 0.56[a] 1.11[b] 0.53[c] Women 0.40[a] 1.0[b] 0.37[c]	p for trend 0.003 p for trend 0.70 p for trend 0.001 p for trend 0.14 p for trend 0.75 p for trend 0.01
Kalandidi et al, 1990 (I)[181]	Greece	1.31[b] 1.01[c]	0.98–1.77 0.64–1.59

continued

101

Table 5.2   continued

Study (Quality Score)	Location	Estimated RR	CI
Mayne et al, 1994 (I)[177]	USA (non-smokers)	0.98[b] 0.70[c]	0.82–1.17 0.50–0.99
Mettlin et al, 1989 (I)[199]	USA	0.5[c]	
Wu et al, 1985 (I)	USA	0.83[b] 0.4[c]	0.36–2.0 0.18–0.91
Harris et al, 1991 (L)[198]	UK	0.45[c‡]	p for trend 0.048
Cohort studies			
Knekt et al, 1991a (H)[185]	N. Europe	Non-smokers 0.68[b] 0.40[c] Smokers 1.34[b] 0.93[c]	
Kromhout et al, 1987 (H)[193]	Europe	0.68[c]	0.35–1.34
Bond et al, 1987 (I)[205]	USA	All 0.49[a] Smokers 0.34[a] All 0.42[c] Smokers 0.27[c]	0.28–0.85 0.13–0.87 0.24–0.74 0.15–0.52
Paganini-Hill et al, 1987 (I)[141]	USA	No relation with vitamin A and β-carotene**	
Shibata et al, 1992 (I)[184]	USA	Men 1.07[c] Women 0.59[c]	0.66–1.74 0.32–1.07
Steinmetz et al, 1993 (I)[182]	USA	0.81[c]	0.48–1.38
Bjelke et al, 1975 (L)[203]	Europe	0.31[a]	
Chow et al, 1992 (L)[158]	USA	0.8[a] 0.9[b] 0.8[c]	0.5–1.2 0.6–1.4 0.5–1.2
Kvale et al, 1983 (L)[183]	Europe	0.62[a]	

[a] Total vitamin A
[b] Retinol
[c] β-carotene
* Odds ratio for case-control studies and relative risk for cohort studies
** After adjusting for smoking
† Low < 7,5000µg/week; high > 15,000µg/week
‡ Low < 1,683µg/day; high > 2,698µg/day

5.3.3.5 Supplementation with β-carotene (20mg/day) for 14 weeks resulted in a reduction in the frequency of micronuclei in sputum cells compared with those given placebo in a group of smokers in the Netherlands who continued smoking during the study[211]. Micronuclei in bronchial exfoliated cells may be an early indicator of DNA damage and smokers have a high frequency of micronuclei in sputum cells. The effect of supplementing males at higher risk of lung cancer, particularly smokers, aged 50–69 with β-carotene (20mg/day) for 6 years was tested in a randomised controlled trial in Finland[212]. This trial found no reduction in the incidence of lung cancer in those receiving β-carotene. Furthermore the study raised the possibility that supplementation with β-carotene

Table 5.3 Age adjusted relative risks (RR) and 95% confidence intervals (CI) for incidence of lung cancer for lowest compared to highest quantiles of serum β-carotene in cohort studies

Study (Quality Score)	Location	Estimated RR	CI
Knekt et al, 1990b (H)[207]	Northern Europe	men 1.3[‡]	0.8–2.4
		men 1.0[‡†]	0.5–1.9
		women 1.8[‡]	0.3–12.0
Comstock et al, 1991 (I)[142]	USA	4.3[a]	1.4–13.4
		1.1[b]	0.4–2.9
		1.3[c]	0.5–3.3
		1.5[d]	0.5–5.2
Nomura et al, 1985 (I)[208]	Hawaii (Japanese)	2.2[†]	0.8–6.0
Stahelin et al, 1984[209]	C Europe	No RR but serum β-carotene significantly lower in cases compared to controls (14.8µg/dl v 23.7µg/dl)	p < 0.05
Connett et al, 1989 (L)[206]	US (men)	2.32	
Wald et al, 1988 (L)[143]	UK	2.44	p for trend 0.008

[a] Squamous cell
[b] Small cell
[c] Adenocarcinoma
[d] Large cell: unspecified
[†] Adjusted for smoking
[‡] After exclusion of the first 2 years of follow-up

increased the risk of lung cancer in this group; the risk of lung cancer was significantly increased by 18% in the those who received β-carotene supplementation compared with those who did not. Mortality due to lung cancer and total mortality were non-significantly higher in those receiving β-carotene supplements. An inverse association between serum levels of β-carotene and subsequent risk of lung cancer was seen in the control group, replicating the findings of previous prospective studies.

5.3.3.6 A variety of suggestions has been put forward to explain the effects of β-carotene seen in this trial: it is possible that the intervention was too short or too late to counteract the damaging effects resulting from a lifetime of exposure to cigarette smoke and other carcinogens; β-carotene may not be the active component of fruit and vegetables and it may have been acting as a non-specific marker for lifestyles that protect against cancer. Whether β-carotene supplementation is harmful in smokers is something that requires careful consideration, although the authors suggested that, in view of the lack of any other evidence that it may be harmful, this finding may have been due to chance. Similar interim findings of non-significantly increased rates of lung cancer and total mortality have since been found in a second intervention trial of β-carotene and retinol supplementation (CARET) in smokers leading the investigators of this trial to discontinue the study after 4 years of intervention[213]. The worse outcome in these studies in those supplemented with β-carotene raises the possibility that a change in the usual balance of carotenoids in the diet (for instance by high dose purified supplements) might lead to potentially adverse perturbations in their absorption, metabolism or function. This raises the possibility that perturbations in carotenoid metabolism might modulate risk of lung cancer. However, similar data were not found in a randomised, double-blind placebo-controlled trial of β-carotene in 22 000 male physicians in the USA. In this trial among healthy men, 12 years of β-carotene supplementation produced no evidence of either benefit or harm in terms of the incidence of lung cancer[214]. These trials, by their design, do not address the question of whether a long-term high level of consumption of fruit and vegetables would reduce the risk of lung cancer in either smokers or non-smokers.

5.3.3.7 Conclusions   Although there is strongly consistent evidence from case-control studies that higher Vitamin A and/or β-carotene intakes are associated with a lower risk of lung cancer, the evidence from prospective studies is only weakly consistent and this has not been confirmed in three intervention trials lasting up to 12 years. There is strongly consistent evidence that higher plasma levels of β-carotene are associated with lower risk of developing lung cancer. It is possible that the associations seen in the observational studies were due to confounding, for example by smoking or by other nutrients associated with β-carotene, or that any protective effect of β-carotene is seen at an earlier stage in the development of lung cancer. Two intervention trials in smokers have found increases in the incidence of lung cancer in those taking β-carotene supplements which emphasises the need to consider the possibility of adverse effects of high doses of single nutrients in the absence of knowledge of the mechanisms operating.

5.3.4 *Other micronutrients*

5.3.4.1 Vitamin E   Serum concentrations of α-tocopherol were measured in three prospective studies: a protective effect of high serum α-tocopherol was seen in one study[142]. In this study, those with the lowest serum α-tocopherol levels had 2.5 times the risk of developing lung cancer as those with the highest levels. No relationship was seen between α-tocopherol levels and risk of lung cancer in either the Multiple Risk Factor Iintervention Trial (MRFIT) study[206] or in a study of 21 720 Finnish men[215]. The effect of supplementing male smokers aged 50-69 with α-tocopherol (50mg/day) or a combination of α-tocopherol and β-carotene for 6 years was tested in the randomised controlled trial in Finland described above[212]. No reduction in the incidence of lung cancer in male smokers receiving either α-tocopherol alone or a combination of α-tocopherol and β-carotene was seen.

5.3.4.2 Vitamin C   Nine case-control and 5 cohort studies reported vitamin C intakes and risk of lung cancer. In 4 case-control studies[169,171,181,187] there was a significantly reduced risk of lung cancer in those with highest intakes of vitamin C. In the other case-control studies there was either no effect[173,174,194] or opposing trends for men and women[176,196] with highest intakes in women leading to increased risk of lung cancer whereas the risk in men was reduced. Of the 5 cohort studies[158,182,184,185,193], one European study[193] showed a significantly reduced risk with higher intakes of vitamin C, a second[185] showed a reduced risk in non-smokers and a non-significantly increased risk in smokers with higher intakes. Steinmetz *et al*[182] showed a non-significantly reduced risk for women with higher dietary intakes of vitamin C (excluding supplements), whereas the risk was increased when supplement intakes were included. Shibata *et al*[184] showed reduced risk for females and no association for males and the fifth

Table 5.4 Estimated odds ratio (OR)* or relative risks (RR)* and 95% confidence intervals (CI) for incidence of lung cancer for highest compared with lowest quantiles of intake for vitamin C

Study (Quality Score)	Location	Estimated RR	CI
Case control studies			
Jain et al, 1990 (H)[174]	Canada	1.08[d]	0.86–1.36
Kalandidi et al, 1990 (I)[181]	Southern Europe non-smokers	0.67	0.42–1.05
Koo, 1988 (I)[187]	Hong Kong Chinese women	0.47	0.23–0.98
Goodman et al, 1992[a] (I)[77]	Hawaii		*p* for trend
	men	1.1	0.07
	women	0.8	0.02
Hinds et al, 1984 (I)[196]	Hawaii		
	males	0.6	0.3–1.3
	females	1.4	0.5–5.0
	smokers	1.1	0.6–2.5
Le Marchand et al, 1989 (I)[176]	Hawaii		
	males	0.5[c]	0.3–0.9
	females	2.5[c]	0.0–5.0
Byers et al, 1987 (I)[194]	USA		*p* for trend
	males	0.8	0.7
	females	0.9	0.5
Fontham et al, 1988 (I)[171]	USA	0.67	0.53–0.84
Candelora et al, 1992 (I)[169]	USA	0.5	0.3–1.0
Cohort studies			
Kromhout, 1987[b] (H)[193]	N Europe	0.36	0.18–0.75
Knekt et al, 1991a (H)[185]	N Europe		*p* for trend
	non-smokers	0.3	< 0.01
	smokers	1.2	0.4
Steinmetz et al, 1993 (I)[182]	USA		
	females[d]	0.81	0.46–1.43
	females[e]	1.41	0.87–2.30
Chow et al, 1992[a] (L)[158]	USA		
	white males	0.8	0.5–1.2
Shibata et al, 1992 (L)[184]	USA		
	males	1.11	0.68–1.81
	females	0.56	0.31–1.02

[a] Relative risks of death among lung cancer patients
[b] Risk ratio of 25 year lung cancer mortality
[c] Total vitamin C
[d] excluding supplements
[e] including supplements

Stahelin et al, 1984[209] vitamin C was lower in cases than controls

study[158] showed a non-significantly reduced risk in US males with higher intakes (see Table 5.4).

5.3.4.3 <u>Selenium</u> A number of prospective studies have reported inverse association between serum selenium levels and lung cancer, although most of the findings were not significant. A large nested case-control study in Finland found a strong, significant inverse association between serum selenium and lung cancer[216] and another found a significant inverse association with respiratory cancer[217]. The Netherlands Cohort Study found an inverse association between toenail selenium and lung cancer in over 120 000 men and women over 3 years[218]. Toenail selenium is a marker for long term selenium intake. Willet *et al*[219] found a non-significant association between serum selenium and lung cancer, although the number of cases was low; and the relationship with total cancer was significant. A further 5 nested case-control studies found non-significant inverse relationships[217,220–223] and 3 studies have found non-significantly increased risks with higher selenium levels[224–226].

5.3.4.4 <u>Folate</u> Bronchial metaplasia is frequently considered as a putative pre-cancerous lesion of lung cancer. Folate supplements (10mg/day) for 4 months in a group of smokers with bronchial metaplasia resulted in a greater atypia reduction rate compared with controls[227]. Vitamin B_{12} supplements, however, showed no effect.

5.3.4.5 <u>Conclusions</u> There is insufficient evidence to draw conclusions on vitamin E, selenium and folate and inconsistent evidence for vitamin C in relation to risk of lung cancer.

5.3.5 *Meat and fish*

5.3.5.1 Seven case-control studies have examined the relationship between meat or types of meat and risk of lung cancer and three (one in men only)[173,199,228] have found significantly higher intakes of meat, mostly processed meats such as bacon or sausages, in cases compared with controls (see Figure 5.19). A fourth (high scoring) study in non-smokers found a non-significantly higher risk associated with red meat intake[180]. Two other studies found no significant differences in intake between cases and controls[181,187] and another, in China, found significantly lower pork intakes in lung cancer cases[190]. This study also found significantly higher intakes of fish in cases compared with controls, whereas another in Hong Kong found significantly lower fish intakes in cases[187]. Two studies (both low scoring) have looked at liver intakes, one found higher intakes[197] and another found non-significantly lower intakes[229] in cases compared with controls.

5.3.5.2 Of seven prospective studies which have examined meat intake and subsequent lung cancer risk, four[98,158,192,230] have found higher risks in those with the highest consumption compared with those with the lowest (see Figure 5.20) but in one study[230] the higher risks were in smokers only. However, with the exception of a significant trend in Japanese women[98], none of the other results are statistically significant[158,192,230]. No relationship between beef or pork

Figure 5.19   Odds Ratios (95% CI) for incidence of lung cancer for highest compared with lowest consumption of meat in case-control studies

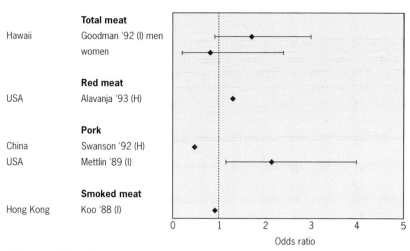

Sunkaranayan '94, red meat OR 12.49; Kalandidi '90 'no relationship'

Figure 5.20   Relative risks (95% CI) for incidence of lung cancer for highest compared to lowest consumption of meat in cohort studies

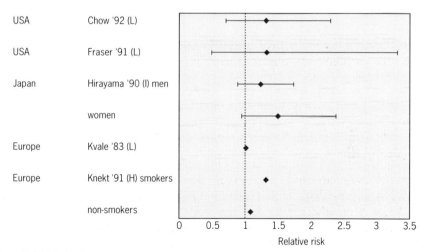

Bond '87 Liver RR 2.52 (CI 0.5-13.5); Shekelle '91 'no relationship'

intake and risk of lung cancer was seen in a study in US men[231] and no relationship was seen by Kvale et al[183] or Knekt et al[230] in non-smokers. Two studies[158,192] looked at poultry consumption and the risk of lung cancer; one found a small inverse association[158] and one found a positive association[192] between higher consumption of poultry and risk of lung cancer. All four studies[98,158,183,230] which examined fish consumption and subsequent risk of lung cancer found no association. Two studies have examined liver consumption and lung cancer risk and neither found a significant association[205,231].

5.3.5.3   <u>Conclusions</u>   The evidence that higher total meat consumption is associated with a higher risk of lung cancer is weakly consistent. However, the majority of studies are not statistically significant. This suggests that any increase in risk is small if one exists at all. Alternatively, these findings might be accounted for by confounding by other diet or lifestyle factors, for example smoking and social class. There is no evidence for a protective effect of consuming higher amounts of fish.

5.3.6. <u>Conclusions</u>   *Lung Cancer and Diet*

Smoking is the most important cause of lung cancer. The potential for confounding by smoking is great in particular as it is difficult to characterise precisely exposure to tobacco smoke. There is weakly consistent evidence for a weak association between higher total meat consumption and increased risk of lung cancer. There is moderately consistent evidence that higher vegetable consumption, and weakly consistent evidence that higher fruit consumption, are associated with lower risk of lung cancer. The strongly consistent negative association between serum β-carotene and lung cancer has not been confirmed as causal by intervention studies.

5.4   Colorectal Cancer

5.4.1   *Introduction*

5.4.1.1   Colorectal cancer is the second most common cancer in Western societies, affecting up to 6% of men and women by the age of 75. Risks increase markedly with age, but there remains at least a 15 fold range in age standardised incidence throughout the world[232]. Countries with the highest risk include Australia, New Zealand, the USA and parts of Northern Europe, and those with the lowest risk include rural Africa, China and India[232]. Epidemiological studies suggest that at least 15% of colorectal cancers are accounted for by dominantly inherited susceptibility genes[233,234]. Genes responsible for two forms of inherited colorectal cancer have been identified. Germline mutations in APC gene cause familial adenomatous polyposis coli, which affects about 1 in 7000 individuals. Hereditary non-polyposis colon cancer (HNPCC) accounts for about 2–4% of colorectal cancer in Western countries[235] (see section 7.2.5).

5.4.1.2   Migrant studies and secular changes in incidence rates both show that environmental factors contribute to geographical differences. Migrants from low risk areas rapidly acquire the incidence rates of a high risk population, for example Japanese migrants to Hawaii, Southern Europe migrants to Australia[236,237]. In Japan itself, there have been striking changes. Whereas rates were once low, age-specific colorectal cancer incidence rates have increased markedly since 1960, and are approaching those recorded in Britain. However, death rates from large bowel cancer in younger (30–40 year old) Japanese are falling[104]. The secular trends in colorectal cancer incidence have been accompanied by increasing westernisation of the diet, so that meat consumption has increased ninefold since 1950, and fat intakes threefold. Rice (and probably starch) consumption fell by one third, but there was little change in non starch polysaccharide (NSP) (dietary fibre) intakes over this time[238,239]. However, due to the low content of non-starch polysaccharides (NSP) in rice, Japanese intakes of NSP have never been high. In the UK there was a decline in colorectal cancer rates during the 1940s and 1950s, which has been attributed to the wartime increase of NSP intakes[30,240].

5.4.2   Meat and fish

5.4.2.1   Much of the international variation in large bowel cancer incidence between countries can be correlated with dietary differences, especially meat and fat consumption[29,241–243] (see Figure 4.1). Reviews of case-control studies conducted in widely varying circumstances and populations, including USA, Japan, Canada, Australia, France and Belgium, all conclude that the majority indicate

Figure 5.21   Odds Ratios (95% CI) for incidence of colorectal cancer for highest compared to lowest consumption of meat in case-control studies

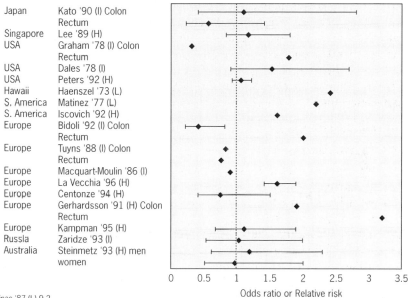

Europe Vlajinac '87 (L) 9.2

Figure 5.22   Odds Ratio for incidence of colorectal cancer with number of servings of meat per week in case-control studies

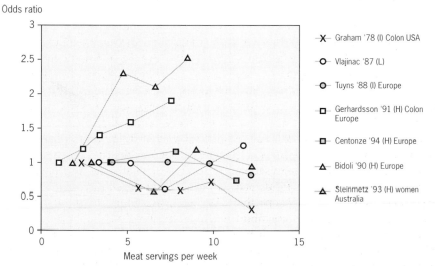

Includes only European, N. American and Australian studies

109

an increased risk of colorectal cancer in individuals who reported consuming more meat (as well as protein and fat)[244–246]. Figure 5.21 shows the odds ratios for high intake to low intake of meat for a number of case-control studies. More than half the studies show an increased risk with the highest intakes. Figure 5.22 shows the odds ratios for developing colorectal cancer against the number of servings of meat per week in case-control studies in Europe, North America and Australia. In general at 7 servings or more per week there is either no association or a greater risk of colorectal cancer.

5.4.2.2   Various indices of meat consumption have been measured in 9 prospective studies[98,99,247–253] reporting on colorectal cancer. Figures 5.23a and 5.23b

Figure 5.23a   Relative risks (95% CI) for incidence of colorectal cancer for highest compared to lowest total meat consumption in cohort studies

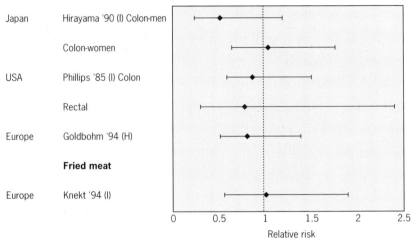

Heilbrun et al, 1989 did not give RR but reported 'effects not significant'

Figure 5.23b   Relative risks (95% CI) for incidence of colorectal cancer for highest versus lowest consumption of different meats in cohort studies

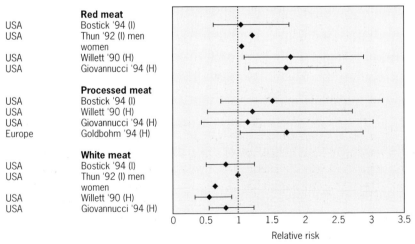

Heilbrun '89 no RR; Goldbohm '94 no RR for red and white meats

110

show the relative risks (RR) for those studies which reported RR. Two studies have found no significant effects of total meat consumption[249,251] and one study found an inverse association[98] with the risk of colon cancer in men but not in women and in rectal cancer in both men and women although these were not significant. Differences in the type of meat and the method of preparation of meat might account for some of the differences between studies. Two high scoring studies have found significantly higher risks of colorectal cancer with higher red meat consumption with relative risks of 1.7 (CI 1.2–2.6)[248] and 1.8 (CI 1.1–2.9)[253] and with the frequency of servings per week (see Figure 5.24). The intake of meat in the top quintile of consumption in the Giovannucci et al[248] study was 129g/day (median) and in the Willett et al[253] study was greater than 134g/day. Four other studies have found no significant association between red meat consumption and risk of colorectal cancer[247,249,250,252] and one study found no association between fried meat consumption and risk[99]. Two high scoring studies[249,253] have found significantly higher risk with higher consumption of processed meats and two other studies[247,248] have found non-significantly higher relative risks. The relative risks in these studies ranged from 1.2[248,253] to 1.7[249]. Women eating more poultry were at significantly lower risk in one study[253] but no significant association was seen in four other studies[247,248,250,252].

Figure 5.24   Relative Risks for incidence of colorectal cancer with number of servings of red meat per week in cohort studies

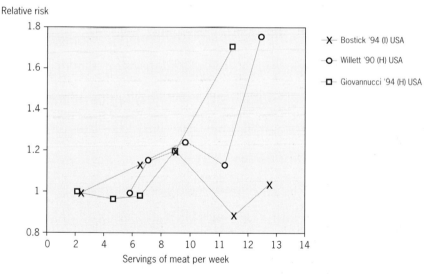

5.4.2.3   Six of the above prospective studies also reported fish consumption. Willett et al,[253] showed a significant positive trend with higher total fish consumption and increased risk of colorectal cancer; however the relative risks of those with the higher consumption were close to unity (RR 1.06 (CI 0.4–3.1)). Four studies showed no significant effect of fish consumption and colorectal cancer [247–250]. Although a study of Japanese found a statistically non-significant higher risk of colorectal cancer in men and rectum cancer in women with higher intakes of all types of fish[98].

5.4.2.4 Adenomas (adenomatous polyps) are premalignant lesions and the risk of cancer increases with the size and number of polyps[254,255], although the risk of malignant transformation within an individual adenoma is low. The combination of individual 'fast acetylation' of aromatic amines and high meat consumption seems to confer greater risk of developing adenomatous polyps (see section 7.13.4.10). However, high meat intakes did not increase the risk of individuals classified as slow acetylators[256]. The majority of case-control studies of dietary factors have yielded non-significant associations. Two prospective studies of a possible relationship between adenomatous polyps and foods and/or macronutrients have been reported[257,258]. The prospective study of Giovannucci et al[257], in male health professionals, found that increased intake of red meat was associated with an increased risk of adenoma (p value for trend 0.03) although the relative risk of those in the upper fifth compared with those in the lowest fifth of consumption was only 1.23 (CI 0.70–2.14). No significant association was seen in the other study[258] (see Table 5.5).

Table 5.5 Summary of trends in risk from adenomatous polyps case-control and cohort* studies by highest v lowest quantile of consumption of meat, fat, vegetables and fibre

Food Group	Significant Positive Association	Significant Inverse Association	No Significant Association
Meat	*Giovannucci et al 1992[257] (red meat) Kono et al 1993[776]	Neugut et al 1993[330] (chicken)	Neugut et al 1993[330] (red meat) Macquart-Moulin et al 1987[432] Sandler et al 1993[455] Benito et al 1993[368]
Fat	Hoff et al 1986[304] Sandler et al 1993[455] (women) *Giovannucci et al 1992[257] (Total fat, SFA, MUFA) Little et al 1991[600] (PUFA)	Neugut et al 1993[330] (men)	Neugut et al 1993[330] (women) Sandler et al 1993[455] (men) Macquar-Moulin et al 1987[432] *Stemmermann et al 1988[258]
Vegetables		Hoff et al 1986[304] *Giovannucci et al 1992[257] Sandler et al 1993 (women)[455] Benito et al 1993[368]	Macquar-Moulin et al 1987[432] Neugut et al 1993[330] Sandler et al 1993[455] (men)
Fibre		Neugut et al 1993[330] (men) Little et al 1991[600] *Giovannucci et al 1992[257]	Neugut et al 1993[330] (women) Hoff et al 1986[304] Sandler et al 1993[455]

5.4.2.5 Conclusions There is inconsistent evidence from cohort studies and weakly consistent evidence from case-control studies of an effect of total meat consumption on risk of colorectal cancer. There is moderately consistent evidence from cohort studies of a positive association between the consumption of red or processed meat and the risk of colorectal cancer with the higher scoring studies tending to find a significant effect of increased risk although the strength of the association is small. No prospective study has found a significantly lower risk of colorectal cancer with higher intakes of red meat or processed meat. The relative risks in all studies are less than 2. There is moderately consistent evidence that poultry (white meat) and fish consumption are not associated with risk of colorectal cancer.

5.4.3 Fat

5.4.3.1 Most case-control studies report an increased risk of colorectal cancer in individuals reported consuming more fat but this often disappears after adjusting for energy intake[259].

5.4.3.2 Total fat intake has been measured in eight prospective cohort studies of colorectal cancer[247–249,252,253,260–262], and in only one[253] was there a significant positive association between trends in fat intakes and large bowel cancer (see Figure 5.25). The majority of studies showed no significant effects, and one suggested decreased risk with increased fat intake[262]. However, with the exception of Stemmerman et al[262], studies in which relative risks have been reported suggest an elevation of relative risk for individuals with the highest fat intakes, although confidence intervals generally include 1.0 and in all but one study the relative risks are close to unity (see Figure 5.25). The evidence from cohort studies for an association between higher fat intake and increased risk of colorectal cancer is, therefore, moderately consistent, though the relative risk of colorectal cancer is likely to be close to unity.

Figure 5.25   Relative risks (95% CI) for incidence of colorectal cancer for highest compared with lowest consumption of total fat in cohort studies

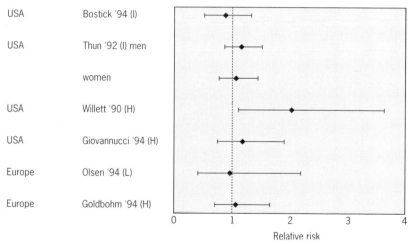

Stemmerman '84 and Garland '85 gave no RR

5.4.3.3 The prospective study of adenomatous polyposis by Giovannucci et al[257], in male health professionals showed a positive association with fat intake (including saturates and monounsaturates but not polyunsaturates). Stemmerman et al[258] found no association between total fat and incidence of adenomatous polyposis. Case-control studies were inconsistent (see Table 5.5). Reduction in fat intake was not associated with an overall reduction in polyp numbers, although larger polyps were less common in an intervention trial in Australia[263]. The combination of a low fat diet and 25g per day wheat bran led to a significant reduction in the frequency of large polyps in the same trial[263]. No significant difference in polyp recurrence was seen in another trial after 2 years on a low fat, high fibre diet[264].

5.4.3.4 <u>Conclusions</u> There is weakly consistent evidence that higher total fat intakes are associated with a higher risk of colorectal cancer. Although the majority of studies are in the direction of higher risks with higher fat consumption, in most the relative risks are close to one and do not reach statistical significance, and in no case is the relative risk greater than 2.

5.4.4 *Fruits and vegetables*

5.4.4.1 Vegetarians are generally at lower risk of colon cancer[265,266]. In the UK, regional differences in colorectal cancer mortality are strongly related to consumption of vegetables excluding potatoes[267]. A consistent inverse association between risk of colon cancer and vegetable consumption is seen in case-control studies. Twenty-three out of 28 studies reporting results for vegetables showed a significant inverse association[268]. In a meta analysis of case-control studies, risk estimates for vegetables alone (0.48) were similar to those based on fibre intake (0.58)[245]. Figure 5.26 shows the odds ratios for risk of colorectal cancer for consumers with high intakes compared with low intakes of total vegetables in case-control studies. All of the high scoring studies showed a reduced risk with higher consumption.

Figure 5.26   Odds Ratios (95% CI) for incidence of colorectal cancer for highest compared to lowest consumption of total vegetables in case-control studies

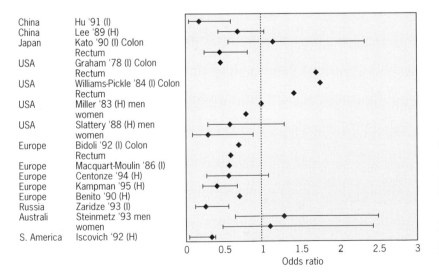

5.4.4.2 Six prospective studies have investigated vegetable consumption and four have found significantly lower risks associated with higher vegetable consumption[184,252,269,270] (see Figure 5.27), but one[184] was in women only, and men had an increased risk. The relative risks are generally between 0.9-0.5. None has reported significantly higher risk with higher consumption, although two have found non-significantly higher risks[184,271]. The Iowa Women's Health Study[270] found an inverse association for consumption of all vegetables but no dose-response pattern was evident and the effect was weakened when adjusted for energy intakes. However, average reported consumption of all vegetables and fruit was substantially higher in this survey than the US average. The most striking association in this study was an inverse association for garlic consumption. Fruit and vegetable consumption was unrelated to risk in the male Health Professionals Study[248], although garlic also showed the strongest evidence of an inverse relationship in this study. Willett et al[253] did not report vegetable consumption, although a failure to find significant effects with "vegetable fibre" probably indicates no significant effects.

Figure 5.27 Relative risks (95% CI) for incidence of colorectal cancer for highest compared to lowest consumption of total and green vegetables in cohort studies

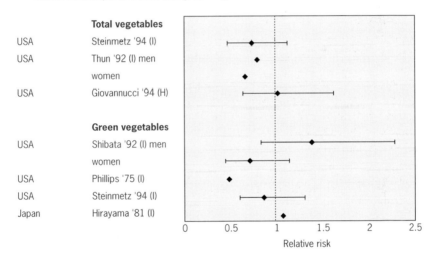

5.4.4.3 There is a weak trend towards reduced risk with higher intakes of fruits in case-control studies but this is least apparent in the higher scoring studies (see Figure 5.28). Four prospective studies have examined fruit consumption; Shibata et al[184] found a significantly lower risk in women but not men with higher fruit consumption; Steinmetz et al[270] found a non-significantly lower risk; Giovannucci et al[248] found no effect; and Phillips[269] a higher risk with higher fruit consumption (see Figure 5.29).

5.4.4.4 Conclusions There is moderately consistent evidence from case-control studies, especially higher scoring studies, that higher consumption of vegetables is associated with a lower risk of colon cancer, but the evidence from cohort studies is only weakly consistent. The relative risks for highest consumption versus lowest consumption are generally between 0.9–0.5. There is only limited and inconsistent evidence of an effect of fruit consumption.

Figure 5.28   Odds Ratios (95% CI) for incidence of colorectal cancer for highest compared to lowest consumption of fruit in case-control studies

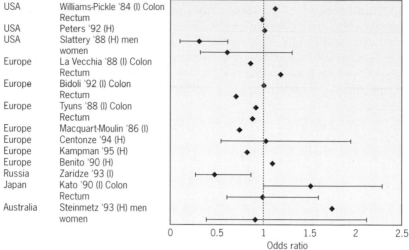

* Steinmetz '93 men 95% Confidence interval 0.88-3.46

Figure 5.29   Relative risks (95% CI) for incidence of colorectal cancer for highest compared to lowest consumption of fruit in cohort studies

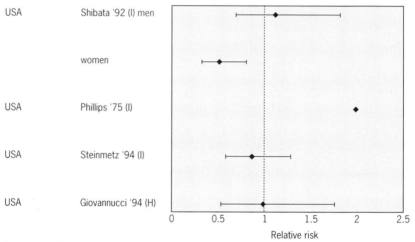

5.4.5   *Non-starch polysaccharides (dietary fibre), starch and sugar*

5.4.5.1   As pointed out in 5.2.6.1 assessment of fibre or non-starch polysaccharides (NSP) intake in epidemiological studies has been difficult due to the lack of consistency in the definition of dietary fibre and the use of different methods of analyses. Fibre is not a single chemical substance because it represents a complex of different types of polysaccharides with different physiological effects. The definition of fibre and laboratory techniques for its analysis have evolved considerably in the last 20 years. Thus the earlier studies focused on the effects of "crude" fibre whereas others used indices of "dietary" fibre[272] intake or of the intake of NSP. These different definitions may have influenced the findings both of case-control and of cohort studies.

5.4.5.2 Dietary fibre intakes have been negatively correlated with colon cancer mortality rates in 38 countries[275]. However, the correlations with fibre intakes became non-significant when adjusted for meat and fat. Within the UK, where meat consumption and fat intakes are high, a protective effect of dietary fibre was seen after controlling for fat, beef and protein suggesting that dietary fibre was independently associated with colorectal cancer[267,274]. Significant inverse relations between colorectal cancer and intakes of dietary fibre and NSP were also obtained from two studies of geographical areas at differing risk of colorectal cancer within Scandinavian populations, and in Germany[275,276].

5.4.5.3 Since the early 1970s more than 20 case-control studies on diet and colorectal cancer have been conducted[277] in widely varying circumstances and populations, including USA, Japan, Canada, Australia, France and Belgium. In most studies, a negative relationship with disease risk was found with intakes of total carbohydrates, dietary fibres, and dietary fibre from cereals and vegetables[244,245,268,278,279]. The degree to which the results of case-control studies may have been influenced by the definition of fibre and its chemical analysis in foods is illustrated by results from the case-control study on colon cancer by Slattery et al[280], who included values for different types of fibre. A protective effect was found only for "crude" fibre. However, there was no clear association between colon cancer risk and "dietary" fibre, or fibre as measured by the neutral detergents method[277].

5.4.5.4 Eight prospective studies[248-250,252,253,261,270,281] have assessed fibre or fibre-containing foods, and three[250,252,261], detected a significant inverse trend between dietary fibre and colorectal cancer incidence (see Figure 5.30). Only one low scoring study by Heilbrun et al[250] demonstrated a higher risk in the rectum but not the colon. Two high scoring large cohort studies found non-significant inverse trends which were attenuated when adjusted for energy and other

Figure 5.30   Relative risks (95% CI) for incidence of colorectal cancer for highest compared to lowest consumption of fibre in cohort studies

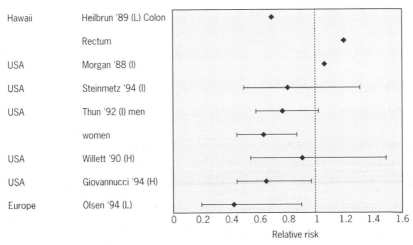

Goldbohm et al 1994 did not give RR

117

risk factors[248,270]. The study in male health professionals found a significantly lower risk in those with the highest vegetable consumption compared with the lowest[248], in line with a previous analysis in this cohort which had found a lower risk of adenomatous polyps in those reporting a higher intake of fibre or fibre-containing foods[257] (see Table 5.5). The Nurses' Health Study found that fibre was protective in high fat consumers[253]. No study has reported bowel cancer risk using analyses of dietary fibre as NSP. Freudenheim *et al*[282,283] separated fibre from cereals or from vegetables and fruits in an analysis of the Western New York study on colon and rectal cancers. After adjustment for total fat intake, colon cancer risk significantly decreased with increased intake of cereal fibre (in both males and females) as well as with fibre from fruits and vegetables (in males). Rectal cancer risk decreased with increasing intakes of fibre from fruits and vegetables, but no effect was observed for cereal fibre. It was concluded that the effects of cereal fibre on risk differ from those of fibre from fruits and vegetables and that they do not have the same effect in the colon as in the rectum.

5.4.5.5 Some reviews of case-control studies have attempted to show that any inverse association between fibre intake and cancer risk is due to the effects of fibre *per se*, rather than to other components of plant foods. Trock *et al*[245] concluded that the data did not permit a clear distinction between the effects due to other components of plant foods, but Howe *et al*[279] concluded that intake of fibre-rich foods after adjusting for vitamin C and β-carotene was inversely related to cancers of both the colon and rectum. Conversely, the estimated effects for vitamin C and β-carotene were considerably reduced by adjustment for fibre intake.

5.4.5.6 Intervention studies so far have been confined to assessing the effect of intervention on recurrence of polyps in high risk groups of patients with familial adenomatous polyposis (FAP), and to patients with adenomatous polyps. In an intervention study of FAP patients, rectal polyp recurrence was inhibited to a greater extent by vitamins C and E with supplements of bran than by supplements of these vitamins alone[284], but supplements of either 30g/day bran or 25g/day wheat bran had no effect on polyp recurrence in two trials in Australia[263,285]. However, the combination of a low fat diet and 25g/day wheat bran for 4 years did lead to a significant reduction in the frequency of large adenomas[263].

5.4.5.7 When accurately measured, the amount of NSP found in diets worldwide is much less than starch, the other major polysaccharide in food. However information on starch intake is rarely reported in the literature. In a study of individual surveys of food consumption in 12 countries, a strong inverse association between colorectal cancer incidence and starch intake was found which remained after controlling for meat and fat consumption[152]. A positive association with protein and fat was found as was a weak negative association with NSP.

5.4.5.8 Measurement of starch intakes has only rarely been attempted in case-control studies; one study showed a significant reduction in risk with starch, and two others showed no effect [280,286,287]. A review of case-control studies reported that a positive association with sucrose intake and risk of colorectal cancer was seen in a number of studies but most were not significant[247]. One prospective study found a higher risk of colon cancer in women consuming more sucrose although the relative risk of the highest consumers compared with the lowest consumers was not significant[247].

5.4.5.9 Conclusions There is moderately consistent evidence that higher intakes of dietary fibre are associated with a lower risk of colon cancer. Although the majority of studies have not found significantly lower risks, the evidence is largely in the direction of lower risk with higher intake. The relative risks for highest consumption versus lowest consumption are generally between 0.9–0.5. This may indicate a protective effect of diets characterised by high consumption of plant foods (in particular cereals, vegetables and fruits) and low consumption of meats and fat or it might indicate a specific protective effect of dietary fibre. There are insufficient data on starch or sucrose and the risk of colorectal cancer to draw any conclusions.

5.4.6 Vitamins A, E and C and carotenoids

5.4.6.1 Using pooled data from five prospective cohorts, the relative risk of those in the top quartile of serum vitamin E adjusted for serum cholesterol was not significantly lower than those in the bottom quartile (RR 0.7 (CI 0.4–1.1)), and there were no significant trends in risk across quartiles[288]. Relative risks were significantly reduced (RR 0.3 (CI 0.1–0.8)) when only those patients with an interval of between 5 and 7.5 years from blood collection to diagnosis were included, suggesting an effect of pre-existing disease. At longer intervals the relative risk increased to 1.2 (CI 0.4 to 3.3). The authors concluded that the evidence for any protective effect was weak[288]. The Iowa Womens Study found a significant reduction in relative risk of colon cancer for women aged less than 60 years who had taken vitamin E supplements, although no effects were found for dietary vitamin E alone[289]. People who take vitamin supplements may differ from those who do not in many other ways as well. Nevertheless, no relationship was seen between intakes of vitamins A and C and β-carotene, whether from diet or supplements, and subsequent risk of colon cancer in this cohort. There are few prospective data on levels of plasma vitamin C in relation to cancer. Only the Basel prospective study[290] has assessed plasma vitamin C levels in relation to cancer, but the cohort size was too small to permit a separate analysis for colon cancer.

5.4.6.2 Intervention trials in patients with adenomatous polyps using very large supplements of vitamins A (30 000 IU), vitamin C (1g) and vitamin E (70mg) have shown reduced proliferation in upper crypt compartments compared with those given placebos[291] but there was no significant effect on polyp recurrence in patients given 400mg doses of vitamins C and E compared with those given a placebo of lactose[292]. A multicentre trial from the USA has shown that supplements of 25mg β-carotene and/or 1g vitamin C with 400mg vitamin E had no effect on polyp recurrence[293]. Supplements of 20mg β-carotene increased polyp recurrence, particularly large polyps, in a study in Australia[263,285]. A trial in patients with Familial Adenomatous Polyposis (FAP) found that rectal polyp recurrence was inhibited to a greater extent by supplements of vitamins C and E with bran than by supplementation with these vitamins alone[284].

5.4.6.3   An intervention trial in 29 000 Finnish males at high risk of lung cancer, principally smokers, found no significant difference in colorectal cancer rates in those receiving α-tocopherol (vitamin E) supplements (50mg/day) or β-carotene supplements (20mg/day) for between 5 and 8 years[212].

5.4.6.4   Conclusions   There is inconsistent evidence from epidemiological studies that the vitamins C and E and β-carotene are associated with risk of colorectal cancer and insufficient evidence to conclude that vitamin A (retinol) is associated with risk of colorectal cancer. Intervention trials in people with FAP or adenomatous polyps have generally failed to find a protective effect of supplements of vitamins C, E and β-carotene on polyp recurrence. Although such interventions are not conclusive, the evidence that higher intakes of these vitamins would reduce the risk of colorectal cancer is not compelling. The findings of increased risk of large adenomas in two intervention studies cautions against the widespread use of β-carotene supplements.

5.4.7   Other micronutrients

5.4.7.1   Folate and methionine   Interest in large bowel dysplasia and hence cancer risk began with a retrospective case-control study in which folate supplementation was associated with a non-significantly lower incidence of dysplasia in ulcerative colitis patients who are at high risk of colon cancer[294]. In a later study, risk of dysplasia in ulcerative colitis was inversely associated with red cell folate levels[295]. No prospective study has reported on the role of folate in colorectal cancer, but relative deficiency has been implicated in adenomatous polyps. Giovannucci et al[296] found significant inverse trends in risk with higher folate intake, with relative risks of 0.71 (CI 0.56–0.89) for colorectal polyps in individuals in the top quintile of folate intake. The level of folate intake in this quintile would not have been achievable from dietary sources and must have been largely derived from supplements. Folate from food alone was not significantly related to adenomas. Combinations of high alcohol and low methionine and low folate diets were significantly associated with a higher risk of colon cancer[297].

5.4.7.2   Meat is the major source of dietary methionine. Despite the positive association found between adenomas and meat consumption[257] this study demonstrated inverse associations with methionine intake[296].

5.4.7.3   Calcium   Potter et al[246] have reviewed the epidemiological evidence on calcium intake and risk of colon cancer and suggest that a protective association is evident. However, a reduction in risk at high levels of calcium intake (>2g/day) was reported in only three out of 9 case-control studies from 1985 to 1992[246]. To date, six prospective studies have reported calcium intake in relation to risk of colorectal cancer[260,289,298–301]. All are suggestive of a lower risk with higher intakes but relative risks are generally not significant (see Figure 5.31). Relative risks in the study of Slob *et al*[300] refer to all gastrointestinal cancers (including stomach), because there were too few cases for a separate analysis. However, women who died of colorectal cancer had reported lower calcium consumption than the rest of the population. Bostick *et al*[289] were unable to detect significant differences in multivariate analyses of a cohort study. Univariate analysis did not show a significant protective effect at dietary levels of calcium intake (800mg), but cases had consumed 209mg calcium per day from supplements whereas controls had consumed 283mg per day, and this difference was statistically significant. The Netherlands Cohort Study found no association with total dietary calcium but an inverse trend with calcium from unfermented dairy products[301]. Several intervention studies with calcium are currently in progress in polyp patients at high risk of colon cancer. One study[302] has reported that oral calcium supplementation (4.5g calcium carbonate/day) showed only minor non-statistically significant reduction of epithelial cell proliferation in the rectum and had no effect in the colon in those at risk of hereditary non-polyposis colorectal cancer. Overall therefore, the results are moderately consistent that higher intakes of calcium are associated with lower risk of colorectal cancer but this may reflect consumption of calcium rich food sources, principally dairy products, rather than calcium itself (see 1.5.6).

Figure 5.31   Relative risks (95% CI) for incidence of colorectal cancer with lowest compared to highest intakes of calcium in cohort studies

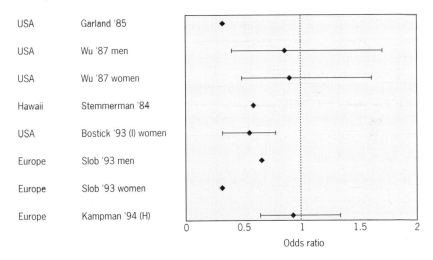

5.4.7.4   <u>Vitamin D</u>   Vitamin D is classically associated with calcium homeostasis but a more fundamental role in controlling cell growth and differentiation has recently emerged. Garland *et al* 1985[260] and 1989[303] found significant protective effects in colon cancer for both dietary vitamin D and serum 25-hydroxyvitamin D in two separate cohorts. Later epidemiological evidence is less consistent, with a non-significant effect for vitamin D shown in one cohort and in two case-control studies in which results have so far been reported[246].

5.4.7.5   <u>Iron</u>   Four case-control studies have measured iron intake, three in polyp patients and one in rectal cancer patients. They have shown no significant

121

effects, or inverse trends[304] but supplemental intakes may not have been recorded[305]. Of the three epidemiological studies which have measured iron status, only the study of Nelson et al[305] assessed serum ferritin levels, which reflect body stores. In this case-control study of patients with both colon cancer and adenoma there was no significant increase in risk associated with increased iron stores in cancer patients (who may have reduced stores due to gastrointestinal bleeding), but patients with adenoma at the upper end of the distribution in ferritin levels had a significant elevated odds ratio of 4.3 (CI 2.00–10.1). The results remained significant after adjusting for alcohol intake and excluding individuals with high serum ferritin levels in excess of 400ng/ml. Two studies have measured transferrin saturation, although levels can be elevated secondarily to chronic inflammation. The study of Stevens et al[306] was based on a relatively small cohort of the NHANES study and separate analyses for colon cancer were not possible. Elevated transferrin saturation levels were associated with increased risk of all sites incidence and mortality. In a large Finnish cohort, elevated risks of 3.04 (CI 1.64–5.62) for colorectal cancer and cancer of all sites 1.43 (CI 1.16–1.77) were evident in those individuals classified into the upper distribution of transferrin saturation[307]. However, although high iron stores are associated with increased risk, they may not be related to increased iron intake and data on intake from prospective studies is required to confirm a role for iron in colorectal cancer.

5.4.7.6   Conclusions   There is insufficient evidence to draw conclusions on the effect of other micronutrients on the risk of colorectal cancer.

5.4.8   Conclusions   *Colorectal Cancer and Diet*

There is moderately consistent evidence that diets with less red and processed meat and more vegetables and fibre are associated with reduced risk of colorectal cancer. Evidence is inconsistent for vitamins A, C and E, and β-carotene.

5.5   Prostate Cancer

5.5.1   *Introduction*

5.5.1.1   Prostate cancer is the third most common cancer in UK men. As the prevalence of latent 'prostatic cancer' seems to be of the same order in countries with high and low clinical cancer rates, a promoting or enhancing role for endogenous or exogenous factors in high risk populations is considered probable. Dietary differences and changes do not explain the virtually two-fold higher incidence in blacks than whites in the United States. A history of sexually transmitted disease is a strong predictor of risk in both blacks and whites.

5.5.1.2   International comparisons suggest an association between increased consumption of animal products and decreased consumption of cereals and potatoes and prostate cancer[161,308]. Within Japan increased prostate cancer rates over time have been associated with increased fat consumption[309]. Studies of migrants to Australia[310] and Japanese migrants to the USA[311] suggested that rates move toward the host country rates.

5.5.2 *Meat and fish*

5.5.2.1 Of 6 case-control studies which looked at meat intakes, 5 found significantly higher risks associated with higher meat consumption[312-316] and a sixth found a non-significantly higher risk[317]. Relative risks were generally around 2.0 for highest consumption compared with lowest consumption. Ewing and Bowie[313] found a relative risk of 2.25 (CI 0.62–10.15) in those consuming meat once a day compared with those consuming meat less than twice a week. A study in Los Angeles found lower risk with more frequent poultry consumption[314].

5.5.2.2 Of 8 prospective studies of diet and prostate cancer which examined meat consumption, three found significantly higher risks of prostate cancer associated with higher meat or red meat consumption[318-320], two found non-significantly higher risks for total meat[98,321], one found non-significantly lower risks associated with total meat consumption[322], one found non-significantly lower risks associated with red meat[323] and one found no difference with fried meat[99] (see Figure 5.32). Two studies found non-significantly higher risks associated with higher processed meat consumption[319,322]. One study found a significant positive trend with fish consumption[319] but most have found no significant effects of poultry or fish[98,318,323]. A review by Key[324], of 11 case-control and prospective studies, reported a significant summary relative risk of 1.34 (CI 1.16–1.55).

Figure 5.32 Relative risks (95% CI) for incidence of prostate cancer for highest compared to lowest consumption of meat in cohort studies

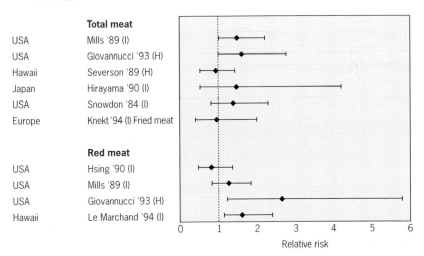

5.5.2.3 <u>Conclusions</u> There is weakly consistent evidence that total meat and moderately consistent evidence that red meat consumption are associated with higher risk of prostate cancer. Although the evidence is largely in the direction of higher risk with higher meat consumption, in the majority of studies it does not reach statistical significance. The data relating to poultry, fish or processed meat consumption on risk of prostate cancer are insufficient to draw conclusions.

5.5.3 *Fat*

5.5.3.1 Of 10 case-control studies which reported fat intakes, 4 found a significantly higher risk associated with higher total fat, animal fat and saturated fatty acids intake[312,315,325,326]. One other study found significantly higher risks in those aged over 70 years but not in younger men[327] and one found a positive non-significant association in men aged 70 years and over[199]. Three other studies failed to find an association[313,328,329]. Ross *et al*[314] found a significant positive association for total fat intake in US Blacks and a non-significant positive association in US Whites (see Table 5.6).

5.5.3.2 Four prospective studies have examined the effects of dietary fat on prostate cancer risk[318–320,322] (see Table 5.6). A study in 14 000 Seventh Day Adventist men found a small positive association between animal fat consumption and risk of prostate cancer, but this was not significant[319]. A much larger study in nearly 48 000 male health professionals found non-significantly higher relative risks in those consuming higher amounts of total fat and animal fat[318] (see Table 5.6). After adjusting for intakes of other fatty acids, only higher intakes of α-linoleic acid were significantly associated with a higher risk of prostate cancer. A study in 20 000 men in Hawaii found a marginally significant higher relative risk in men consuming more high fat animal products (RR 1.6 CI 1.0-2.4)[320]. Severson *et al* [322], found a non-significantly lower risk associated with higher consumption of total fat and no association with saturated and unsaturated fats.

5.5.3.3 <u>Conclusions</u> The limited data are weakly consistent that higher total fat intakes are associated with higher risks of prostate cancer.

5.5.4 *Fruits and vegetables*

5.5.4.1 In case-control studies, higher consumption of green vegetables and fruit, vegetable protein, yellow-green vegetables, cooked green vegetables, spinach and carrots have all been associated with lower risk in four intermediate scoring studies[133,314,315,331]. A high scoring study in Northern Italy found a non-significantly higher risk with more frequent consumption of fresh fruit[317]. A high scoring study in Japanese men in Hawaii found that risk was significantly higher in men aged over 70 who consumed a lot of papaya[322].

5.5.4.2 Of the prospective studies of diet and prostate cancer, three intermediate scoring studies have found higher consumption of fruits and/or vegetables associated with subsequently lower risk[156,319,333] (see Figures 5.33 and 5.34). The Japanese study[156] found an inverse association with yellow-green vegetables for men aged under 75 years, whereas the study in Seventh Day Adventists[319] found lower risk associated with beans, fresh fruit, dried fruit, green salad, tomatoes and nuts, although only tomatoes and beans were significant after adjusting for the consumption of other foods. The Health Professionals Follow-up study[333] found tomatoes, tomato juice, tomato sauce and pizza to be inversely associated with risk of prostate cancer. A positive association with fruit intake was found among Japanese men in Hawaii[322]. However Hsing *et al*[323] found a

124

Table 5.6 Estimated odds ratio (OR)* or relative risks (RR)* and 95% confidence intervals (CI) for incidence of prostate cancer for highest compared to lowest quantiles of intake for fat and fatty acids in epidemiological studies

Study (Quality Score)	Location/subjects	Estimated OR or RR	CI and/or Significance
Case-Control			
Kolonel et al, 1988[327] (H)	Hawaii	Total fat 1.5	0.9–2.3 NS
	Men $\geq$ 70 yrs	SFA 1.7	1.0–2.8 p=0.02
		UFA 1.3	0.8–2.0 NS
	Men <70 yrs	Total fat 1.0	0.6–1.7 NS
		SFA 1.0	0.6–1.9 NS
		UFA 1.2	0.7–2.0 NS
West et al, 1991[325] (H)	USA	Total fat 2.9	1.0–8.4 p=0.05
	Men 68–74 yrs	SFA 2.2	0.7–6.6 NS
		MUFA 3.6	1.3–9.7 p<0.05
		PUFA 2.7	1.1–6.8 p<0.05
Whittemore et al, 1995[326] (H)	Blacks <84 yrs	Total Fat 1.3	0.7–2.2
(Los Angeles, San Francisco, Hawaii,	Whites <84 yrs	Total Fat 1.4	0.9–2.3
Vancouver and Toronto)	Chinese/Americ	Total Fat 4.0	1.3–12.8
	Japanese/Americ	Total Fat 1.6	0.9–3.0
	Blacks <84 yrs	SFA 1.6	0.7–3.8
	Whites <84 yrs	SFA 1.1	0.5–2.5
	Chinese/Americ	SFA 3.1	0.4–26.1
	Japanese/Americ	SFA 4.0	1.3–12.8
Mettlin et al, 1989[199] (I)	USA		
	Men >69 yrs	Animal fat 1.2	0.6–2.3 NS
	Men <69 yrs	Animal fat 1.5	0.7–3.1 NS
Ross et al, 1987[314] (I)	USA		
	Blacks	Total fat 1.9	p<0.05
	Whites	Total fat 1.6	NS
Walker et al, 1992[315] (I)**	South Africa		
	Blacks	Total fat 2.6	1.6–4.0 p<0.01
Ohno et al, 1988[328] (L)	Japan		
	Men 50–79 yrs	Total fat 0.8	NS
Bravo et al, 1991[312] (L)	S. Europe	Diets rich in animal	
	50–88 yrs	fats 2.56	1.30–5.05 Sig
		Diets rich in veg-	
		etable fats 1.26	0.58–2.71 NS
Kaul et al, 1987[329] (L)	USA	Total & SFA	NS
	Black men	Weak +ve association	
	30–49 yrs	Linoleic acid	NS
		strong-ve association	
	50+ years	Total & SFA	NS
		Weak -ve association	
		Linoleic acid	
		strong-ve association	p<0.04
Ewings & Bowie, 1996[313] (I)	UK	Fat on meat 1.28	0.78–2.13 NS

continued

Table 5.6   continued

Study (Quality Score)	Location/subjects	Estimated OR or RR	CI and/or Significance
Cohort studies			
Le Marchand et al, 1994[320] (I)	Hawaii	High fat animal products 1.6	1.0–2.4
Giovannucci et al, 1993[318] (I)	USA	Total fat 1.79	1.04–3.07 p trend 0.06
		Animal fat 1.63	0.95–2.78 p trend 0.08
		SFA 1.68	0.41–2.21 p trend 0.04
		α-linolenic 3.4	p trend 0.002
Mills et al, 1989[319] (I)	USA Seventh Day Adventists	Animal fat 1.35	0.81–2.23
Severson et al, 1989[322] (I)	Hawaii Japanese Men	Total fat 0.87 SFA 1.00 Unsat fat 1.09	0.58–1.31 NS 0.68–1.46 NS 0.75–1.60 NS

*   Odds Ratio for case-control studies and relative risk for cohort studies
** Comparison between fat intake ≥25% energy and <25% energy.

non-significant increased risk with higher intakes of cruciferous vegetables and non-significant decreased risk with higher intakes of fruits.

5.5.4.3 <u>Soya products</u> Soya products have been suggested as being possibly protective against prostatic cancer because of their high content of isoflavones, a type of phytoestrogen (see Chapter 8). However, no significant difference in intake of miso soup was seen between men with prostatic cancer and those with benign hyperplastic disease or with hospital controls[334]. Severson *et al,*[322]

Figure 5.33   Relative risks (95% CI) for incidence of prostate cancer for highest compared to lowest consumption of fruit in cohort studies

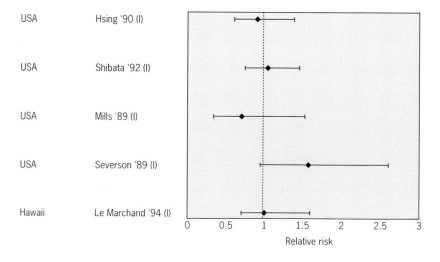

Figure 5.34   Relative risks (95% CI) for incidence of prostate cancer for highest compared to lowest consumption of vegetables in cohort studies

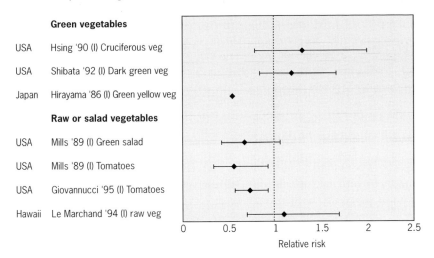

showed a weak inverse association with tofu consumption but no effect with miso soup in a group of 8 000 Hawaiian men followed for almost 20 years. No significant association was seen between soyabean soup and prostate cancer risk in a cohort of Japanese men[309] Mills et al[319] found that the use of vegetarian protein products (meat substitutes such as soy products and gluten) were associated with a non-significant decrease in the risk estimate for prostate cancer in the cohort of Adventist men.

5.5.4.4   Conclusions   The limited evidence is moderately consistent that higher vegetable consumption, especially raw and salad vegetables, is associated with a lower risk of prostate cancer. The evidence for an association between consumption of fruit and risk of prostate cancer is inconsistent. There are insufficient data on the intakes of soya products to reach a conclusion on the association of soya products with risk of prostate cancer.

5.5.5   Vitamins A, E and C and carotenoids

5.5.5.1   Three case-control studies found reduced risk associated with increased intakes of β-carotene[199,314,328] (two intermediate and one low scoring) and one intermediate scoring study found increased risk associated with increased intakes of vitamins A and C in men over 70 years at interview[316]. Four studies found a positive association with vitamin A and prostate cancer[325,335–337]. In another case-control study[338] no association was seen with vitamins C and E and β-carotene but there was an inverse association with energy adjusted retinol.

5.5.5.2   Some prospective studies have suggested that the association of β-carotene with risk may be different in different age groups; for example, Hsing et al[339] reported an elevated relative risk of borderline significance in younger men but a strongly protective association in older men. Another study found no relationship between foods rich in vitamin A or β-carotene and future risk of prostate cancer[141]. The mean age of residents in this study in a retirement home

127

was 74 years. The Health Professionals Follow-up Study[333] found no association between prostate cancer incidence and dietary retinol or β-carotene, α-carotene, lutein and β-cryptoxanthin but a significant inverse association with lycopene intake (RR 0.79, CI 0.64–0.99). Three prospective studies have measured serum concentrations of different antioxidant vitamins and related these to subsequent risk of prostate cancer. Of these, one study found a higher risk of prostate cancer with low serum vitamin A concentrations which increased with time between serum collection and diagnosis[340], one found no relationship between β-carotene, vitamin C or lycopene and subsequent risk of prostate cancer[142] and the third found no relationship between serum concentrations of vitamin E and carotene and subsequent risk of prostate cancer[215].

5.5.5.3   The Finnish intervention trial in 29 000 middle-aged male smokers found a significant, one third reduction in rates of prostate cancer in those who received supplements of α-tocopherol (50mg/day) compared with those who did not[212]. However, this was not a hypothesis under test, and many comparisons were made in this study and it is possible that this effect might have arisen by chance. Those receiving β-carotene supplements (20mg/day) had increased rates of prostate cancer compared with those who did not. Again, this effect might have arisen by chance.

5.5.5.4   Conclusions   The evidence that intakes of vitamins A, C and E and β-carotene are associated with risk of prostate cancer is inconsistent.

5.5.6   Conclusions   *Prostate Cancer and Diet*
There is moderately consistent evidence that higher red meat consumption and weakly consistent evidence that higher total meat consumption and higher total fat consumption are associated with increased risk of prostate cancer. There is moderately consistent evidence that higher vegetable consumption, especially raw and salad vegetables, is associated with reduced risk of prostate cancer but the evidence that consumption of fruits, and intakes of vitamins A, C and E and β-carotene, are associated with prostate cancer is inconsistent.

5.6   Bladder Cancer

5.6.1   *Introduction*
5.6.1.1   The three major factors which have been implicated in bladder carcinoma are smoking, occupation and bilharzial infection. Occupational exposures in the rubber and dyestuffs industries have now largely been eliminated but excess risk has been reported from the leather, painting and other industries using organic chemicals. Many of these studies have not controlled for tobacco use. A role of diet and nutrition in bladder carcinogenesis is plausible since many substances or metabolites, including carcinogens, are excreted through the urinary tract[341].

5.6.2   *Meat*
5.6.2.1   Of the 2 case-control studies identified which examined meat, neither found a significant relationship with meat consumption, although a marginally significant lower risk was seen with higher meat consumption in one high

scoring study[342] and a non-significantly higher risk was seen in another high scoring study[343]. Of the 2 prospective studies of meat and bladder cancer, one low scoring study reported significantly higher risks of bladder cancer with higher consumption of beef and pork; however the food frequency questionnaire was very limited and only mentioned 8 foods so the results of this study are probably unreliable[344]. A large Japanese cohort[156] found lower risk of bladder cancer associated with increased meat consumption.

5.6.2.2   Conclusions   There is insufficient evidence to draw conclusions on meat consumption and risk of bladder cancer.

5.6.3   Fat

5.6.3.1   Of the three case-control studies which examined sources of fat in the diet, two high scoring studies reported higher risks of bladder cancer with higher intakes of saturated fats, butter and cream[342] or with fried foods[343]. A third low scoring study found no relationship with fat[345].

5.6.3.2 Conclusions There is insufficient evidence to draw conclusions on fat consumption and risk of bladder cancer.

5.6.4   Fruits and vegetables

5.6.4.1   Of the 8 case-control studies identified which considered various types and measures of fruit and vegetable consumption, 7 studies found lower risk of bladder cancer with higher consumption of green vegetables, carrots, dark green vegetables, vegetables and fruit or fruit juice[133,345–350] with relative risk estimates between 0.5 and 0.7 for the highest versus the lowest consumption level but not all were significant.

5.6.4.2   Three prospective studies were identified which reported diet and bladder cancer and, of these, one intermediate scoring study found lower risk with daily consumption of green-yellow vegetables[156], another intermediate scoring study found a lower risk with cooked green vegetables (RR 0.5) and with fruit juice (RR 0.3)[351] and a low scoring study found no relationship[344]. In a review of epidemiological studies, La Vecchia & Negri[341] concluded that there is suggestive evidence that a diet rich in fresh fruit and vegetables is a correlate–or an indicator–of reduced bladder cancer risk.

5.6.4.3   Conclusions   The limited evidence is moderately consistent that consumption of vegetables and fruit is inversely associated with risk of bladder cancer.

5.6.5   Vitamins A, C, E and carotenoids

5.6.5.1   Case-control studies have tended not to find any association between bladder cancer and vitamins A, C and β-carotene. Nomura et al[348], found no relation between carotenoids or vitamin A and risk of bladder cancer, although they did note an inverse association with vitamin C in women. No relationship between vitamin A, carotenes and vitamin C and bladder cancer risk was seen in a study in Hawaii[352]. However, a study in New York found lower risk of bladder cancer associated with higher intakes of vitamin A[336].

5.6.5.2   One prospective study found a lower risk of bladder cancer in those with high β-carotene intakes[141]. However, 3 prospective studies (all intermediate scoring) which measured serum concentrations of β-carotene and vitamin E found no relationship with subsequent risk of bladder cancer[142,210,353]. One study found lower risk associated with higher lycopene concentrations[142]. Supplementation with either 50mg vitamin E or 20mg β-carotene for between 5 and 8 years did not reduce rates of bladder cancer in 29 000 male smokers in Finland[212].

5.6.5.3   Conclusions   There is insufficient evidence to draw conclusions on vitamins A, C, E and β-carotene intake in relation to risk of bladder cancer.

5.6.6   Coffee and tea

5.6.6.1   Coffee consumption has been associated with higher risk of bladder cancer in some[345,348,350] but not all[355] case-control studies. IARC reviewed 22 case-control studies and found a weak positive association in 16 studies, of which the findings were significant in 7[356]. It was concluded that the data were consistent with a weak positive relationship between coffee consumption and bladder cancer but the possibility that it is due to bias or confounding cannot be excluded. Coffee was classified as being possibly carcinogenic to the human urinary bladder[356].

5.6.6.2 A case-control study in Japan found higher risk of bladder cancer associated with cocoa consumption and lower risk associated with black tea consumption[349]. However, in a prospective study of Japanese men in Hawaii, no relationship was seen between black tea consumption and subsequent bladder cancer[357]. IARC found no consistent association between tea consumption and risk of bladder cancer[356].

5.6.6.3   Conclusions   There is insufficient evidence to draw conclusions on coffee and tea consumption in relation to risk of bladder cancer.

5.6.7   Conclusions   Bladder Cancer and Diet

There is moderately consistent evidence from limited data that fruit and vegetables are inversely associated with risk of bladder cancer but there is insufficient evidence to associate other dietary factors with risk of bladder cancer.

5.7   Gastric Cancer

5.7.1   Introduction

5.7.1.1   Early infection with *Helicobacter pylori*—leading to chronic atrophic gastritis and eventual gastric neoplasia—has been recognised by IARC as carcinogenic, with a relative risk of around six[358]. This observation would explain, at least in part, the higher incidence of this cancer in poor populations in which infection by this bacterium occurs at an early age.

5.7.1.2   Smoking is also accepted as a risk factor for stomach cancer. Several prospective studies have observed a modest excess risk, with a dose response relationship, of stomach cancer among smokers[359,360].

5.7.1.3 Gastric cancer incidence rates vary approximately ten-fold internationally. The highest rates are seen in Japan, China and parts of South America and the lowest rates are seen in the United States, Canada, Australia and parts of sub-saharan Africa[12,260]. Migrant studies suggest that populations moving from high to low risk countries maintain their high risk of cancer while their children have lower risks[237,361]. Incidence rates are higher in men than in women (Parkin et al, 1992) and in lower socio-economic classes than in more affluent classes[362].

5.7.1.4   Internationally there has been a steady decline in gastric cancer mortality in most countries[263], with rates starting to decline later in Japan. There are still substantial international differences and these have been related inversely to differences in consumption of animal products and positively to consumption of cereals and fish[161,364–366] in ecological studies. Comparisons within Japan[367,368] suggested associations with higher consumption of pickled vegetables and salted fish, which is supported by a positive association within China between salt sales data and gastric cancer mortality[369]. Gastric cancer mortality rates in 65 rural counties in China were correlated negatively with the consumption of green vegetables but not with fruit[360] also an association with low levels of plasma ascorbic acid and selenium was suggested[370]. Time trends suggested that the decline in gastric cancer mortality was associated with an increased consumption of milk, meat, fish, fat and sugar, and with a decline in consumption of cereals and salted fish in Japan (Tominaga et al 1982) and Chile (Zaldivar 1977), increased consumption of fruits and vegetables in Poland (Jedrychowski et al 1986) and increased consumption of fruit in Japan (Hirayama, 1975). Studies in Japanese migrants to the USA and Canada (reviewed by MacDonald 1966) suggested that rates did fall in the migrant groups, but still remained higher than the general population, but their offspring acquire a risk close to those of the host countries (Kono & Hirohata 1996).

5.7.2   *Salt and Salty Foods e.g. salted meats, fish and vegetables*

5.7.2.1   Sixteen case-control studies of gastric cancer and salt or salty foods were identified. Of these, 11 found a positive association between consumption of salty foods or the addition of salt to food and the risk of gastric cancer[375–380,382–389], although 2 studies were not significant for salty meat[378,388] and two studies for salty fish[375,389] (see figure 5.35). One study in Japan[381] found no association between salted/dried fish and gastric cancer but a significant positive association between consumption of salted vegetables and gastric cancer. A study in Sweden[390] found no association between intake of salty foods and risk of gastric cancer. Many of these studies were in populations with generally high salt intakes, eg China, Japan, Puerto Rico, Uruguay, but seven were in European countries. Nine studies[375,376,379,382,385,386,389,391,392] estimated salt intake, frequency of use of table salt or use of household salt. The odds ratios were generally in the region of 1.5–2.0. However the study by Graham et al,[379] in New York found odds ratios for highest intake of table salt of 3.1 (CI: 1.65–5.79) in

131

men and 4.7 (CI: 2.26–9.55) in women, Coggan et al[377] found odds ratios of 3.0 (CI: 1.3–7.1) for salty foods and table salt and Nazario et al[385] found odds ratios of 6.7 (CI: 2.7–16.8) for the highest quartile of salt intake.

5.7.2.2   Four prospective studies[359,393–395] were identified which reported on salty foods and/or table salt and risk of gastric cancer. Two measured salted vegetables in Japanese populations[394,359] and found no significant association with risk of gastric cancer in those with the highest frequency of consumption. Nomura et al[394] also measured ham or bacon and table salt/soy sauce and found a non-significant increased risk with ham and bacon and no association with table salt. A study on Norwegian men in the US found a non-significantly higher risk in those consuming more salted bacon/pork[395]. Kneller et al[395] also measured consumption of salted fish and found a significantly higher risk, RR 1.9 (CI: 1.0–3.6) with the highest levels of consumption. The IARC concluded that Chinese salted fish is carcinogenic to humans, based mainly on the evidence for an effect on nasopharyngeal cancer[10].

5.7.2.3   It has been suggested that high salt intakes irritate the gastric mucosa, resulting in superficial gastritis and ultimately chronic atrophic gastritis (see 7.5.5.2). However, infection with *Helicobacter pylori* is now recognised to be the prime cause of chronic atrophic gastritis (see 7.5.5.1) and this was not taken into account in the case-control studies discussed above. No difference in urinary sodium excretion was seen in a case-control study in the UK of 134 people found to have intestinal metaplasia (a putative precancerous lesion) on endoscopy compared with 133 controls who were found to be without either intestinal metaplasia or chronic atrophic gastritis[396]. This study found that 83% of people with intestinal metaplasia were seropositive for *H. pylori* compared with only 23% of people without[397].

5.7.2.4   Conclusions   Although the majority of case-control studies show higher intakes of salt both from salty foods and added table salt in gastric cancer cases and the few prospective studies identified showed moderately consistent evidence that high intakes of salty meat and fish are associated with higher risk of gastric cancer, this does not generally relate to foods commonly consumed in the UK. Furthermore these studies did not take account of *H. pylori* infection which is an important potential confounder. Therefore it is not possible to draw a conclusion about the association of salt and the risk of gastric cancer relevant to the UK. There are no data pertaining to any possible role of diet and nutrition in increasing susceptibility to *H. Pylori* infection.

5.7.3   *Fruits and vegetables*

5.7.3.1   There is a large body of evidence relating consumption of fruit and vegetables with risk of gastric cancer. Of the 37 case-control studies reviewed, 23 found reduced risks with higher consumption of fruits and vegetables[66,189,375,377,378,381,382,388,389,392,398,406,408–410] and no studies have found significantly increased risks with higher consumption of fruit although two South East Asian studies[383,384] found small increased risks with increased consumption of total vegetables and green/yellow vegetables respectively (see Figures 5.35, 5.36 and 5.37). This association has been observed in populations from several European countries, North and South America, China and Japan. Most of the studies have adjusted for relevant covariates, especially some indication of socio-economic status, although relatively few have adjusted for consumption of other dietary variables. The effect has been seen for all types of fruit and vegetables including raw (salad) vegetables, cooked vegetables, fresh fruit, dried fruit and citrus fruit. In general, the estimated relative risk decreased with increasing number of servings per week for both fruit and vegetables (see Figures 5.38 and 5.39).

Figure 5.35   Odds Ratios (95% CI) for incidence of gastric cancer for highest compared to lowest consumption of fruit in case-control studies

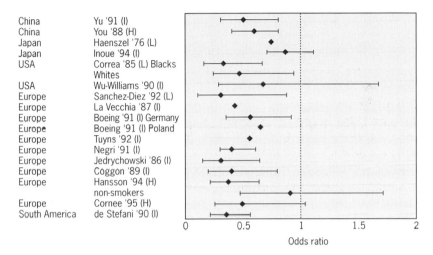

Figure 5.36   Odds Ratios (95% CI) for incidence of gastric cancer for highest compared to lowest consumption of total vegetables in case-control studies

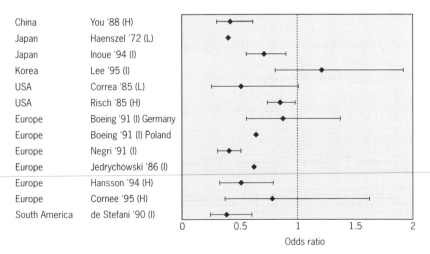

133

Figure 5.37 Odds Ratios (95% CI) for incidence of gastric cancer for highest compared to lowest consumption of green and raw vegetables in case-control studies

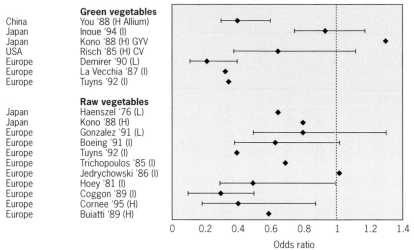

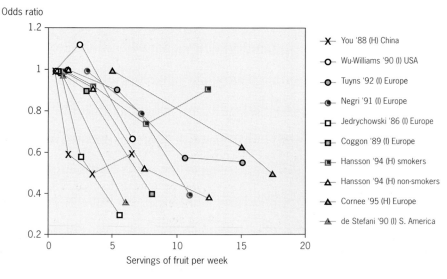

* GYV green yellow vegetables, CV cruciferous vegetables

5.7.3.2 Of six prospective studies reviewed, two found a significantly lower risk with higher fruit and vegetable consumption[411,412], one a non-significantly lower risk for higher fruit and vegetable consumption[413], and two studies in the US found no relationship between fruit and vegetable consumption, or foods rich in vitamin A or carotenes and subsequent gastric cancer risk[395,414] while another, in Japan, found daily fruit consumption associated with a significantly higher relative risk compared with those who ate fruit less than once or twice a week[359] (see Figure 5.40). Data from a European study in the Netherlands shows a lower risk of gastric cancer associated with higher onion consumption but not with leek or garlic consumption[186]. The results from prospective studies show a trend

Figure 5.38 Odds Ratio for incidence of gastric cancer with number of servings of fruit per week in case-control studies

Figure 5.39   Odds Ratio for incidence of gastric cancer with number of total vegetables per week in case-control studies

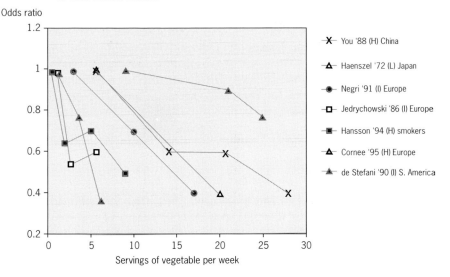

Odds ratio

Servings of vegetable per week

-X- You '88 (H) China

-△- Haenszel '72 (L) Japan

-●- Negri '91 (I) Europe

-□- Jedrychowski '86 (I) Europe

-■- Hansson '94 (H) smokers

-▲- Cornee '95 (H) Europe

-▲- de Stefani '90 (I) S. America

Figure 5.40   Relative risks (95% CI) for incidence of gastric cancer for highest versus lowest consumption of vegetables and fruits in cohort studies

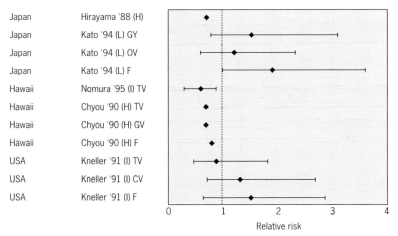

Japan	Hirayama '88 (H)
Japan	Kato '94 (L) GY
Japan	Kato '94 (L) OV
Japan	Kato '94 (L) F
Hawaii	Nomura '95 (I) TV
Hawaii	Chyou '90 (H) TV
Hawaii	Chyou '90 (H) GV
Hawaii	Chyou '90 (H) F
USA	Kneller '91 (I) TV
USA	Kneller '91 (I) CV
USA	Kneller '91 (I) F

Relative risk

GY=Green Yellow vegs; OV=Other vegs; TV=Total vegs; GV=Green vegs; CV=Cruciferous vegs; F=Fruits
Paganini Hill '85 (L) no relationship

towards reduced risk of gastric cancer with higher consumption of fruits and vegetables, especially the high scoring studies.

5.7.3.3   Pickled vegetables   The consumption of pickled or salted vegetables has been associated with a higher risk of gastric cancer in Chinese and Japanese populations in some[380] but not all case-control studies[389,415]. A large prospective study in Japan found a higher risk of gastric cancer associated with regular consumption of pickled vegetables in men but not in women[309] but two other prospective studies in Japan and Hawaii found no association[413,416]. The IARC

135

concluded that pickled vegetables, as traditionally prepared in Asia, are possibly carcinogenic to humans[10].

5.7.3.4 Conclusions The majority of case-control studies show reduced risk of gastric cancer with higher intakes of fruit and vegetables. Data from cohort studies also show that more than half the studies found reduced risks with higher consumption of fruits and vegetables. Therefore, there is moderately consistent evidence that higher intakes of fruit and vegetables are associated with lower risk of gastric cancer. Although it is possible that confounding by *H. pylori* infection may partly account for these findings, the strength, consistency and dose response relationship argue against this.

5.7.4 *Vitamins C, E and carotenoids*

5.7.4.1 In those studies in which nutrient intakes have been calculated, an apparently protective effect is observed with high intakes of ascorbic acid (vitamin C), carotenoids and, in some studies, α-tocopherol (vitamin E). The only consistent results are with ascorbic acid as the apparently protective effects of other nutrients are, in some studies, lessened by adjustment for other nutrients (see Table 5.7). One study looked specifically at the effects of reported vitamin supplementation (usually with vitamins A, C and E) and found that regular use of such supplements was associated with a significantly reduced risk of gastric cancer after adjustment for dietary micronutrient intake[403]. Prospective studies have found that a higher vitamin C index[417] or higher blood levels of vitamin C, β-carotene and/or vitamin E[210,290,418] are associated with a lower risk of gastric cancer. The Basel Prospective Study is the only study in which plasma vitamin C levels have been measured on a relatively large scale (nearly 3000 men)[290]. The relative risk of gastric cancer in men over 60 years with initially lower levels of plasma vitamin C was 4.7 (CI 1.4–15.7). However, the difference in relative risk was reduced and was no longer statistically significant when deaths

Table 5.7 Estimated Odds Ratios (OR) for incidence of gastric cancer for highest compared to lowest quantiles of dietary intake of vitamin C, carotene and vitamin E in case-control studies

Study (quality Score)	Location	Estimated OR for Vitamin C intake	Estimated OR for Carotene intake	Estimated OR for Vitamin E intake
Boeing et al, 1991[b] (H)[375]	N. Europe	0.4[a]*	0.8[a]	N/A
Buiatti et al, 1990 (H)[860]	S. Europe	0.5[a]*	0.6[b]	0.6[a]*
Hansson et al, 1994 (H)[403]	N. Europe	0.4[a]*	0.5[a,b]*	0.6[a]*
You et al, 1988 (H)[389]	China	0.5*	0.5*	N/A
Gonzalex et al, 1994 (I)[932]	S. Europe	0.6[c]	0.7	1.0
La Vecchia et al, 1994[745]	S. Europe	0.4[a]*	0.3[a,b]*	1.3[a]
Ramon et al, 1993[386]	S. Europe	0.4[a]*	0.5[a,d]	0.8[a]

[a] Analysis not adjusted for other micronutrients
[b] Reported as β-carotene
[c] Trend test significant (over all intake categories)
[d] Reported as vitamin A from fruit and vegetables
* Statistically significant (highest intake group compared with lowest intake group)

in the first 2 years of follow-up were excluded from the analysis. This might suggest that the low levels of plasma vitamin C were a consequence of preexisting, but undiagnosed disease rather than a cause of gastric cancer. Higher serum β-carotene levels, but not retinol or vitamin E levels were associated with a lower risk of gastric cancer in a Japanese nested case-control (high scoring) study[412].

5.7.4.2   The results of two randomised vitamin supplementation trials have been published[212,419]. The first trial took place in rural China among 30 000 adults aged 40-69 years. A multisupplement of β-carotene (15mg/day), α-tocopherol (30mg/day) and selenium (50mg/day), given for 5 years significantly reduced incidence and mortality rates of gastric cancer by about 20%. There was no effect on gastric cancer of three other multisupplements consisting of retinol/ zinc; riboflavin/niacin and ascorbic acid/molybdenum. It has been suggested that secular changes in intakes of ascorbic acid might have reduced the difference in plasma levels between the intervention and placebo groups sufficiently to negate the effect of supplementation and, because of this, a possible influence of ascorbic acid on risk of gastric cancer cannot be excluded. In addition, the intake of most of these micronutrients in this region is normally very low; it is possible that the effects seen in this study may be limited to those with low intakes of these nutrients. The relevance of this trial to the UK is uncertain, therefore. The second intervention trial was in Finland in 29 000 male smokers aged 50–69[212]. This trial found no effect on gastric cancer rates of supplements of either β-carotene (20mg), α-tocopherol (50mg) or both together given for between 5 and 8 years. This trial is discussed in more detail in section 5.3.3.

5.7.4.3   Conclusions   There are few studies reporting dietary intake and blood levels of vitamin C, β-carotene and vitamin E. From these there is strongly consistent evidence that higher levels of vitamin C and moderately consistent evidence that higher intakes of carotenoids are associated with lower risk of gastric cancer. The evidence for vitamin E is inconsistent. Evidence from intervention studies suggest that reduced risk of gastric cancer with a multisupplement of β-carotene, α-tocopherol and selenium may be limited to those with low intakes of these nutrients.

5.7.5   Conclusions   *Gastric Cancer and Diet*

The major predisposing factor to gastric cancer is *Helicobacter pylori* and this has not been taken account of in the studies we have considered. There is moderately consistent evidence that diets rich in salted meats and fish and salted and pickled vegetables are associated with increased risk of gastric cancer but these foods are not characteristic of the UK diet. There is moderately consistent evidence that higher intakes of fruits and vegetables are associated with lower risk of gastric cancer and this is reinforced by the strongly consistent evidence that higher dietary intakes of vitamin C and moderately consistent evidence that higher dietary intakes of carotenoids are associated with lower risk of gastric cancer. Any effects of supplementation with vitamins C and E, β-carotene and selenium appear to be limited to those with initial intakes much lower than those usually encountered in the UK. Although it is possible that confounding by

H. pylori infection may account for these findings, the strength and consistency and dose response relationship argue against this.

5.8 Cervical Cancer

5.8.1 *Introduction*

5.8.1.1 Infection with the human papillomaviruses (HPV) is accepted as the main cause of cervical cancer[420]. Risk factors for cervical cancer include early age at first intercourse, multiple sexual partners and smoking.

5.8.1.2 There are relatively few studies on diet and cervical cancer. In addition, the recent discovery of human papillomaviruses (HPV) as the main cause of cervical cancer means that studies which have not taken this into account may give misleading results. Within China, cross-sectional studies have found higher rates of cervical cancer associated with lower consumption of green vegetables and animal foods, and serum selenium levels, and higher serum ferritin and body mass indices[415]. Declining rates of cervical cancer have been associated with increased consumption of foods from animals[309]. In a study of five ethnic groups in Hawaii[311], cervical cancer showed no relationship with any of the nutrients examined, including fat, protein and vitamins A and C.

5.8.2 *Fruits and vegetables*

5.8.2.1 Of the six case-control studies[421–426] (4 high, 1 intermediate and 1 low scoring) which measured fruit and vegetable consumption, all found a reduced risk of cervical cancer associated with increased fruit and vegetable consumption, although only two[421,423] found a statistically significantly lower risk. A large Japanese prospective cohort found lower risk of cervical cancer associated with higher consumption of green and yellow vegetables[156].

5.8.2.2 Conclusions   There are few studies which have examined the relationship between fruit and vegetable consumption and cervical cancer incidence. The evidence is strongly consistent that higher intakes of fruit and vegetables are associated with reduced risk of cervical cancer but are too limited to draw firm conclusions. In addition possible confounding by infection with Herpes Virus has generally not been taken into account.

5.8.3 *Vitamins A, C, E and carotenoids*

5.8.3.1 Dietary intakes of vitamin A and/or carotenoids were inversely associated with cervical cancer in 7 of 10 case-control studies[422,423,425,427–430]. Two showed no association[424,431]. One study in 257 cases in the Netherlands[421] found higher risk of cervical cancer associated with higher intakes of β-carotene, despite having found apparently protective effects of fruits and tomatoes. Results from blood levels of carotenoids are more consistent. In a review of case-control studies, Portischman & Brinton[436] found that, in general, reduced risks associated with higher serum levels have been observed in most studies. An intervention trial in about 600 women with cervical dysplasia in the Netherlands found that β-carotene supplements (10 mg/day) for 3 months had no effect on the risk of progression of the dysplasia[421].

5.8.3.2 Dietary vitamin C was inversely associated with cervical cancer in 9 case control studies[421,423–425,428,431,433–435], although the effect was only significant in three of the studies[423,425,435] and disappeared in some studies when adjusted for other factors[424,431].

5.8.3.3 Only two case-control studies[423,434] have been identified which reported on dietary vitamin E in relation to cervical cancer; both found a reduction in overall risk for high compared with low intake of vitamin E after adjusting for smoking, although only Verrault *et al*[423] showed a significant reduction in risk with higher intake of vitamin E (OR 0.7, CI 0.4 -1.1; OR 0.4, CI 0.2-0.9 respectively). Slattery *et al*[434] found that the reduction in risk with higher intakes of vitamin E was greater in smokers than non-smokers. A small case-control study in the UK showed a significant inverse association with blood α-tocopherol and risk of cervical cancer[436]. However, a large study in Latin America[439] failed to show an effect. Blood data from cohort studies are also conflicting. In Finland, serum α-tocopherol was inversely associated with cervical cancer[437] but no association was found in the Washington County cohort study[438].

5.8.3.4 Conclusions There are few studies, especially cohort studies, which have examined the relationship between antioxidant vitamins and cervical cancer. Evidence for dietary vitamin A and /or carotenoids and blood carotenoids are weakly consistent and for dietary vitamin C are moderately consistent for a reduced risk of developing cervical cancer with higher intakes. The very limited evidence for dietary and blood levels of vitamin E are moderately consistent for a reduced risk of developing cervical cancer with higher intakes but insufficient to draw firm conclusions.

5.8.4 *Folates*

5.8.4.1 All of the eight case control studies identified which have examined a relationship between folates intake and cervical cancer have found a higher risk of cervical cancer in women with low folates, whether measured as folates intake or red blood cell or serum folate levels[423–425,428,431,433,435,440], although only one[435] for red blood cell folate was statistically significant after adjustment for sexual factors. An intervention trial in 235 women with mild or moderate cervical dysplasia found no difference in changes in dysplasia or in biopsy when given either folic acid 10mg/day or vitamin C 10mg/day for 6 months[441]. A previous, smaller trial by the same author had found significant differences in cytology and biopsy scores in women given folic acid 5 mg/day compared with women given vitamin C 5mg/day for 3 months[442].

5.8.4.2 Conclusions There are few studies which have examined the relationship between dietary and blood folates and cervical cancer incidence. The limited evidence is moderately consistent that higher intakes and blood levels of folates are associated with reduced risk of cervical cancer but insufficient to draw firm conclusions.

139

5.8.5 <u>Conclusions</u>   *Cervical cancer and diet*

In general, there are few studies, especially cohort studies, which have looked at diet and cervical cancer. The limited evidence is strongly consistent that higher intakes of fruit and vegetables are associated with reduced risk of cervical cancer, which is reinforced by the also limited evidence showing that higher intakes and/or blood levels of vitamin A and/or carotenoids, vitamins C and E and folates are associated with reduced risk.

5.9 Ovarian Cancer

5.9.1   There are substantial geographical differences in occurrence of ovarian cancer with high rates in North America and Europe and low rates in developing countries and Japan[433].

5.9.2   Ovarian cancer shares many of the risk factors associated with breast and endometrial cancer. Higher risk is associated with late menopause and infertility while parity and oral contraceptive use are protective. These factors explain only a minor proportion of the substantial differences in worldwide ovarian cancer incidence and mortality. New evidence from Barker et al[37] has implicated fetal growth as a factor. Germline mutations in BRCA1 and BRCA2 account for about 5% of ovarian cancer.

Table 5.8   Summary of case-control and cohort* studies of the association with highest v lowest quantile of consumption of meat, fat and dairy products and the risk of ovarian cancer

Food group	Positive association	Inverse Association	No significant association
Meat	La Vecchia et al, 1987[449] (H) Meat RR 1.6 (CI 1.2−2.1) for ≥7 vs <4 portions/week Ham RR 1.9 (CI 1.4−2.5) for ≥4 vs <2 portions/week		*Knekt et al, 1994[99] (I) Fried meat Risch et al, 1994[448] (H) Animal protein
Fat	Risch et al, 1994[448] (H) SFA OR 1.20 (CI 1.03−1.40) for each 10g/ day of intake La Vecchia et al, 1987[449] (H) Total fat RR 2.1 (CI 1.6– 2.9) for highest v lowest quantiles. Shu et al, 1989[450] (I) Total Fat OR 2.3 (CI 1.2−4.4)	Tzonou et al, 1993[451] (H) MUFA OR 0.8 (CI 0.7–1.0)	Tzonou et al, 1993[451] (H) SFA PUFA Slattery et al, 1989[453] (H) SFA Engle et al, 1991[452] (I) SFA Risch et al, 1994[448] (H) PUFA
Dairy products			Engle et al, 1991[452] (I) Dairy foods
Fruit & Vegetables	Negri et al, 1991[133] (H) Fruit RR 1.5 (CI 1.2–2.0)	Negri et al, 1991[133] (H) Vegetables La Vecchia et al, 1987[449] (H) Engle et al, 1991[452] (I)	
β-carotene		Risch et al, 1994[448] (H) Slattery et al, 1989[453] (H)	Negri et al, 1991[133] (H)

5.9.3. Observational population studies have implicated dietary animal fat in the aetiology of ovarian cancer. In Southern European countries, for example, where consumption of meat and dairy fats is increasing, mortality from ovarian cancer is rising[444]. Most of the information on diet and ovarian cancer has come from case-control studies. Results from cohort studies in Seventh-Day Adventists, mostly lactovegetarian, in California[445], Mormons in Utah[447] and British nuns with low intakes of meat and fats[446], have been inconsistent.

5.9.4 *Fat, meat and dairy products* In seven case-control studies, three reported a positive association with dietary saturated fatty acids[448–450], three found no effect[451–453] and one suggested that monounsaturated fatty acids were protective[451]. Meat consumption was associated with increased risk in a study carried out in Northern Italy[449] (see Table 5.8). Lactose intake from consumption of milk products rather than animal fat has been proposed as a risk factor but this was not confirmed in a small case-control study[452]. In one study[454] oral contraceptives gave greater protection to women consuming over 11g lactose daily. A prospective study in Finland, with only a small number of cases, found a non-significantly higher risk of ovarian cancer in those with the highest intakes of fried meat compared with those with the lowest[99].

5.9.5 Conclusion There are too few studies which have examined the relationship between meat, fat and dairy products and ovarian cancer to draw conclusions.

5.9.6 *Fruits and vegetables* Fruit and vegetable consumption was recorded in three case-control studies. All reported a significant inverse association between vegetables and ovarian cancer with an approximate halving of risk at the highest levels of consumption[133,449,452]. One study found a small but significantly higher risk at the highest fruit intake (RR 1.5; CI 1.2-2.0)[133]. β-carotene was inversely associated with risk in two studies[448,453] but not in a third[133]. Two studies reported an inverse association with crude fibre[451] and vegetable fibre[448] while one study reported no effect[453].

5.9.7 Conclusions There are two few studies which have examined the relationship between fruits and vegetables and ovarian cancer to draw conclusions.

5.9.8 Conclusions *Ovarian Cancer and Diet*

There is insufficient evidence to draw conclusions on the association between consumption of fat, meat, dairy products, fruit and vegetables and risk of ovarian cancer.

5.10 Endometrial cancer

5.10.1 Endometrial cancer is more common in unmarried and nulliparous women but the most important associated risk factor is obesity (see Chapter 6), possibly acting through increased endogenous production of oestradiol. Early hormone replacement therapy regimes consisting of unopposed oestrogen led to an increase in this cancer, a finding consistent with a promoting effect.

5.10.2   *Dietary factors*   While a large number of studies have examined total energy intake and body weight on the occurrence of endometrial cancer, few have investigated the effects of patterns of diet. Three case-control studies published in 1993[456–458] controlled for total energy intake, unlike some earlier studies which had suggested that increased risks for endometrial cancer were associated with higher intakes of fat and protein of animal origin. All studies found higher calorie intakes among cases than controls, which were statistically significant in two[457,458]. Higher risk was also associated with higher consumption of meat, eggs, and fresh fish[458], meat, eggs, added fats and oils[457] and cholesterol[456]. Significantly lower risks were associated with higher consumption of vegetables, and fruit in all studies and with complex carbohydrates in one[457]. Barbone *et al.*[456] also found a significant positive association with dairy product consumption. A prospective study in Finland, with only a small number of cases, found a non-significantly higher risk of endometrial cancer in those with the highest intakes of fried meat compared with those with the lowest[99].

5.10.3   Conclusions   *Endometrial Cancer and Diet*

There is insufficient evidence to draw conclusions on the role of aspects of the diet and endometrial cancer.

5.11   Pancreatic cancer

5.11.1   *Introduction*

5.11.1.1   Tobacco use is the most important known risk factor for pancreatic cancer. The attributable risk from smoking is between 20 and 40% in males and 10 to 20% in females. The disease carries a very poor survival, with high mortality rates within one year and death occurring within five years for all but 5% of cases. However, there is inconsistency between incidence and mortality trends. This may be due to problems of either diagnosis, registration and/or death certificate imprecision.

5.11.1.2   There are large international differences in rates of pancreatic cancer. The international differences are associated positively with consumption of sugar, eggs, milk, meat and energy from animal sources, and negatively with beans and vegetables[29,162,459]. Within Germany regional differences in rates of pancreatic cancer have been associated with protein intake[276]. Hirayama[460] has suggested that the trends in pancreatic cancer in Japan were related to increased animal fat intake.

5.11.2   *Meat and fish*

5.11.2.1   Of seven case-control studies[461–467] which looked at meat consumption, all four studies reporting on total meat consumption have reported higher risks of pancreatic cancer with higher intakes of total meat[463–465,461], two of which were significant. Three reported higher risks with higher beef consumption[463,466,467]. However, Falk *et al*[462] found no association for men and a

142

Figure 5.41 Odds Ratios (95% CI) for incidence of pancreatic cancer for highest compared to lowest consumption of meat in case-control studies

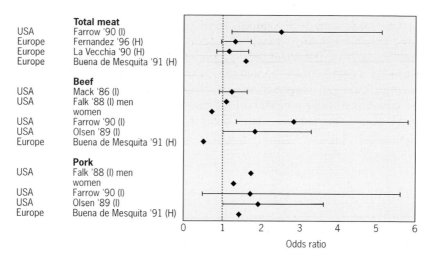

decreased risk for women with higher consumption of beef, and a high scoring European study[461] found a lower risk with higher consumption of beef. All four studies reporting on consumption of pork and pork products found a higher risk of pancreatic cancer with higher consumption[461–463,467]. The relative risks were generally between 1 and 2 but Farrow and Davis[463] reported higher relative risks for both total meat and beef (see Figure 5.41). Processed meat was associated with a higher risk in one American study[468] (RR 1.8; CI 1.0–3.4) but not in another[466] (RR 0.9; CI 0.6–1.4). Poultry was associated with a significantly higher risk in one study[463] but not in two others[467,469] and fish was associated with significantly higher risk in two studies[461,462] but not in a third[468].

5.11.2.2 Two prospective studies reporting on pancreatic cancer and diet[460,106] have found a higher risk of pancreatic cancer with higher meat consumption, and a European study[99] found no effect of consumption of fried meat when the risk was adjusted for sex and age only but a non-significant higher risk when adjusted for sex, age, BMI, energy intake and other foods (RR 1.54: CI 0.53–4.50).

5.11.2.3 The Kaiser-Permanente study (intermediate score), which took blood measurements on 175 000 people found increased levels of serum iron were associated with increased risk of pancreatic cancer[470].

5.11.2.4 Conclusions Though based on limited data, the evidence is moderately consistent that higher total meat and red meat (beef and pork) consumption is associated with higher risk of pancreatic cancer. The evidence that consumption of poultry, fish and processed meat are associated with risk of pancreatic cancer is inconsistent.

5.11.3 *Fat*

5.11.3.1 Only two case-control studies[459,471] (one high and one intermediate scoring) out of eight[459,463,469,471–475] found higher total fat intakes associated

143

with higher risk of pancreatic cancer. And the combined data from the five case-control studies carried out under the auspices of the IARC SEARCH program[476] in Canada, the Netherlands, Australia, and Poland, show no evidence for any positive association with total fat, and saturated, monounsaturated and polyunsaturated fatty acids after adjusting for energy intakes.

5.11.3.2 Conclusions There are few studies to draw conclusions on the association of total fat, saturated, monounsaturated and polyunsaturated fatty acids intakes with risk of pancreatic cancer. The limited data available are weakly consistent that higher total fat intakes are not associated with higher risk of pancreatic cancer.

5.11.4 *Fruits and vegetables*

5.11.4.1 Of 6 case-control studies which reported fruit consumption and risk of pancreatic cancer[133,461,462,464,467,468], five[133,462,464,467,468] found higher intakes of fruits associated with a lower risk of pancreatic cancer and three were significant (see Figure 5.42). The other study[461] found a non-significant small increase in risk. All three case-control studies[133,461,469] reporting consumption of green vegetables and risk of pancreatic cancer found a significant decrease in risk with higher consumption (see Figure 5.43). Two European studies, one high scoring[461] and one intermediate scoring[468] reported on consumption of carrots and risk of pancreatic cancer, the first found an increased risk with higher consumption whereas the second found a significantly decreased risk with higher consumption of carrots. Two USA studies[466,478] reported total fruit and vegetable consumption with risk of pancreatic cancer and both found significantly reduced risks with higher consumption. Of the two prospective studies which measured consumption of fruit and vegetables, one found lower risk in those consuming more beans, lentils, peas and dried fruit[106], one found lower risk with fresh fruit and vegetables[479]. No studies have reported evidence of significant positive associations for higher intakes of fruit and vegetables.

Figure 5.42   Odds Ratios (95% CI) for incidence of pancreatic cancer for highest compared to lowest consumption of fruit in case-control studies

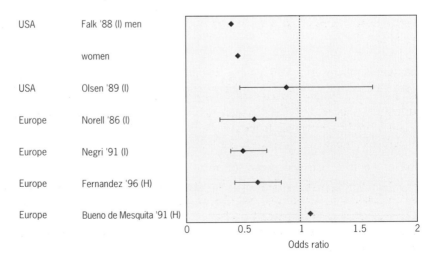

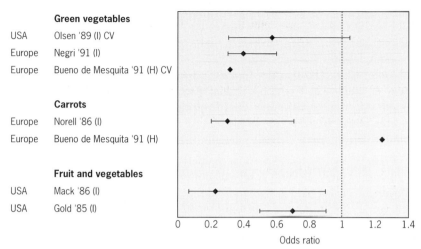

Figure 5.43   Odds Ratios (95% CI) for incidence of pancreatic cancer for highest compared to lowest consumption of vegetables in case-control studies

CV cruciferous vegetables

5.11.4.2   Conclusions   The limited data relating fruit and vegetable consumption and pancreatic cancer are strongly consistent that higher intakes of fruit and vegetables are associated with reduced risk of pancreatic cancer.

5.11.5   Vitamins C, E, carotenoids and fibre

5.11.5.1   Seven case-control studies, including the five in the IARC SEARCH programme have found that higher intakes of vitamin C were associated with lower risk of pancreatic cancer[459,461,462,469,473–475]. Four of the IARC SEARCH studies[459,461,469,473] also measured β-carotene intake but only two found a lower risk with higher intakes of β-carotene and the combined analysis of all four studies showed a non-significant decreased risk with increased intakes of β-carotene. One prospective study measured intakes of vitamin C and β-carotene, both of which showed a non-significant lower risk with increased intakes[466]. Two prospective studies which measured serum antioxidants found a lower risk of pancreatic cancer associated with higher levels of α-tocopherol[215] or lycopene and selenium[480].

5.11.5.2 Four out of five case-control studies in the IARC SEARCH programme have found that higher intakes of dietary fibre were associated with lower risk of pancreatic cancer[459,461,469,473], three of which were significant. The combined analysis of all five studies found relative risk of 0.42 (CI 0.30–0.58) in the upper quartile of intake compared with the lowest.

5.11.5.3   Conclusions   There is limited, moderately consistent evidence that higher intakes of vitamin C and dietary fibre are associated with lower risk of pancreatic cancer. The limited evidence for intakes of β-carotene is inconsistent and the data on serum antioxidants and the risk of pancreatic cancer are insufficient to draw conclusions.

5.11.6   *Coffee and Tea*

5.11.6.1   IARC reviewed 21 case-control studies and 6 prospective studies of coffee consumption and pancreatic cancer. No prospective study found a significant positive association with higher coffee consumption. The IARC concluded that the data were suggestive of a weak relationship between high levels of coffee consumption and pancreatic cancer, but the possibility that this is due to bias or confounding was tenable[356]. They reviewed 6 case-control studies and 4 prospective studies of tea drinking and pancreatic cancer. One case-control study found a positive association, one prospective study found an inverse association and the others found no association[356].

5.11.6.2   <u>Conclusions</u>   There is moderately consistent evidence for a weak relationship between high levels of coffee consumption and increased levels of pancreatic cancer and no relationship between levels of tea consumption and pancreatic cancer, but the possibility of bias or confounding remains.

5.11.7   <u>Conclusions</u>   *Pancreatic Cancer and Diet*

There is moderately consistent evidence that higher total and red meat consumption and high levels of coffee consumption are associated with increased risk of pancreatic cancer. The evidence for an association with total fat and fatty acid intakes is insufficient to draw conclusions. There is moderately consistent evidence that higher intakes of fruit and vegetables, vitamin C and dietary fibre are associated with lower risk of pancreatic cancer but the evidence for intakes of β-carotene is inconsistent.

5.12   Oesophageal cancer

5.12.1   *Introduction*   Most cancers of the oesophagus are caused by alcohol and tobacco use, a dose response relationship being demonstrated for alcohol and cigarettes as well as the duration of exposure. There is evidence that alcohol and tobacco interact in a multiplicative fashion. Alcohol and tobacco account for about 80–90% of oesophageal cancer in Europe. However, in Asia, under nutrition is probably a more important cause of oesophageal cancer.

5.12.2   There are substantial international differences in rates of oesophageal cancer which have been associated with poor diets, including low fat diets[161,481–483], and it has been suggested that specific vitamin and mineral deficiencies may play a part[484]. Extensive studies in Iran[485–488], and studies in Japan[367] and South Africa[489,490] have suggested an inverse association with fruit and vegetable consumption. Lu and Qin[369] reported a positive association between sales of salt and rates of cancer within China. Migrant studies of Japanese to the USA[361] and Poles to the UK[491] suggest that rates decline toward the host country rates over time.

5.12.3   *Fruits and vegetables*

5.12.3.1   Available evidence from ecological studies suggests that oesophageal cancer is associated with low intakes of fruits and vegetables[492].

146

Figure 5.44   Odds Ratios (95% CI) for incidence of oesophageal cancer for highest compared to lowest consumption of total and citrus fruits in case-control studies

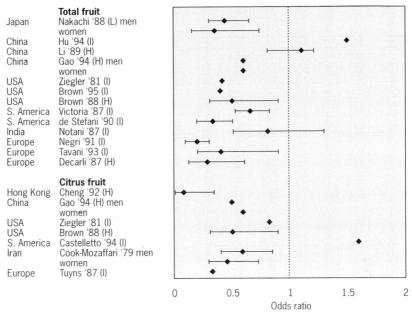

95% Confidence intervals for Hu '94 (0.8-2.9) and Castelletto '94 (0.8-3.1)

Figure 5.45   Odds Ratios (95% CI) for incidence of oesophageal cancer for highest compared to lowest consumption of total and raw vegetables in case-control studies

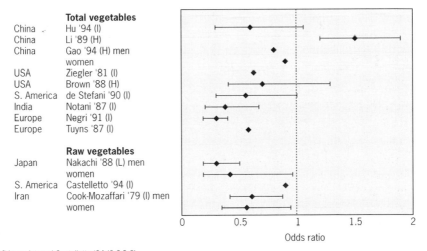

95% confidence interval Castelletto '94 (0.3-2.6)

5.12.3.2   Twenty-five case-control studies were identified which reported on fruit and/or vegetables and oesphageal cancer. Of the 13 studies reporting on total fruit intake, 11[133,493–504] found lower risk with higher consumption of total fruit and all except one were significant (see Figure 5.44). One high scoring study[499] found a non-significant increased risk and one intermediate scoring study[498] found a significantly increased risk with higher consumption of total fruit. Six[165,493,497,505–507] out of the 7 case-control studies which reported on citrus fruit consumption found a significant decreased risk with higher consumption (see Figure 5.44). The seventh study[505] found an increased risk with higher consumption of citrus fruit in a South American population. Twelve case-control studies[133,493,496–501,503,505–507] reported on total vegetables or raw vegetables and risk of oesophageal cancer. All except one Chinese study[499] found a decreased risk with higher consumption of vegetables (see Figure 5.45). The study in China[499] found that most measures of diet were associated with increased risk, suggesting an overall effect of eating more food.

5.12.3.3   Relatively few cohort studies have reported dietary data in relation to oesophageal cancer. Daily consumption of green and yellow vegetables was associated with a three-fold reduction in risk compared with those consuming no green and yellow vegetables in a large prospective cohort from Japan[156]. A retrospective cohort study in Linxian, China, also found that frequent consumption of fresh vegetables was associated with decreased risk[508]. However, the relevance of these studies to UK eating patterns is not clear.

5.12.3.4   Pickled vegetables   Consumption of pickled vegetables was associated with a higher risk of oesophageal cancer in a case-control study in Hong Kong[165] but not in two other studies in China[499,509]. The IARC concluded that pickled vegetables, as traditionally prepared in Asia, are possibly carcinogenic to humans[10].

5.12.3.5   Conclusions   The evidence that higher consumption of fruits and vegetables reduces the risk of oesophageal cancer is strongly consistent, but the relevance to the UK where there are no prospective data is unclear.

5.12.4   *Various micronutrients*

5.12.4.1   Case-control studies analysing for β-carotene, vitamin E or vitamin C intakes have tended to find inverse associations with intakes of these nutrients and risk of oesophageal cancer[133,495,503,507,510–512]. However, higher retinol intakes are consistently associated with higher risk of oesophageal cancer[495,512,513,507], although Prasad *et al*[515] found no relationship between serum vitamin A and oesophageal cancer.

5.12.4.2   Four intervention trials have been identified: one trial tested the prevention of oesophageal cancer in a high risk population[514] while 2 trials tested the prevention of oesophageal cancer in those with precancerous lesions such as oesophageal dysplasia or chronic oesophagitis[516,517] and one tested the prevention of precancerous lesions in a high risk population[518–520]. Supplementation with a combination of retinol (15mg/day), riboflavin (200mg/day) and zinc (50mg/day) for 13 months had no effect on the prevalence of precancerous lesions such as oesophagitis, atrophy or dysplasia in a high risk population in China, although blood micronutrient levels improved in both groups[518,519,520]. However, the prevalence of micronucleated cells was significantly lower in the treatment group compared with the placebo group. A large trial in China in 3300

148

people with oesophageal dysplasia found no effect on the incidence and a non-significant reduction in mortality of oesophageal cancer after taking a multi-vitamin and mineral supplement containing 14 vitamins and 12 minerals for 6 years[516]. One trial has shown that supplementation with 600mg calcium daily for 7 months inhibits basal cell hyperplasia or dysplasia[517].

5.12.4.3 Supplementation for almost 6 years with four combinations of supplements: retinol (5000IU/day) and zinc (22.2 mg/day); riboflavin (3.2 mg/day) and niacin (40 mg/day); ascorbic acid (120mg/day) and molybdenum (30 µg/day); or β-carotene (15mg/day), selenium (50 µg/day) and α-tocopherol (30mg/day) resulted in no significant reductions in either the incidence or mortality rates from oesophageal cancer in 30 000 people in a high risk region of China[419]. The interpretation of these trials in China has been impaired by the improvement in nutritional status affecting all the population including the controls. Therefore, the negative findings of the study should be regarded with caution. The trials may also have been too short to show any effect on incidence or mortality. If these nutrients have a protective effect in the early stages of carcinogenesis, an effect on short-term mortality would not be expected to be seen, nor would an effect on the progression of precancerous lesions to carcinoma be expected.

5.12.4.4 Conclusions Although higher dietary intakes of antioxidant nutrients, β-carotene, vitamin C and vitamin E, are associated with a lower risk of oesophageal cancer in case-control studies, the results from intervention trials have not demonstrated any effect on either the prevalence of pre-cancerous lesions or on the incidence and mortality of oesophageal cancer. It is possible that the apparent effect is due to confounding by other factors. The evidence is inconsistent.

5.12.5 *Meat and fish*

5.12.5.1 The evidence from case-control studies that meat consumption is related to oesophageal cancer is conflicting. Of 12 case-control studies[493,494,496,497,499,500,501,503,504,506,507,511], which cited odds ratios for total meat, 2 studies in China and Brazil[499,504] found a significantly higher risk associated with higher total meat consumption and a further 3 studies[493,497,501] found non-significantly higher risks (see Figure 5.46). Three other studies found significantly higher intakes of barbecued meats in cases compared with controls[496,505,521] (see Figure 5.46). However, five studies found significantly lower risks with higher fresh meat consumption[495,500,503,505,507] and others have found a non significant lower risk[494,511]. A number of studies have found non-significantly lower risks in those with higher intakes of poultry or fish[497,506,522] but two found significantly higher risks associated with canned fish[503,507]. Consumption of Chinese salted fish was associated with a higher risk of oesophageal cancer in a study in Hong Kong, although the effect was weakened when consumption of pickled vegetables was taken into account[165]. The IARC concluded that Chinese salted fish is carcinogenic to humans, based mainly on the evidence for an effect on nasopharyngeal cancer[10].

Figure 5.46   Odds Ratios (95% CI) for incidence of oesophageal cancer for highest compared to lowest consumption of total and barbecued meat in case-control studies

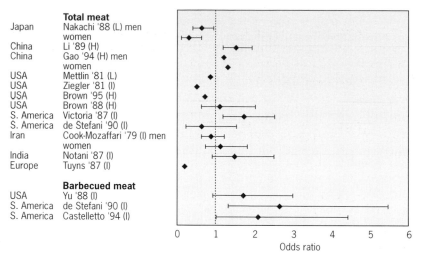

	Total meat	
Japan	Nakachi '88 (L) men	
	women	
China	Li '89 (H)	
China	Gao '94 (H) men	
	women	
USA	Mettlin '81 (L)	
USA	Ziegler '81 (I)	
USA	Brown '95 (H)	
USA	Brown '88 (H)	
S. America	Victoria '87 (I)	
S. America	de Stefani '90 (I)	
Iran	Cook-Mozaffari '79 (I) men	
	women	
India	Notani '87 (I)	
Europe	Tuyns '87 (I)	
	Barbecued meat	
USA	Yu '88 (I)	
S. America	de Stefani '90 (I)	
S. America	Castelletto '94 (I)	

Decarli '87 reported 'cases less than controls' but no OR given

5.12.5.2   Of two prospective studies, in China and Japan, the Chinese study[508] found a significantly increased risk associated with increased pork consumption and the Japanese study[98] found no significant effect of meat consumption. The Japanese study found a significantly lower risk in men with higher fish consumption[98].

5.12.5.3   Conclusions   The evidence relating meat consumption to oesophageal cancer, from case-control and prospective studies, is inconsistent. Furthermore, the relevance of the evidence to meat as commonly eaten in the UK is limited.

5.12.6   Conclusions   *Oesophageal Cancer and Diet*

There is strongly consistent evidence from case-control studies that higher intakes of fruits and vegetables are associated with lower risk of oesophageal cancer but there are no data, particularly prospective, relevant to the UK. Higher dietary intakes of antioxidant nutrients are also associated with lower risk of oesophageal cancer. However, results from intervention trials supplementing with various micronutrients have not demonstrated a reduction in risk. The evidence relating meat consumption to oesophageal cancer is inconsistent.

5.13   **Malignant Melanoma**

5.13.1   The majority of skin cancers in Great Britain are not malignant melanomas. However, skin cancers other than malignant melanomas were not considered by the Working Group because there has been no suggestion that they are related to diet. The incidence of malignant melanoma of skin, while relatively low, accounting for 1–2% of all cancer in Great Britain, is increasing rapidly. The major recognised risk factor is intermittent, but usually intense, solar exposure leading to sunburn, particularly in childhood. The number of palpable benign pigmented naevi is a marker of risk as are a light skin and a tendency to freckle easily.

5.13.2   Dietary factors have been suggested as modifying the response to UV damage. Several case-control studies have been carried out but the results have been weak and inconclusive. The most consistent, but not universal, findings have been an inverse risk with vitamin E[523,524].

5.13.3   Conclusions   There are too few studies to reach any firm conclusions concerning a relationship between dietary factors and risk of malignant melanoma.

5.14   Laryngeal cancer

5.14.1   Laryngeal cancer is a rare cancer in Great Britain, though the incidence is about five times higher for men than for women. The major risk factors are smoking and alcohol consumption.

5.14.2   *Fruits and vegetables*

5.14.2.1   Riboli, Kaaks and Estéve[525] reviewed twelve case-control studies, carried out between 1956 and 1995. The foods and nutrients measured in the studies varied considerably, with only six reporting consumption of fruits and vegetables. High consumption of fruit was found to be associated with a significant decrease in risk of laryngeal cancer in four studies[501,526–528]. In these studies, there was evidence of a linear increase in risk from the lowest to the highest consumption level. A fifth study in China[529] found a reduced risk with consumption of citrus fruits while it was less marked for total fruit consumption. The study in south western Europe[528] found that high intake of fruit, vegetables, vegetable oil, fish and low intake of butter and preserved meats were associated with reduced risk of both epilaryngeal and endo-laryngeal cancers, after adjustment for alcohol, tobacco, social status, and non-alcohol energy intake. The risk (odds ratio) for cancer of the endo-larynx for those consuming less than 70g fruit per day compared with those consuming more than 250g per day was 1.39 (CI 1.04–1.87) after adjusting for alcohol, tobacco and energy intake, and for cancer of the hypopharynx/epilarynx was 1.84 (CI 1.26–2.69).

5.14.2.2   Total vegetable consumption was found to be associated with a significant reduction in risk in three case control studies[468,527,528]. Results from a fourth study[526] indicated an increased risk with 'infrequent intake of vegetables' and in a study in China[529] low consumption of some dark green vegetables and of garlic was associated with a significant increase in risk.

5.14.2.3   Conclusions   There is limited, moderately consistent evidence that higher intakes of fruits and vegetables are associated with reduced risk of laryngeal cancer.

5.14.3 Conclusions *Laryngeal Cancer and Diet*

The major risk factors for laryngeal cancer are smoking and alcohol consumption. There is limited, moderately consistent evidence that higher intakes of fruits and vegetables are associated with reduced risk of laryngeal cancer. There is not enough evidence to draw conclusions about other dietary factors.

5.15 Oral and Pharyngeal cancer

5.15.1 The major risk factors for oral and pharyngeal cancer are smoking and chewing of tobacco and betel nut, accounting for about three-quarters of all these cancers. Alcohol also increases risk of these cancers.

5.15.2 *Fruits and vegetables.* Winn[530] reviewed the literature on diet and oropharyngeal cancer. Eight of 12 case-control studies of fruit consumption found lower risks associated with higher consumption, with risk reductions ranging from 20 to 80% in those with high levels of consumption, compared with those with the lowest consumption. An association with vegetables was less clear cut. No association was found in 7 studies, a moderate effect was found in one study and 5 studies showed an apparent protective effect with some vegetables in certain population subgroups. Consumption of pickled vegetables during weaning and childhood was associated with a higher risk of nasopharyngeal cancer in three case-control studies in Hong Kong, China and Tunisia but the effect tended to disappear when consumption of salted fish or other foods was taken into account[514]. The IARC concluded that pickled vegetables, as traditionally prepared in Asia are possibly carcinogenic to humans[10].

5.15.2.1 Conclusions The evidence from case control studies is weakly consistent that high fruit consumption and inconsistent that high vegetable consumption are associated with reduced risk of oropharyngeal cancer but no cohort studies were identified.

5.15.3 *Vitamin A and β-carotene* Intervention trials with retinoids and β-carotene suggest both may have a limited role in preventing the recurrence of primary cancers and stabilising leukoplakia, which is thought to be a predisposing factor for oro-pharyngeal cancer.

5.15.3.1 Conclusions There is not enough evidence to reach any firm conclusions about the relationship between vitamin A and β-carotene and oral and pharyngeal cancer.

5.15.4 *Chinese salted fish* Chinese salted fish consumption, particularly during childhood, is consistently associated with a higher risk of nasopharyngeal cancer in case-control studies. IARC concluded that Chinese salted fish is carcinogenic to humans[10].

5.15.4.1 Conclusions There is strongly consistent evidence that consumption of salted fish is associated with increased risk of pharyngeal cancer, but such fish is rarely consumed in the UK.

5.15.5 Conclusions *Oral and Pharyngeal Cancer and Diet*

The effects of diet appear to be modest when compared with those for smoking and alcohol consumption. There is weakly consistent evidence that higher consumption of fruits is associated with a reduced risk of oral and pharyngeal cancers but the evidence for vegetables is inconsistent.

5.16 Testicular cancer

5.16.1 The incidence of testicular cancer has been increasing throughout this century. Undescended testis is a major factor associated with testicular cancer and the increase in the incidence of these tumours has been associated with a parallel increase in undescended testis, though this accounts for less than 10% of the disease[531]. No associations have been found between cancer risk and weight, height or BMI[532].

5.16.2 An association between testicular cancer and high fat intakes has been suggested in cross-sectional studies[29] and with consumption of dairy products[533] but few case control studies of the effects of diet on this cancer have been carried out. In a recent case-control study in the UK[534] the odds ratio for the association of undescended testis and testicular cancer was 7.19 (CI 2.36–21.9). The same study found that for each extra quarter pint of milk consumed the risk increased by 1.39 (CI 1.19–1.63).

5.16.3 Conclusions *Testicular Cancer and Diet*

There is not enough evidence to reach any conclusions about the relationship between dietary factors and risk of testicular cancer.

6. Energy Balance, Obesity and Development of Cancer

6.1 Introduction

6.1.1 Comparisons of energy intake in the absence of data on energy expenditure or energy balance are difficult to interpret. High energy intakes are not necessarily associated with obesity and the converse, mainly as a result of under-reporting or incomplete collection of food intake data from food frequency questionnaires, is often the case in cross-sectional studies. Nevertheless, energy intake is often used as a marker of energy expenditure. Furthermore positive or negative energy balance is usually slight in comparison to absolute intakes, and can occur at any level of energy intake and/or expenditure. In addition, energy balance maintained at a high level of energy expenditure might have different physiological effects to energy balance maintained at lower levels of energy expenditure. However, information on energy intake and energy expenditure in the same people is rarely available. Obesity is a marker of long term positive energy balance, and measures of obesity can help to interpret data on energy intakes. Systematic epidemiological reviews of specific cancer sites and measures of obesity were carried out and are reported in this chapter.

6.1.2 Physical activity is an important determinant of energy expenditure. In addition, heavy competitive exercise induces profound, but transient, changes in sex hormone levels both in women and in men[535]. In female athletes menarche may be delayed and in adult women amenorrhoea can occur, both of which lead to reduced life time exposure to oestrogens. However, it is unclear how far ordinary, moderate exercise might reduce oestrogen exposure. Moderate physical activity may reduce susceptibility to weight gain. Despite the relationships of physical activity with energy expenditure, obesity, changes in sex hormone levels and age at menarche, physical activity was considered to be outside the scope of this report and so no systematic review has been carried out but reference has been made to it where relevant.

6.2 Breast cancer

6.2.1 *Energy intake and physical activity* No relationship between energy intake and breast cancer has been observed in 6 prospective studies of diet and either pre-menopausal or post-menopausal breast cancer[55,101,121,125,126,536], one study[122] found an inverse relationship. The relative risks are equally distributed around 1.0 and none are statistically significant. In human studies identified which have investigated the effects of physical activity on risk of breast cancer, one found a significantly lower rate in those who had been college athletes compared to those who had not[538]; one reported a significantly higher prevalence of breast cancer in women in sedentary jobs compared to those in high activity

154

occupations but did not adjust for socio-economic status or age at first pregnancy[539] and the third found no significant difference in risk of breast cancer
between women who had played sports for more than 5 hours per week 35–50
years previously and those who played less[540]. Shephard[541] in a review of exercise and cancer concluded that two well-controlled studies (one US and one
Canadian) show that regular physical activity confers a statistically significant,
but small, measure of protection against breast tumours; a third study is weakly
supportive and positive; less well-controlled studies show little evidence of benefit. Lee I-M[542] in another review stated that a possible explanation for discrep-
ant findings might be that physical activity is inversely related to breast cancer
risk in younger, but not older, women, although the biological basis for this
remains unclear.

6.2.2 *Overweight, obesity and pre-menopausal breast cancer* Of 25 case control studies in pre-menopausal women, 2 found a significantly higher risk of
breast cancer in obese or overweight women compared to normal weight
women[82,543]; 7 found non-significantly higher risks[80,89,544–548]; 5 found no
association[549,550–553]; 7 found non-significantly lower risks associated with
overweight or obesity[117,554–559] and 4 found significantly lower risks[560–563] (see
Figure 6.1). Of 8 prospective studies in pre-menopausal women, 2 found non-significantly higher risks of breast cancer in women with a BMI over 27 compared
to women with a BMI less than 23[96,564]; one found a non-significantly lower
risk associated with increasing BMI[565] and 5 found significantly lower risks in
women with a BMI over 27 compared to those with a BMI less than 22[566–570]

Figure 6.1   Odds Ratios (95% CI) for incidence of premenopausal breast cancer for highest
compared to lowest BMI in case control studies

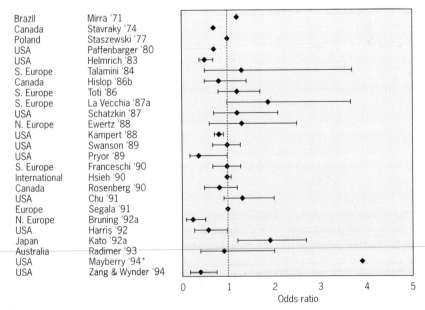

*Upper 95% CI=11.6

155

Figure 6.2   Relative risk (95% CI) for incidence of premenopausal breast cancer for highest versus lowest BMI in cohort studies

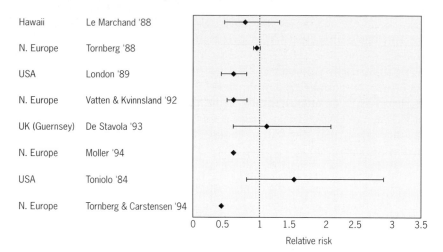

(see Figure 6.2). The evidence for an association between BMI and pre-menopausal breast cancer is therefore inconsistent.

6.2.3   *Overweight, obesity and post-menopausal breast cancer*   Of 29 case control studies in post-menopausal women, 12 found either a significant positive association between higher BMI and risk of breast cancer or significantly higher relative risks in overweight or obese women compared to normal weight women[80,82,113,544-546,548,549,551,552,555,571]; 11 found non-significantly higher risks[89,547,550,553,557,558,560,563,572-574] and 6 found non-significantly lower risks[117,543,544,556,559,561] (see Figure 6.3). Of 13 prospective studies, 12 found a positive association between BMI and risk of breast cancer or higher risks in overweight or obese women compared to normal weight women[96,121,564-567, 570,575-579], although only 4 were statistically significant[96,566,570,575] (see figure 6.4). One study found a non-significantly lower risk[124]. The relative risks were around 1.1–1.2 in most studies. There is therefore strongly consistent evidence for a positive association between BMI and post-menopausal breast cancer, although the relative risks are small. There is increasing evidence that central obesity is particularly associated with higher risks of post-menopausal breast cancer. Some case-control[562,580,581] and prospective studies[578,582,583] have found a higher risk of breast cancer with various measures of central obesity. However, not all were statistically significant and others have found no association[571,579,584-586].

6.2.4   Obese women generally have higher levels of available oestrogen than normal weight women[562,587-591] which might explain the higher risk associated with obesity (see section 7.13.2). In addition, some studies[592-599] but not all studies[108,556,588,600-604] have found a higher prevalence of oestrogen receptor positive tumours in post-menopausal women. However, a number of studies have found that in pre-menopausal women, a higher prevalence of oestrogen receptor positive tumours was associated with lower BMI[588,597]. In one study, women with breast cancer were found to have a higher prevalence of insulin resistance, which

156

Figure 6.3   Odds Ratios (95% CI) for incidence of post menopausal breast cancer for highest
compared to lowest BMI in case control studies

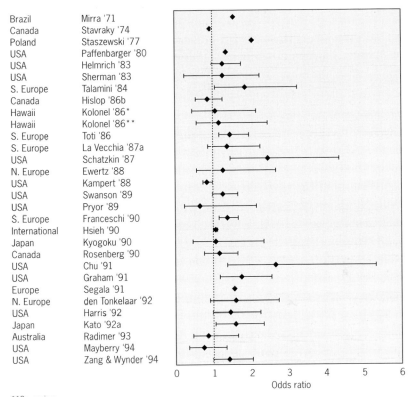

Brazil	Mirra '71
Canada	Stavraky '74
Poland	Staszewski '77
USA	Paffenbarger '80
USA	Helmrich '83
USA	Sherman '83
S. Europe	Talamini '84
Canada	Hislop '86b
Hawaii	Kolonel '86*
Hawaii	Kolonel '86**
S. Europe	Toti '86
S. Europe	La Vecchia '87a
USA	Schatzkin '87
N. Europe	Ewertz '88
USA	Kampert '88
USA	Swanson '89
USA	Pryor '89
S. Europe	Franceschi '90
International	Hsieh '90
Japan	Kyogoku '90
Canada	Rosenberg '90
USA	Chu '91
USA	Graham '91
Europe	Segala '91
N. Europe	den Tonkelaar '92
USA	Harris '92
Japan	Kato '92a
Australia	Radimer '93
USA	Mayberry '94
USA	Zang & Wynder '94

Odds ratio

*Japanese; **Caucasians

Figure 6.4   Relative risk (95% CI) for incidence of post menopausal breast cancer for highest
versus lowest BMI in cohort studies

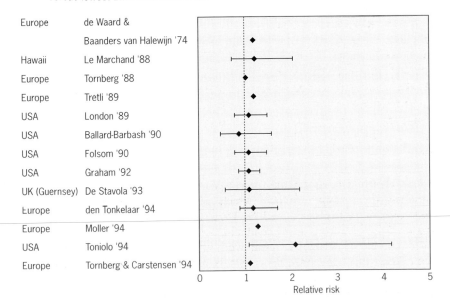

Europe	de Waard & Baanders van Halewijn '74
Hawaii	Le Marchand '88
Europe	Tornberg '88
Europe	Tretli '89
USA	London '89
USA	Ballard-Barbash '90
USA	Folsom '90
USA	Graham '92
UK (Guernsey)	De Stavola '93
Europe	den Tonkelaar '94
Europe	Moller '94
USA	Toniolo '94
Europe	Tornberg & Carstensen '94

Relative risk

157

is also associated with central obesity. A link between central obesity, hyperinsuli-naemia, decreased sex hormone binding globulin synthesis and increased oestrogen availability and breast cancer has been proposed[562]. This requires further research.

6.2.5 *Weight gain* There is evidence that weight gain in adulthood is associated with higher risks of post-menopausal breast cancer, with most[124,548,555,558,559,565,567,578,605–607] but not all[543,574] studies finding higher risks in those who gained weight, particularly if they were lean in early adulthood. The relative risk for a weight gain of more than 10kg was in the order of 2.0 in at least three of the studies.

Figure 6.5   Estimated odds ratio (OR) or relative risk (RR) and 95% confidence intervals (CI) for the incidence of premenopausal breast cancer by body height in case-control studies

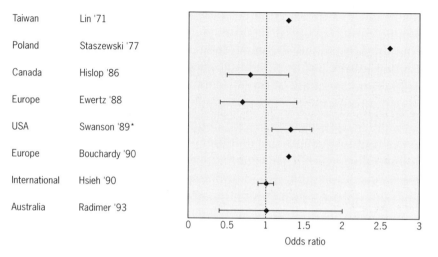

* All women; Adami '77 No OR but stated 'not significant'

Figure 6.6   Estimated odds ratio (OR) or relative risk (RR) and 95% confidence intervals (CI) for the incidence of post menopausal breast cancer by body height in case-control studies

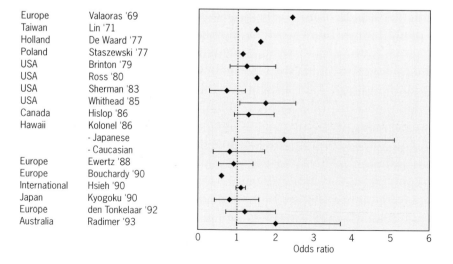

6.2.6 *Height* Most [549,552,556,559,571,573,608–614] but not all[547,555,572,574,615–617] case-control studies and most [96,564–567,576,577,618] but not all[579] prospective studies have found a small positive association between height and risk of post-menopausal breast cancer (see Figures 6.5 and 6.6). Although the majority of these studies are not statistically significant, recent findings from the Netherlands Cohort Study[619] have shown a significant positive and graded association between height and risk of post-menopausal breast cancer, with a relative risk of 2.37 in women 175cm or above compared to those less than 165cm. The relationship between height and risk of pre-menopausal breast cancer is less clear with the majority of case-control and prospective studies failing to show an association (see Figures 6.7 and 6.8). A recent case-control study has shown a significant positive association between height and risk of pre-menopausal breast cancer which was strengthened in women who were also of lower body weight. Risk of the disease was twice as high in women who were tall and thin as compared with women who were heavy and short[614].

6.2.7 Conclusions

There is no evidence of a relationship between energy intake and risk of pre- or post-menopausal breast cancer. The evidence for a relationship between risk of pre-menopausal breast cancer and BMI is inconsistent and there is no clear association with height. There is strongly consistent evidence for a positive association between BMI and post-menopausal breast cancer with relative risks between 1.1 and 2.0. There is increasing evidence that central obesity and weight gain in adult life are associated with higher risks of post-menopausal breast cancer. There is also evidence that taller women are at greater risk of post-menopausal breast cancer.

Figure 6.7   Relative risk (RR) and 95% confidence of the incidence of premenopausal breast cancer by body height in cohort control studies

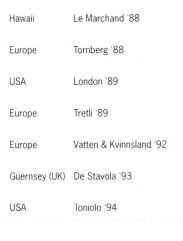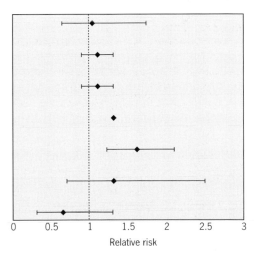

Figure 6.8   Relative risk (RR) and 95% confidence of the incidence of premenopausal breast cancer by body height in cohort studies

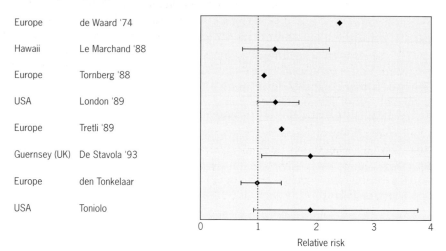

Europe	de Waard '74
Hawaii	Le Marchand '88
Europe	Tornberg '88
USA	London '89
Europe	Tretli '89
Guernsey (UK)	De Stavola '93
Europe	den Tonkelaar
USA	Toniolo

Relative risk

6.3   Colorectal cancer

6.3.1   *Energy intake and physical activity*   No significant association between energy intake and colorectal cancer has been observed in the majority of prospective studies of diet and colorectal cancer, although most have relative risks less than 1.0[248,249,299,620]. One study found a significantly lower risk of colon cancer in those with the highest energy intakes[247]. Consistent protective effects of increased energy expenditure, in case-control and cohort studies are reported in a review by Potter *et al*[246]; however, it did not include the studies of Paffenberger *et al*[540] which failed to find relationships with physical activity in either dockworkers or college alumni.

6.3.2   *Overweight, obesity and colorectal cancer in men*   Of 7 case-control studies in men, 4 found a significant association between BMI and colon and colorectal cancer[563,621-623]. Three found no association[182,624,625]. Of 12 prospective studies, 10 found a higher risk of colon or colorectal cancer associated with higher BMI although not all were statistically significant[208,251,252,298,575,626-630]. One found no association[631] and another found a significantly lower risk in those with higher BMI[632]. The relative risks were around 1.5 to 2.0. The evidence for an association between BMI and risk of colon cancer in men is therefore moderately consistent.

6.3.3   *Overweight, obesity and colorectal cancer in women*   Two of the 5 case-control studies in women found a higher risk of colon or colorectal cancer associated with higher BMI, although only one was significant[621,622], 2 found non-significantly lower risks associated with higher BMI[623,633] and one found no association[625]. Of 9 prospective studies in women, one found a significantly higher risk of colon or colorectal cancer associated with higher BMI[247], 5 found non-significantly higher risks[252,298,575,626,634] and 3 found no association[251,627,631]. The relative risks were between 1.0 to 1.5. The evidence for an association in women between BMI and risk of colon cancer is therefore weakly consistent.

160

6.3.4   Although the effect of physical activity on risk of colorectal cancer is usually attributed to reduced transit time through the large gut[622], there is no effect of physical activity on transit time in studies in which food intake has been controlled[635]. Increased serum triglycerides and glucose have been suggested to be common factors in the putative link between diet, obesity and lack of exercise, and increased risk of colon cancer. Higher levels of serum triglycerides were found to be associated with increased risk of polyp recurrence, and higher levels of circulating insulin or glucose may be associated with increased neoplastic cell growth[264].

6.3.5   Conclusions

There was no evidence for a significant association between energy intake and risk of colorectal cancer, although most prospective studies had relative risks less than 1 with higher intakes (possibly reflecting higher levels of physical activity). The evidence for a positive association between BMI and risk of colon cancer in men is moderately consistent with relative risks in the range of 1.5 to 2.0 and in women is weakly consistent.

6.4   Prostate cancer

6.4.1   *Overweight, obesity and prostate cancer*   Some[563,636,637] but not all[315,316,327,638,639] case control studies and some[208,321,575,626,640] but not all [606,629,631] prospective studies have found higher risks of prostate cancer in men with higher BMI or relative weight, though not all studies were significant. The relative risks were around 1.5. The evidence for an association between BMI and risk of prostate cancer is inconsistent.

6.4.2   Conclusions

The evidence for an association between energy expenditure, BMI and/or relative weight and risk of prostate cancer is inconsistent.

6.5   Endometrial cancer

6.5.1   *Energy intake*   There is some evidence from case-control studies that higher energy intakes are associated with a higher risk of endometrial cancer. Of 3 prospective studies[456–458], all found higher risks associated with higher energy intakes, although only 2 were statistically significant[457,458].

6.5.2   *Overweight, obesity and endometrial cancer*   All   case-control studies[405,547,563,641–651] and all [332,570,652,653] but one[586] prospective studies have found a positive association between higher BMI and risk of endometrial cancer. Most studies show a two to three fold increase in risk and a number of studies have found a dose response relationship with increasing weight or BMI. Case-control studies tend to find higher relative risks than prospective studies but they are probably biased by the common use of hospital based controls who may have experienced recent weight loss. There is, therefore strongly consistent evidence that higher body weight and higher BMI are associated with increased risk of endometrial cancer.

6.5.3   As with breast epithelial tissue, oestrogen strongly stimulates mitosis in endometrial epithelial cells (see section 7.12.5). Consistent with the higher risk of endometrial cancer with increasing overweight, obese women generally have higher levels of available oestrogen than normal weight women[562, 587–591].

6.5.4   Conclusions

There is moderately consistent evidence from epidemiological studies that higher energy intakes and strongly consistent evidence that higher body weight and higher BMI are associated with higher risk of endometrial cancer.

6.6   Other cancers

6.6.1   *Overweight, obesity and other cancers*   There are too few studies to draw conclusions on the risk of ovarian cancer, pancreatic cancer or testicular cancer. Some [570,575,654], but not all[655] studies have suggested that obesity is associated with a higher risk of ovarian cancer, particularly in pre-menopausal women. Most studies have found no association[452,563,584,656]. Studies of gastric cancer and lung cancer tend to find a lower risk with increasing body weight or BMI but this is more likely to be a consequence of the disease or due to confounding, for example by smoking, than being a causal factor[208,398,415,477,563,657,658].

6.6.2   Conclusions

There are too few studies to draw conclusions about the relationship between body weight, height and BMI with ovarian, pancreatic, and testicular cancers. There is evidence for lower incidence of lung and gastric cancers with higher body weight or BMI but this is likely to be a consequence of the disease or due to confounding, for example by smoking.

6.7   Overall Conclusions

6.7.1   There is no evidence of a relationship between energy intake and risk of pre- or post-menopausal breast cancer and colorectal cancer. There is moderately consistent evidence that higher energy intakes are associated with higher risk of endometrial cancer.

6.7.2   The evidence for a relationship between risk of pre-menopausal breast cancer and BMI is inconsistent but there is strongly consistent evidence for a positive association between BMI and post-menopausal breast cancer with relative risks between 1.1 and 2.0. There is increasing evidence that central obesity and weight gain in adult life are associated with higher risks of post-menopausal breast cancer. The evidence for a positive association between body weight and BMI with risk of endometrial cancer is strongly consistent as is the evidence for a positive association between BMI and risk of colon cancer in men with relative risks in the range of 1.5 to 2.0. There is moderately consistent evidence from prospective studies and inconsistent evidence from case control studies for a positive association between BMI and risk of colorectal cancer in women.

6.7.3   There is no clear association between height and pre-menopausal breast cancer but there is evidence that taller women are at greater risk of post-menopausal breast cancer.

7. Biological Processes in Human Cancer

7.1 Introduction

7.1.1   The purpose of this Chapter is to summarise some of the knowledge of the biological processes underlying the development of cancer, and to discuss the ways in which diet might influence these processes. Newcomers to the field of the molecular biology of cancer are referred to Yarnold *et al* [659] for a simple but comprehensive review. The first part of the chapter deals with mechanisms of carcinogenesis and cancer as a genetic disease. The second part reviews some of the ways in which diet and dietary components might influence and participate in these mechanisms.

7.1.2   *Cellular basis of cancer*

7.1.2.1   The timing and rate of cell division, as well as the number of divisions preceding programmed cell death (apoptosis), are strictly regulated in normal cells. The uncontrolled and excessive tissue growth, and spread to distant sites in the body that typifies cancers arises as a result of disturbances in the processes regulating the cell cycle, cellular architecture, and the way in which cells recognise their position and function in space and time. Malignant cells (cells that compose cancers) fail to respond to some or all of the factors that regulate cell division, cell growth, cell differentiation and apoptosis (programmed cell death) and there is also some loss of structural and functional specialisation.

7.1.3   *Multistep nature of cancer*

7.1.3.1   The development of cancers is a complex multistep process[660–663]. Each step may itself be the result of alterations in a number of cellular mechanisms, rather than a discrete abnormality. Much of the understanding of the processes underlying the development of cancers is based on experiments *in vitro* and in animals and led to the concepts of 'initiation', 'promotion' and 'progression'[664]. Although still widely used, the distinction between these stages has become increasingly blurred as knowledge has increased. Nevertheless, classification of substances that cause cancer ('carcinogens') by their biological activity, and which embody these concepts, can still be useful. 'Complete' carcinogens induce all stages of cancer development. Some substances ('initiators') are capable only of inducing the beginning of the sequence. At the experimental level, an initiator is a mutagen. A promoter is an agent that enhances the yield of tumours in an animal exposed to a low dose of an initiator. Progression is the complex process involved in the development of malignancy from benign tumours, expressed as the capacity to invade and disseminate. Many experiments have used single chemicals, often in very high doses. While these experiments can give insight into the processes underlying the development of cancers, their direct relevance to

163

human cancer is limited. The experimental conditions in such tests are particularly important in determining their results. It is possible to devise experiments which can indicate carcinogenic potential of many substances, but the relevance of the results of such tests to cancer in humans requires careful interpretation[26].

7.1.4 *Cancer as a genetic disease of somatic cells*

7.1.4.1 It is now generally accepted that cancer is a genetic disorder of somatic cells and that an accumulation of genetic changes underlies the process by which a normal cell can give rise to a cancer. The number and kinds of genes that have to be mutated in order to establish the full cancer phenotype is still under investigation and may vary from one type of cancer to another, but is probably at least 2 in inherited cancer predispositions, and not less than 5 or 6 in most types of sporadic cancer[665,666].

7.1.4.2 *Somatic mutation and clonal evolution* In the 'somatic-mutation' model of cancer it is proposed that a single cell acquires a mutation in a regulatory gene that confers a selective growth advantage over its normal neighbours. This single cell divides to produce a clone of mutant offspring. The mutant clone expands by further cell divisions and one of its cells acquires a mutation in a second regulatory gene and thereby produces a clone carrying mutations in two regulatory genes. A cell in this doubly mutant clone then acquires an advantageous mutation in a third regulatory gene and produces a clone that is even more aberrant in its capacity for autonomous growth. This process of 'clonal evolution' continues until a clone appears that has accumulated enough mutant genes to enable it to express the full malignant phenotype[667,667]. Most cancers that have been examined are clonal in composition and their cells carry mutations in growth-regulatory genes, or have lost such genes. This supports the theory that clonal evolution driven by somatic mutation and Darwinian selection is a crucial mechanism in carcinogenesis.

7.1.4.3 *Serial accumulation of independent mutations during carcinogenesis* Direct evidence for the importance of genes whose products mediate signal transduction, control the cell cycle, maintain genomic stability, and mediate apoptosis and cellular senescence has been obtained from studies of the occurrence of mutations in successive histopathological stages that mark progression from normal tissue to a fully malignant tumour[661,663,667]. The most well-documented and widely-quoted example is colorectal cancer, which appears to require for its development 7 independent genetic events in the same cell lineage (see Figure 7.1). This illustrates the multistep nature of carcinogenesis and gives a flavour of the complexity of the process. Similarly consistent associations between mutations in specific regulatory genes and histopathological stages of carcinogenesis are seen in other cancers, including those of the skin, brain and stomach.

7.2 Genes involved in cancer

7.2.1 *Introduction* Several types of gene have been identified as undergoing mutation in cancer and its precursor lesions[659,661,663,669,670]. Such genes are often referred to as 'cancer genes'. This is a useful short-hand, but it must be borne in mind that a cancer gene is a mutant version of a normal gene and that proteins encoded by 'cancer genes' are abnormal or are absent.

164

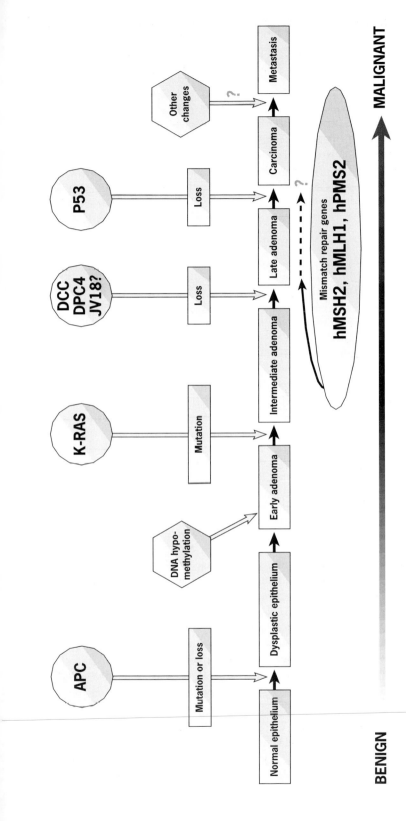

Figure 7.1   Genetic changes accompanying human colorectal carcinogenesis (modified from Kinzler and Vogelstein, 1996[235]). APC, DCC, DPC4, JV18, P53 and mismatch repair genes are tumour suppressor genes, both alleles of which are inactivated by mutation or loss, requiring mutation only in one allele. Inactivation of mismatch repair genes enhances the mutation rate and increases the risk of further mutation of other critical genes in pathway to malignancy. 'Other changes' refers to genetic events known to occur in some advanced colorectal cancers and to other, unknown, changes.

7.2.2 *Oncogenes* Oncogenes are mutant forms of a large family of genes– 'proto-oncogenes'–that control cell growth and proliferation[659,669,671–676]. The gene products of proto-oncogenes include growth factors, growth factor receptors, and other proteins which regulate cellular activity and control transcription or replication of DNA. In cancers, only one of the two homologous proto-oncogene alleles in a diploid cell is mutated, and its gene product – a protein – acquires new and abnormal properties. Thus, oncogene mutations are 'dominant' at the cellular level, since their effects are exerted despite the presence in the cell of a normal homologous wild-type allele. An example of the participation of oncogene activation at an early stage in carcinogenesis is shown in Figure 7.1. However, proto-oncogene activation may be important throughout carcinogenesis.

7.2.3 *Tumour-suppressor genes* Tumour-suppressor genes are involved in carcinogenesis when they are deleted or inactivated[669,677,678]. Unlike oncogene mutations, which act dominantly and lead to new functions, tumour-suppressor genes affect cell behaviour adversely only when both alleles are inactivated by mutation or genetic rearrangement. Such mutations are recessive at the cellular level, since they exert their effects only in the absence of the gene product. There is a growing catalogue of tumour suppressor genes[659], for example p53, BRCA1 and BRCA2. Figure 7.1 provides an example of the role of tumour-suppressor genes in colorectal carcinogenesis.

7.2.4 *Genomic instability and mismatch-repair genes* Cancers often display signs of genomic instability. Mutation or loss of genes (e.g. p53) that maintain the stability of the genome is a common event in human cancer. DNA replication is normally remarkably accurate, with error frequencies of less than 1 mutation per billion base-pairs per cell division. However, errors do occur but are corrected either by enzymes which 'proof-read' the nascent chain before it is elongated or by enzyme complexes that repair remaining mismatches (inappropriate base-pairing between mother and daughter strands).

7.2.5 The absence of genes for various components of the mismatch-repair system substantially increases the risk of mutation at each round of DNA replication. Germline mutations in such genes predispose to hereditary non-polyposis colon cancer (HNPCC)[235]. Every somatic cell in an individual with a germline mutation in one of these genes contains only one intact copy (see section 7.3.1 below). Loss of this copy due to a second genetic accident results in a cell lineage with a greatly enhanced mutation rate and a high risk of acquiring further mutations that lead to cancer. Mismatch-repair genes therefore act as tumour-suppressors. HNPCC is one of the commonest of human genetic disorders, and accounts for between 2% and 4% of all colorectal cancer. The discovery that heritable defects in mismatch-repair are causally related to a common cancer is powerful evidence for the central role of mutation in the genesis of cancer.

7.3 Germline versus somatic mutation of cancer genes

7.3.1 Mutations in genes involved in carcinogenesis can occur in germ cells (sperm or ova) or in somatic cells. Somatic mutations are passed from one cell generation to the next, whereas germline mutations are passed from parents to

166

offspring. A germline mutation in a 'cancer gene' results in an individual who is heterozygous for that gene–every somatic cell contains one functional (wildtype) copy and one inactive (mutant) copy. Such an individual has a heritable predisposition to cancer, the site at increased risk being determined, *inter alia*, by the gene that is mutated and in some cases by the location and nature of the mutation within the gene. Cancer predisposition genes are predominantly of the tumour-suppressor type probably because the loss of function of the mutant allele is compensated for by the remaining wildtype allele, allowing normal development of the embryo. A somatic cell in an individual who is heterozygous for a cancer predisposition gene may lose its remaining functional copy by mutation or loss. Such a cell will then possess a selective growth advantage, since it can no longer produce the tumour-suppressing protein encoded by the tumour-suppressor gene. This 'second hit' is the trigger for the events leading to development of cancer in that individual (the 'first hit' is the germline mutation). Inherited disposition to cancer is estimated to account for between 1% and 5% of the total cancer burden, but its study contributes disproportionately more to understanding the processes underlying carcinogenesis.

7.3.2 *Genotype and phenotype* The cancer predisposition genes discussed above are highly penetrant; most affected individuals will develop the cancer that is characteristic of the inherited genetic defect. However, even among these people, the relationship between the genotype (the mutation) and the phenotype (the clinical manifestation of cancer) can be very complex. This is not surprising, bearing in mind that other somatic mutations are required before cancer can develop. These complex relationships between genotype and phenotype in hereditary cancers suggest the intervention of modifying genes and of environmental factors (which may include diet) in the development of cancer.

7.4 Genotype, phenotype and environmental factors

7.4.1   The bulk of human cancer (at least 95%) is known by cancer geneticists as 'sporadic' and cannot be explained by genetic predispositions attributable to germline mutations of high penetrance. Rather, sporadic cancer is the outcome of a complex interplay between genetics, environment and the play of chance. It is impossible, at present, to disentangle the relative contributions that each of these factors makes to the risk of cancer in an individual or within a given population.

7.4.2 *Metabolic polymorphisms and susceptibility to cancer* Polymorphic alleles are defined as allelic variants at a single genetic locus which are present in more than 1% of the population. There are numerous examples of metabolic polymorphisms in the human population, their effects being manifest by large differences in response to the same drug by different individuals[679]. There is a 10–200-fold range over which metabolic polymorphisms exert their effects. Definitive studies of the quantitative effects of these pharmacogenetic polymorphisms on human cancer are not yet available.

7.5 Sources of genetic damage—genotoxic agents

7.5.1   The concept that cancer is a genetic disease of cells implies the presence and activity of processes and agents that cause genetic damage. Such processes and agents are described as 'genotoxic', a term that embraces 'mutagenic' and includes the ability to cause damage to the genetic apparatus, including DNA and chromosomes. Carcinogens fall into two distinct classes–genotoxic carcinogens and non-genotoxic carcinogens–discussed in section 7.9.

7.6 Endogenous and exogenous processes and agents

7.6.1   A broad distinction can be made between genotoxic effects caused by endogenous processes and those caused by exogenous agents taken into the body, for example, in the diet, and by smoking, drug abuse, medical treatments and occupational exposure (see Figure 7.2).

7.6.2   *Endogenous genotoxic processes and agents*   Lindahl[680] has reviewed the various chemical and enzymatic processes that may account for spontaneous mutation. These include spontaneous chemical degradation of DNA in the aqueous *milieu* of the cell, mismatch and proof-reading errors during DNA replication, and mutation resulting from the biomethylation of DNA.

7.6.3   *Biomethylation of DNA*   In vertebrates newly-replicated DNA is modified by the enzymatic methylation of the 5′ position of cytosine by a methyltransferase that conveys a methyl group from *S*-adenosylmethionine (SAM) to form 5-methylcytosine (5mC)[681–683]. About 3% of cytosines in mammalian DNA are methylated. Methylation occurs in both DNA strands, is symmetrical and the pattern of methylation is stably inherited during cell division. This global methylation of DNA is believed to compartmentalise the genome into active and inactive regions so that gene expression can be regulated during development[684–688].

7.6.3.1   5-Methylcytosine is easily oxidised to form thymine. Because cytosine ('C') pairs with guanine ('G') and thymine ('T') pairs with adenine ('A'), a base-pair-substitution mutation (CpG → TpG) would occur at the next round of DNA replication. This mutation occurs about ten times as frequently as other transitions and accounts for a high proportion of point mutations in the human germline[689]. Thus, although it plays an essential role in gene-regulation, the chemical instability of 5mC can also be thought of as a source of endogenous mutation[690]. CpG → TpG transitions are very common in the p53 gene in human cancers. It is estimated that about half of all cancers which occur in the UK and the USA contain p53 mutations[690]. This gene may be particularly vulnerable to endogenous mutation[692].

7.6.3.2   In vertebrates, the pattern of DNA methylation is believed to play a crucial role in the control of gene expression, embryonic development, genomic imprinting and X-chromosome inactivation in somatic cells[684,685,693]. Changes in the pattern and intensity of methylation are often the earliest and most consistent molecular abnormalities to be seen in human neoplasms[684,694,695] (see also Figure 7.1). Both hypomethylation (under-methylation) and hypermethylation (over-methylation) have been observed in tumour tissue or neoplastic cells[684,696], and the precise role of methylation in human cancer is poorly understood. How diet may modulate DNA methylation and influence cancer risk is discussed later (section 7.11.4).

168

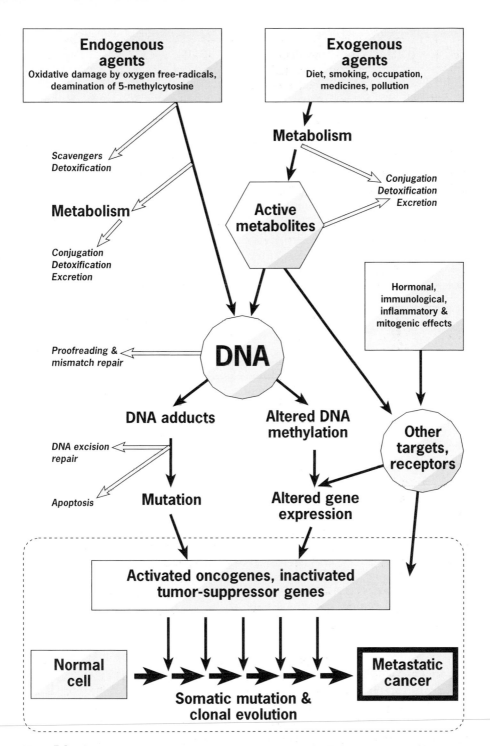

Figure 7.2 Pathways of events that occur during carcinogenesis. The open arrows and italic text denote defence mechanisms that maintain the integrity of normal tissues against carcinogenic influences. The dark green arrows denote pathways that favour carcinogenesis.

7.6.4   *Free radical mediated damage*   Free radical mediated damage is another cause of endogenous genetic toxicity. Free radicals are highly reactive atoms or molecules which are produced by normal oxidative metabolism during a variety of pathological processes, including inflammation, tissue reperfusion after vascular blockage and damage by UV light and ionising radiation. They can damage proteins, lipids and DNA by oxidation. Individual free radicals vary considerably in their reactivity and half-life in biological systems. The hydroxyl radical is the most reactive, degrading any molecule within diffusion distance, and is considered to be the ultimate radical species responsible for damaging DNA. Thymine oxidation products have been detected in human urine[697–699] and appear to result from the removal of oxidised DNA bases during DNA repair[697]. It has been estimated that each human cell undergoes between 10^3 and 10^4 oxidative modifications to the thymine in its DNA each day[700]. There is evidence that this oxidative damage is involved in some of the events of cancer induction and progression[701,702].

7.6.4.1   Defence mechanisms protective against the potentially damaging effects of these reactive molecules include the antioxidant enzymes (e.g. superoxide dismutases, catalases, peroxidases, glutathione transferase, glutathione reductase and glutathione peroxidase), the iron binding proteins (such as ferritin and transferrin) and other antioxidant compounds including essential nutrients (e.g. vitamins C and E) present in the diet. The trace elements selenium, zinc and manganese are essential for the activity of the antioxidant enzymes. Lack of availability of these elements, either for reasons of deficiency in the diet or failure of absorption, might impair protection from free radical activity.

7.6.4.2   Dietary antioxidants include vitamins C and E, carotenoids such as β-carotene, lycopene and lutein, and flavonoids, such as quercetin, luteolin and kaempferol. The water soluble ascorbic acid (vitamin C) acts as a first line of defence against water soluble free radicals[705], reacting rapidly with superoxide and hydroxyl radicals, but only poorly with hydrogen peroxide[703,704]. Ascorbate is also thought to be involved in the regeneration of other reducing agents, such as α-tocopherol (vitamin E) depleted from membranes by oxidation[706]. Ascorbate may also have a role as a chemical defence against endogenous genotoxins. For example, at acid pH ascorbate prevents the formation of N-nitroso mutagens produced in the presence of nitrite[707]. The fat soluble carotenoids, including ß-carotene, have been shown to be highly effective radical trapping agents and thus potentially to be capable of reducing oxidative damage to DNA[708,709]. Though β-carotene is the most prevalent dietary carotenoid, others e.g. lycopene are more effective radical trapping agents[710]. In membranes α-tocopherol is the major radical trap, reacting rapidly with peroxyl radicals[711]. It also quenches singlet oxygen[712] and scavenges superoxide radicals[713]. Like ascorbate, α-tocopherol has been shown to provide protection against endogenous genotoxins[707]. Glutathione has a role in scavenging free radicals by donating hydrogen atoms, and may protect against DNA damage[714]. There are many other dietary antioxidants[715]. These include carnosol and carnosic acid from rosemary[716], caffeine[717], the flavouring agent, vanillin[718] and diallyl polysulphides from aged garlic extracts[719] in addition to the carotenoids and flavonoids mentioned above.

7.6.4.3 Under certain circumstances, many antioxidants can have pro-oxidant properties. Thus, in the presence of free iron, ascorbic acid can induce oxidative damage. Other antioxidants that inhibit lipid peroxidation, e.g. the flavonoid quercetin, may be pro-oxidant in relation to DNA. The ultimate effect of a particular compound will therefore depend on a number of factors, including the level of intake, and cannot easily be predicted. It is not always clear under what conditions an antioxidant will develop pro-oxidant properties and thereby induce potentially adverse effects.

7.7 Exogenous genotoxic agents: carcinogens

7.7.1 Genotoxic carcinogens fall into a wide range of chemical classes and vary greatly in terms of their potency, the range of tumours they induce and their modes of action[660]. However, a property common to a wide variety of otherwise disparate carcinogens is their ability to form chemical bonds with DNA, to produce entities known as 'DNA adducts' (see Figure 7.2). These play a major role in the mode of action of chemical mutagens and carcinogens[660,674,720–724]. Generally, a single chemical will give rise to several different DNA adducts.

7.7.2 *Metabolic activation*   Some genotoxic carcinogens (for example, several alkylating agents used in cancer chemotherapy) are intrinsically reactive and can form DNA adducts directly, either with DNA in solution in a test-tube, or with DNA in a living cell. However, most genotoxic carcinogens are metabolically activated to become adduct-forming by enzymes whose normal function is the metabolism, detoxification and elimination of potentially toxic substances. The inactive molecule is the 'pro-carcinogen', its intermediate metabolites are 'proximate carcinogens', and the metabolite that actually reacts with DNA is the 'ultimate carcinogen'. Many pro-carcinogens from a variety of chemical classes undergo such metabolic activation. They include polycyclic aromatic hydrocarbons, aromatic amines, alkyl and arylnitrosamines and many natural products such as mycotoxins (*e.g.* aflatoxins) and plant products (*e.g.* safrole, cycasin)[720].

7.7.2.1 Enzymes with these functions fall into two main classes, 'phase 1' and 'phase II'. Most phase I enzymes are members of the cytochrome P450 superfamily of enzymes–'mono-oxygenases'. These perform oxidative metabolism by inserting one atom of oxygen into a relatively inert and usually non-polar substrate. Cytochrome P450s catalyze the biosynthesis and degradation of many normal biochemical substrates, including steroids, fatty acids, prostaglandins, leukotrienes, biogenic amines and plant metabolites. Phase I enzymes often activate pro-carcinogens. Phase II enzymes, such as glutathione-S-transferase, conjugate reactive intermediates formed by oxidative metabolism with various endogenous molecules, such as glucuronides, glutathione or sulphate, to polar, hydrophilic products that are more readily excreted from the cell and from the body[725,726]. Phase II enzymes tend to reduce cellular exposure to carcinogens. There is some evidence that genetic susceptibility to cancer may in part be determined by genetic polymorphisms of such enzymes (see section 7.4.2).

7.7.3 *Consequences of DNA adduct formation* The biological consequences of adduct formation depend to a large extent on the nature of the adduct and its precise location in the DNA molecule. Adduct formation can lead to base-substitution, deletion and addition, and therefore to point mutation. The distribution of point mutations within a gene is not random, but occurs at 'hotspots' determined, *inter alia*, by the base sequence of the given gene and by the chemical structure and reactivity of the adduct-forming agent[727-729].

7.8 DNA Repair

7.8.1 Living organisms have evolved a complex battery of defences against damage inflicted by genotoxic agents. These include 'guardians of the genome', such as p53, the DNA editing and proof-reading systems exemplified by the mismatch-repair enzymes referred to in section 7.2.4, and excision repair, referred to below.

7.8.2 The response of the organism to DNA damage is just as important to the final outcome as the nature of the primary damage[730]. Having sustained DNA damage a cell may respond in several ways. For example, it might repair the damage by excising it, to restore the DNA exactly as it was, in which case mutation will not occur, the repair being 'error-free'. The cell might die because the presence of adducts provoke apoptosis (programmed cell death), or prevent DNA replication, functions mediated by the p53 protein. However the cell may possess repair mechanisms which are sufficient to allow it to survive and divide despite a burden of pre-mutational lesions[730].

7.8.3 *Genetically determined cancer-prone conditions and DNA repair* Several rare recessively inherited disorders are associated with both an increased predisposition to develop cancer and with DNA-repair deficiencies or increased chromosome fragility. For example, patients with xeroderma pigmentosum are defective in excision repair of UV-induced DNA damage and develop multiple skin tumours when exposed to sunlight. Bloom's syndrome, Fanconi's anaemia and ataxia telangiectasia are all associated with chromosomal instability, DNA-repair defects and an increased risk of cancer[731].

7.9 Non-genotoxic carcinogens

7.9.1 There is a substantial number of substances that, when tested in laboratory rodents, induce cancer in a single organ, sex or species, and are devoid of genotoxic activity. Such non-genotoxic carcinogens tend to produce neoplasms only at doses that evince organ-specific or generally toxic effects that are accompanied by cell proliferation (mitogenesis) in tissues or organs that are normally quiescent. This is in sharp contrast to genotoxic carcinogens, which generally produce tumours in a number of different organs or tissues, in both sexes, in a range of strains and species, and often at doses lower than those that produce obvious organ-specific or general toxicity. There is no general hypothesis to account for the mechanisms underlying non-genotoxic carcinogenesis. Instead, a variety of different mechanisms must operate, each depending on the nature of the substance involved. The only common factor linking otherwise disparate non-genotoxic carcinogens is their ability to stimulate sustained cell proliferation.

Substances that are not themselves genotoxic may nevertheless enhance muta-genesis by stimulating mitogenesis in cells which have suffered endogenous DNA damage[732,733], and cellular hyperproliferation may make an important con-tribution to carcinogenesis[734–742].

7.10 Other endogenous factors that may influence development of cancer

7.10.1 Local characteristics, or characteristics specific to particular tissues, can predispose to cancer, by influencing physiological processes which interfere with the normal control of the cell cycle. For instance, increased mitosis, character-istic of cancer cells, can predispose to cancer development. There are many stim-uli for mitosis, such as growth factors, hormones and inflammation. Disturbances of the immune system can influence the likelihood of survival of a cell express-ing novel antigens due to genetic change. Chronic inflammation results in increased cellular proliferation and a number of local biochemical changes, which can also increase the likelihood of the development of cancer. Certain tis-sues are sensitive to specific hormones, and some cancers which arise in them are thought to develop at least in part from hormonal stimulation of abnormal cell proliferation.

7.11 Mechanisms by which diet and its components might influence carcinogenesis

7.11.1 Under certain circumstances, components of the diet may directly influ-ence the occurrence of tumours by causing genetic damage, by disturbing cell division and growth, by modulating hormonal and other physiological regulatory processes, or by altering cell differentiation. These actions, which often involve complex signalling systems within and between cells of various types, may also influence the likelihood that a cell already affected by some other carcinogenic agent will develop into a clinically apparent tumour. On the other hand, dietary components may also protect against cancer by a variety of mechanisms[743]. The Working Group recognised that mechanisms can occur throughout life (see 4.1.5.1) and looking for mechanisms in adult life may not be adequate.

7.11.2 *Anticarcinogens* Anticarcinogenic compounds can be classified accord-ing to the stage of the carcinogenic process at which they are thought to act. Blocking agents are compounds which reduce the tumour yield when given to animals immediately before or during treatment with a chemical carcinogen. Suppressing agents inhibit the emergence of tumours when given some time after treatment with a carcinogen, and are thought to act by preventing the pro-gression of initiated cells[743,744,755].

7.11.3 The activity of Phase I and Phase II enzymes (see section 7.7.2.1) can be influenced by various components of the diet. Some substances, such as phenethyl isothiocyanate from brassica vegetables and diallyl sulphone from garlic[934], inhibit Phase I enzymes and could potentially have an anticarcinogenic effect. Brassicas, including cabbages, broccoli, cauliflower and Brussels sprouts, may protect against cancer by virtue of their relatively high glucosinolate content. Glucosinolates are hydrolysed by myrosinase, an enzyme released from damaged plant cells. Some of the hydrolysis products, notably indoles and isothiocyanates, modulate phase I and phase II enzyme activities, possibly influencing several processes related to carcinogenesis, e.g. metabolic activation, DNA-binding and mutagenic activity of promutagens. These compounds have also been shown to reduce tumour formation in rats and mice treated with carcinogens. On the other hand, there is evidence that certain indoles and isothiocyanates are genotoxic *in vitro* and that allyl isothiocyanate induces bladder tumours in male rats[746]. Compounds such as quercetin and flavone induce the Phase II enzyme glutathione-S-transferase, and might be expected to have an anticarcinogenic effect[747].

7.11.4   Lipotropes are major dietary sources of labile methyl groups and include choline and methionine, which are methyl donors, and folic acid and vitamin B_{12} which are methyl transfer factors[748]. Diets low in lipotropes lead to the appearance of hypomethylated DNA in rat hepatocytes and also to increased cell proliferation and turnover, lipid peroxidation, oncogene activation and activation of protein kinase C, all of which can be associated with carcinogenesis[749–751]. Diets severely deficient in lipotropes can induce liver tumours in rats, even in the absence of known exposure to carcinogens[755]. Folate deficiency enhances the development of colonic neoplasia in rats after treatment with a colon carcinogen[752]. Hypomethylation of DNA is one explanation of these results. However, as well as causing methyl-deficiency, low levels of dietary folate can lead to imbalances in intracellular deoxyribonucleotide pools, a mechanism associated with DNA damage and mutagenesis[753,754]. Thus, diets deficient in folate might increase risk of cancer by at least two mechanisms, one involving disturbances in DNA biomethylation and the other due to DNA damage (leading to mutation) provoked by perturbation of nucleotide pools.

7.12   Mechanisms controlling cell proliferation

7.12.1   A number of non-genotoxic carcinogens act at least partly by stimulating cell proliferation. Some anticarcinogenic suppressing agents act by inhibiting cell proliferation. Intracellular signalling mechanisms controlling cell proliferation can be modified by a number of factors, including components of the diet.

7.12.2   *Inhibition of oncogene expression*   *Ras* proteins are involved in the control of cellular proliferation and differentiation. Overexpression of activated mutated *Ras* proteins is characteristic of many tumours. There is evidence that some dietary components can inhibit the activation of *Ras* and so inhibit the development of carcinomas[935]. Quercetin has been shown to inhibit the growth of transformed cells expressing a mutated *Ras* gene[759].

7.12.3   *Inhibition of protein kinase C*   Activated protein kinase C (PKC) triggers increased cell proliferation in a number of systems. Phytate, which has been shown to be a suppressing agent in rats, is proposed to inhibit PKC activation and so suppress cellular proliferation[756,757]. There is evidence that some dietary components can inhibit PKC directly and are anti-tumorigenic[758].

7.12.4   *Modification of fatty acid metabolism*   There is some evidence from animal studies that under certain experimental conditions, n-6 polyunsaturated fatty acids (principally linoleic acid) can promote tumour growth, while n-3 fatty

174

acids (α-linolenic acid and eicosapentaneoic acid (EPA)) can have an opposing effect[760-763]. The long chain polyunsaturated fatty acids, arachidonic acid (derived from linoleic acid) and eicosapentaenoic acid (derived from α-linolenic acid), are metabolised by the enzymes cyclo-oxygenase and lipoxygenase to a range of compounds, including leukotrienes and prostaglandins, which are biologically active, for instance in the inflammatory response. Those produced from arachidonic acid have a greater pro-inflammatory effect than those from eicosapentaenoic acid[764]. Increased metabolism of arachidonic acid via the cyclo-oxygenase and lipoxygenase pathways commonly occurs in experimental models of tumour promotion, although it is not clear whether this is a consequence of the tumour rather than a cause. Inhibition of these enzymes by synthetic inhibitors slows the growth of human tumour cells and inhibits the promotion of colon and mammary tumours in animal models. Aspirin, which inhibits cyclo-oxygenase, has been associated with reduced growth of adenomatous polyps and a lower incidence of colon cancer in man[765]. Flavonoids such as quercetin down-regulate lipoxygenase activity[766]. Although it has been suggested that *trans* fatty acids might interfere with essential fatty acid metabolism, and so predispose to cancer, good experimental evidence in support of this is lacking[767].

7.12.5 *Hormonal stimulation* Hormones and hormone-modifying compounds can predispose to cancer by stimulating cell proliferation, mainly in their normal target tissues and, in some circumstances, in the liver which is the prime site of their metabolism. For example, thyroid cancer in rats following iodine deficiency is due to the consequent increased levels of thyroid stimulating hormone, and oestrogen-induced cell proliferation is thought to play a role in some tumours, for instance of the breast and endometrium. The association between obesity and risk of post-menopausal breast and endometrial cancers is attributed in part to the higher circulating levels of oestrogen in obesity (see 6.5.3).

7.12.6 *Immune system* One role of the immune system is to detect the appearance of novel antigens in the body. Tumour cells may either express new antigens or fail to express antigens found on their normal predecessors. Immune responses can involve destruction of some abnormal cells, restraint of proliferation of others, and stimulation of proliferation of yet others. Escape from these and other controls may facilitate cellular proliferation and tumour formation. The balance between the various components of the immune system depends to some extent on the supply of substrates for the many mediators involved (prostaglandins, cytokines, interleukins). In particular the balance between the supply of particular fatty acids (e.g. the ratio between n-3 and n-6 polyunsaturated fatty acids) can influence immune function. In addition supplies of carbohydrates, amino acids and energy can influence aspects of immunocompetence. The dietary content of these substrates will influence their supply to the tissues and so could lead to disturbances in immune function. Such disturbances can affect antigen recognition, and immune reactions against recognised antigens, for instance against oncogenic viruses, and might therefore influence the development of cancers. Understanding of the relationship between diet, the immune system and cancer is still very limited, and no firm conclusions about its importance and mechanisms can currently be drawn.

7.12.7 *Effects of energy restriction* The spontaneous development of tumours at several sites in laboratory rats and mice increases after about 18 months of life. Several studies in rats and mice have shown that restriction of dietary energy intake, even by as little as about 10–20%, and possibly protein intake, leads to a fall in their rate of weight gain and to a reduction in the incidence of tumours at those sites[768-770]. Many, but not all, of the neoplasms affected are influenced by circulating hormone levels. The minimum degree of energy restriction required to produce an effect and the nature of the "dose-response" relationship, are not certain as a similar reduction in tumour incidence is seen when energy intake is restricted by 15–20% or by 30–40% throughout adult life[768,770-772]. To have this effect, which is seen in both sexes, the reduced energy intake must be maintained throughout life. There is some evidence that dietary energy restriction decreases the rate of cell turnover in many epithelial tissues[773], which would reduce the likelihood that mutations would become fixed. Considerable dietary restriction can lower the activity of Phase I and II enzymes in the liver, which might reduce the activation of potential carcinogens[774] (see 7.7.2.1). This is consistent with separate evidence that severe dietary restriction lessens spontaneous DNA damage and possibly enhances DNA repair[775]. The analogous situation in humans is not clear, though weight gain in adult life is associated with a higher risk of post-menopausal breast cancer (see section 6.2.5). The importance of these mechanisms under normal physiological circumstances and their relevance to human carcinogenesis is not known.

7.12.8 *Cell differentiation* Tumours vary widely in their tendency to spread both locally into adjacent tissues, and more distantly by blood and lymphatic spread (metastasis). More aggressive tumours tend to exhibit lesser degrees of cellular differentiation, that is their cells have lost to a greater or lesser extent the characteristic features, either structural or functional, of their tissue of origin. Cellular differentiation is often characterised by reduced cell proliferation, increased cellular adhesion, reduced invasiveness and the expression of cell-type specific markers[777]. In general, therefore, undifferentiated tumours carry a poorer prognosis than more differentiated ones, but even individual tumours may display substantial cellular heterogeneity.

7.12.9 Although a loss of cellular differentiation is associated with an increased likelihood of local and distant spread, it is not certain whether the degree of cellular differentiation itself influences the behaviour of a tumour or is merely a marker of tumours which, for some other reason, behave more aggressively. A multitude of genes and gene products is involved in the complex processes of cell differentiation. Retinoic acid, a metabolite of retinol, can induce cell differentiation through its ability to alter the expression of the wide variety of genes which contain retinoic acid response elements[777]. However, there is little evidence that this process is influenced by dietary variation in retinol intake within the usual range.

7.13 Processes occurring in specific organs

7.13.1 *Introduction* Though many of the processes described in the previous section could theoretically be influenced by nutritional factors, there is little direct evidence for this. Some processes specific to particular organs may be

176

more responsive to diet or nutritional factors, either because they are exposed to particular environments which can be nutritionally modulated (e.g. bowel contents and the colon) or because they are particularly sensitive to them (e.g. hormone sensitive tissues). This section describes factors which may operate particularly in some organs.

7.13.2   Breast cancer

7.13.2.1   Dietary fat   There is a large body of data from experiments with animal models examining the amount and type of dietary fat on mammary carcinogenesis. These show consistently that rodents fed diets containing 40% of energy as fat develop mammary tumours initiated with chemical carcinogens earlier and more than animals fed diets containing about 10% energy as fat. The effect is shown primarily after initiation and is dependent on an adequate supply of linoleic acid, about 12% total energy. Polyunsaturated n-3 fatty acids do not increase the numbers of tumours formed, and may reduce the enhancing effects of n-6 fatty acids. The mechanisms whereby fats increase tumorigenesis in these animal models are not established. Dietary restriction is known to have a powerful inhibiting effect but the energy contribution of fat does not account for the full effect, nor for differences between types of fat. However, high fat intakes are generally associated with high energy intakes and hormonal involvement has not been identified[755]. It has been argued that over nutrition in early life causes rapid growth that results in early menarche, which in turn increases breast cancer risk, and that over nutrition and high fat consumption in later life results in breast cancer-promoting hormonal imbalance[778]. Despite the enhancing effect of n-6 fatty acids, conjugated linoleic acid isomer has been shown to be a very efficient suppressor of mammary tumours in animal experiments[779]. Milk fat is a good source of conjugated linoleic acid isomer[780].

7.13.2.2   Oestrogen status   There is strong and consistent evidence for higher circulating oestrogen concentrations in populations at high risk of breast cancer. Oestrogen stimulates mitosis in breast epithelial cells. Only free and albumin bound oestrogens are available for tissue uptake as that bound to sex hormone binding globulin (SHBG) is unavailable. After the menopause, circulating oestrogens are derived from the aromatisation in peripheral tissues, particularly adipose tissue, of androstendione produced by the adrenals and the ovary.

7.13.2.3   Circulating levels of oestrogens are higher in Caucasian women (who are at high risk of breast cancer) than in rural Oriental women (who are at low risk of breast cancer)[778,781–785], although one comparison of urban Japanese women and British women found no difference in plasma oestrogen levels[786]. Case-control and prospective studies show that higher oestradiol concentrations, especially free and albumin bound oestradiol, are associated with higher risk of post-menopausal breast cancer. Although not all studies are statistically significant, none of the studies found significantly lower concentrations of oestradiol in breast cancer cases than in controls.

7.13.2.4   There is evidence relating dietary fat intake to circulating oestrogen fractions. Of 9 studies reporting low fat dietary interventions in pre-menopausal women, 4 found significant reductions in one of the oestrogen fractions, oestradiol, oestrone or dehydroepiandrostenidione (DHEA)[787-791]. One study showed a reduction in 16 α-hydroxylation of oestradiol in women on a low fat diet for 2 months but no change in oestrogen production or metabolic clearance rates[792]. Other studies have found no effect of low fat diets (15–25% energy as fat) on circulating oestradiol or oestrone levels[793-796]. Only 4 low fat dietary intervention studies in post-menopausal women have been reported and of these, two found a significant reduction in oestradiol levels[797,798] and another found a marginal, but significant increase in SHBG but no effect on levels on free oestradiol[796]. A third study, in women with breast cancer, found a significant reduction in oestrone sulphate but no difference in free or bound oestradiol or in SHBG levels in women on a diet containing 15–20% energy as fat[799]. Thus, evidence that low fat diets affect circulating oestrogen levels in either pre- or post-menopausal women is equivocal and inconsistent. Furthermore, weight loss was seen in the majority of studies described above, despite efforts to control energy intake, and this may confound the results. The preliminary results of an intervention trial in women with mammary dysplasia found no difference in either the density of dysplasia or the extent of dysplasia after one year in those counselled to follow a low fat diet (15% energy from fat) compared to a control group (36% energy from fat)[794].

7.13.2.5 Reductions in oestrogen levels are more evident in studies in which a combination of high fibre and low fat interventions were used. Three studies in pre-menopausal women which tested the effects of low fat, high fibre diets have found a significant reduction in one or more oestrogen fractions[791,800,801]. One study in post-menopausal women found no effect of a low fat, high fibre diet on oestradiol levels after 2 months[801]. Three dietary intervention studies in pre-menopausal women on high fibre diets have found a significant reduction in circulating oestradiol or oestrone levels[791,802-803]. The study by Rose found significant reductions with wheat bran but not with oat or corn bran.

7.13.2.6 Phytoestrogens (isoflavones and lignans), found in some vegetable products such as soya and linseed, are weakly oestrogenic, but in competition with more potent endogenous oestrogens can have a net anti-oestrogenic effect. They may therefore act as suppressing agents. Soya ingestion reduced mammary tumour growth in two rat models of breast cancer, but a soya product from which the isoflavones had been chemically removed did not[804]. Consumption of 45mg conjugated isoflavones as textured vegetable protein (60g/day) by pre-menopausal women over one month significantly prolonged the length of the follicular phase of the menstrual cycle[152,805]. These effects were not seen when an isoflavone-free soya product was used. However, 10g/day linseed powder given over three menstrual cycles to 18 pre-menopausal women had little effect on their sex steroid hormone metabolism[806]. In post-menopausal women, soya flour supplements over 4 weeks and linseed supplements over 6 weeks significantly suppressed gonadotrophins[876].

7.13.2.7 Several studies have found an association between age at menarche and levels of SHBG in adulthood[562]. Increased breast growth with cell proliferation at the time of puberty might increase risk of cancer. Environmental factors

178

including nutrition at other critical growth periods such as during fetal or infant life might also render breast tissue susceptible to later cancer development.

7.13.2.8 Diet and age at menarche   Age at menarche may be an important determinant of lifetime exposure to oestrogens, and therefore of risk of oestrogen-related cancers such as breast[808]. In most westernised countries there has been a decrease in age at menarche coupled with a marked increase in body size, which have both been attributed in part to nutritional factors[809–811]. It has been proposed that the timing of onset of menarche is closely related to body fat[691]. It has also been proposed that dietary fibre (non-starch polysaccharides) has an independent effect on age of menarche[812,813]. This effect of fibre (non-starch polysaccharides) was supported in a 3 year prospective study of diet and sexual maturation, when plasma gonadotrophin and oestradiol levels, and age of menarche, were significantly related to intakes of dietary fibre after controlling for the effects of body size and energy intake[814]. Use of grains, nuts and legumes was associated with 6 months later menarche and meat with 6 months earlier menarche in a prospective assessment[810]. Delayed puberty has also been attributed to zinc deficiency, arising in part from excessive intakes of phytate associated with fibre containing foods[815]. In one retrospective case-control study, higher cereal fibre consumption in adolescence was associated with a decrease in risk of pre-menopausal and a (not significant) decrease in risk of post-menopausal breast cancer[117].

7.13.2.9 Meat   Heterocyclic amines are produced during cooking of meat (see section 7.13.4.10) and three of these have been shown to be mammary carcinogens in rodent models, one of which, PhIP is the most abundant in human diets. These compounds have been found to produce adducts in mammary tissue of rodents, and are known to be absorbed from the human gastrointestinal tract[816]. In addition N-nitroso compounds (NOC) are formed endogenously in the human colon in response to eating meat[817]. N-nitroso-N-methylurea is a well established mammary carcinogen in rodent models but the effect of endogenous production of NOC on the aetiology of human mammary carcinogenesis has not been investigated.

7.13.3 *Lung cancer*

7.13.3.1 Antioxidants   Animal studies have demonstrated that high doses of retinoids (synthetic vitamin A analogs) could inhibit carcinogenesis in several organs, including the respiratory tract[818]. Significant inverse associations between serum β-carotene level and lung cancer have been observed in various prospective cohort studies. Dietary intake is positively related to serum levels while cigarette smoking and alcohol drinking are associated with reduced serum levels of β-carotene[184]. Micronuclei in bronchial exfoliated cells may be an early indicator of DNA damage and smokers have a high frequency of micronuclei in sputum cells. Supplementation with β-carotene (20mg/day) for 14 weeks resulted in a reduction in the frequency of micronuclei in sputum cells compared to those given placebo in a group of smokers in the Netherlands who continued to smoke during the study[211].

7.13.4.   *Colorectal cancer*

7.13.4.1   Hypotheses involving dietary factors in the aetiology of large bowel cancer mainly concern events in the lumen of the large bowel, and the metabolism of the colonic flora, which in turn is influenced by diet.

7.13.4.2   <u>The colonic flora and fermentation</u>   The colon is host to a large and diverse commensal flora of anaerobic bacteria which has considerable flexibility and potential for metabolic transformations, and which is controlled largely by residues entering the large gut from the small bowel. These in turn are determined by dietary intakes, particularly of carbohydrates.

7.13.4.3   <u>Carbohydrate, stool weight and transit time</u>   Carbohydrate such as starch and non-starch polysaccharides (NSP) entering the large bowel stimulates anaerobic fermentation, leading to an increase in microbial cell mass (biomass). Sugars and oligosaccharides are also substrates for fermentation, but NSP and starch escaping digestion in the small intestine are quantitatively more important.[819]. The stimulation of bacterial growth, together with water binding to residual unfermented NSP, leads to an increase in stool weight, dilution of colonic contents and faster transit time through the large gut[819,820]. Average stool weight is inversely associated with colorectal cancer incidence in different communities[821]. Low stool weight leads to constipation, and both this and use of cathartics are risk factors for colorectal cancer[822].

7.13.4.4   <u>Short chain fatty acids and butyrate</u>   During fermentation, the short chain fatty acids (SCFA) acetate, propionate and butyrate are formed. SCFA influence epithelial function in the large gut[823] where they are absorbed[825]. The sigmoid and distal colon, which are the areas of the gut where most tumours arise[824], are particularly dependent on adequate supplies of butyrate. Butyrate is an anti-proliferative and differentiating agent, modulating gene transcription and inducing apoptosis[826–830]. High starch diets, which increase colonic luminal butyrate, have been shown to reduce proliferative activity in the colons of mice and humans[831,832].

7.13.4.5   <u>Fat, bile acids, pH</u>   High fat diets lead to increased levels of bile acids in the colonic lumen[833]. Bile acids are metabolised by the bacterial flora to the secondary bile acid deoxycholic acid. Deoxycholic acid may promote bowel cancer in rodent systems[834,835,757]. The conversion of primary to secondary bile acids such as deoxycholic acid[836,837] is decreased by the lower pH induced by SCFA produced on diets high in starch and NSP. Deoxycholic acid is less soluble at low pH[838], which might limit any potential adverse effects.

7.13.4.6   <u>Calcium</u>   It has been proposed that, by forming insoluble soaps in the colon, supplements of 1.5-2 g calcium daily might limit damage to the colonic mucosa and so reduce the increased rates of cell proliferation caused by free fatty acids and bile acids arising from a high fat diet[936]. However, several short term intervention trials in patients with polyps have failed to show conclusive results[839–841].

7.13.4.7   <u>Iron</u>   Free iron catalyses the production of hydroxyl radicals and it has been proposed that oxidative damage occurs in the colon, which can be suppressed by the presence of phytic acid, a known chelator of iron[842]. In animal studies very high doses of iron (equivalent to 10-times the human intake) can induce tumours, whose yield is reduced if phytate is added into the diet[843,844]. However, increased iron does not increase lipid peroxidation products in a rodent colon cancer model[845].

7.13.4.8 Faecal mutagens and fecapentaenes Human faeces contain mutagens, and a number of studies have shown alteration by dietary factors[846–848]. Fecapentaenes are directly-acting alkylating mutagens, produced by *Bacteroides* spp, the commonest species in the human colon, probably from phospholipids in food such as meat[849–851]. However, their importance in human bowel cancer is unclear since two studies have shown that colorectal cancer cases have lower fecapentaene excretion than controls[852,853].

7.13.4.9 Meat, ammonia and N-nitrosocompounds Nitrogenous residues from meat and other protein containing foods enter the large bowel where they are substrates for fermentation by proteolytic bacteria leading to increased ammonia production[854]. The amount of ammonia in the colon increases with increasing meat consumption[50,833]. Ammonia at levels found in the human colon enhances cell proliferation and can promote adenocarcinomas in rodents[855–857]. The human colonic lumen is also rich in amines and amides which are substrates for bacterial nitrosation by nitric oxide (NO) to N-nitrosocompounds (NOC) which are found in human faeces[50]. Carcinogenic NOC are alkylators, and alkylative DNA adducts have been detected in human colonic tissue[724,858,859]. Endogenous production of NOC and nitrite is increased with consumption of red meat, but not white meat or fish[817] which is consistent with the epidemiological findings[861] (section 5.4.2).

7.13.4.10 Meat and heterocyclic aromatic amines Cooked meat and some vegetable proteins are sources of heterocyclic amines which have been proposed to increase risk of colon cancer, though their importance is uncertain. Over 20 heterocyclic amines have been isolated from cooked fish, beef, chicken, pork and soybeans. The type of cooking, time, temperature, and type and content of fat all affect the amount and type of heterocyclic amine found. Three have been shown to be large-bowel carcinogens in animal models, but their calculated daily intakes in humans are in the order of 1000 to 5000 times less than those found to induce cancer[862], and the mutations found in colon cancer do not match those produced by heterocyclic amines[863]. Nevertheless, the most abundant heterocyclic aromatic amine, PhIP has attracted particular attention because it induces colon tumours in rats with a high frequency of microsatellite instability similar to that seen in human inherited sporadic colorectal cancers[864]. Another heterocyclic amine, MeIQx, which is carcinogenic in rodents, has been isolated from cooked protein products, particularly red meat, fish and poultry[724]. Preliminary observations suggest that MeIQx does form low levels of DNA adducts in the human colon but the significance of this to human cancer remains to be determined. It has been claimed that the ingestion of dietary heterocyclic amines might cause at most 0.25% of all colorectal cancers in the USA[865]. For conversion to the carcinogenic form, the exocyclic amine of these heterocyclic amines is hydroxylated by cytochrome P450 enzymes. Covalent binding to DNA then occurs. There are organ, species, and individual differences in P450 enzymes so that direct extrapolation from rodent experiments to human risk may be misleading. Comparatively high levels of PhIP adducts have been found in human colonic tissue[866]. The combination of individual 'fast acetylation' of aromatic amines and high meat consumption seems to confer greater risk of developing adenomatous polyps. However, high meat intakes did not increase the risk of individuals classified as slow acetylators[256]. Other genetic changes seen in sporadic colorectal cancer are characteristic of the effects of alkylating agents such as N-nitroso compounds (NOC)[817].

7.13.4.11 n-3 and n-6 fatty acids In animal studies fish oils, which contain large amounts of eicosapentaenoic acid and docosahexanenoic acid, can reduce cell proliferation[867] and reduce aberrant crypt formation[868], probably by modifying the inflammatory response. In humans, the consumption of fish oils has been shown to reduce levels of PGE2, an inflammatory prostaglandin produced from arachidonic acid[869], as well as rectal cell proliferation rates, though there is no clear dose-response relationship[869-871]. In humans, several studies show that use of aspirin, which also inhibits prostaglandin synthesis, is associated with reduced risk of colorectal cancer[765].

7.13.4.12 Animal studies The role of dietary factors has been extensively investigated in animal models of colorectal cancer. Bran, cellulose, energy restriction and n-3 fatty acids are generally associated with less tumorigenesis, although some sources of soluble NSP may enhance tumorigenesis. Fat and n-6 fatty acids generally increase tumorigenesis although the effect is less consistent than in mammary cancers[755].

7.13.5 *Prostate cancer*

7.13.5.1 The incidence of latent prostate cancer is fairly constant across different populations. This suggests that the initiation of prostate cancer is more closely related to endogenous rather than environmental factors, whereas the progression of disease and mortality appear to be more strongly related to environmental factors. Sex hormone levels have been proposed as a possible endogenous factor. However, the evidence that sex hormone levels, within normal ranges, are related to subsequent risk of prostate cancer is weak. Two prospective studies do not support a simple relationship between serum testosterone and risk of prostate cancer[872,873]. One study found a suggestion that the ratio of testosterone to dihydrotestosterone was associated with higher risk of prostate cancer 14 years later but it was of only marginal significance[873].

7.13.5.2 A number of trials has examined the effects of lignans, a type of phytoestrogen found in linseed, and isoflavones on hormone metabolism in men. Supplements of 13.5g linseed/day had no effect on plasma testosterone, free testosterone or SHBG in a group of 6 men in one study[874]. However, 40g linseed/day lead to significant reductions in FSH, total cholesterol and LDL cholesterol in another study[875]. Serum testosterone and dihydro-testosterone (DHT) showed a trend towards reduced levels on the linseed diet but there was no change in total urinary androgen output. A trial using 60g/day textured vegetable protein found no significant hormonal modifications in a group of middle-aged men[875].

7.13.6   Gastric cancer

7.13.6.1   Infection with the bacterium *Helicobacter pylori* is now thought to be the major causative agent in the development of gastric cancer, and has been classified as a human carcinogen by the International Agency for Research on Cancer[358]. The first stage in gastric carcinogenesis is proposed to be the development of superficial gastritis following chronic injury and repair[877]. Subsequent extensive cell loss results in chronic atrophy of the gastric mucosa, and reduced acid secretion. This leads to the development of intestinal metaplasia and increasingly severe forms of epithelial dysplasia, ultimately resulting in intestinal-type gastric cancer. It is likely that individual steps in this sequence have different causes and that carcinogenesis occurs only after a series of distinct exposures[878].

7.13.6.2   The most common cause of chronic atrophic gastritis in the UK is probably infection with *H. pylori*[397,879]. However, it can be caused by a number of factors, including physical irritants such as coal dust[880], severe undernutrition[881], high salt intakes[882], acute viral enteritis[883], ageing[884] and vagotomy, resulting in reduced gastric acid secretion. Chronic atrophic gastritis results in a progressive loss of gastric acid secretion and a rise in gastric pH which permits the colonisation of the gastric lumen with bacterial species which are able to reduce nitrates to nitrites. Nitrites, in reaction with amines, produce N-nitroso-compounds, some of which are carcinogens. In addition, the host response to *H. pylori* infection is chronic inflammation which is accompanied by increased free radical production and potentially, oxidative damage to DNA[885].

7.13.6.3   Concentrations of ascorbic acid in gastric juice are also significantly lower with *H. pylori* associated gastritis than in normal controls[886–888]. This may be a consequence of the decreasing levels of vitamin C found in gastric juice as intragastric pH rises above pH4[889]. Eradication of *H. pylori* results in the re-establishment of normal concentrations of ascorbic acid in gastric juice[886] and to normal levels of free radical production[890]. Vitamin C supplementation has also been shown to reduce the endogenous formation of N-nitroso-proline in a high risk group in China[891]. However, an intervention trial in China failed to find an effect of vitamin C supplementation on rates of gastric cancer of the cardia, although it is not clear whether this type of gastric cancer has the same aetiology as gastric cancer of the antrum, the more common form seen in the UK. There are a number of ongoing intervention trials testing the hypothesis that *H. pylori* eradication, and/or vitamin C supplementation in people with intestinal metaplasia will slow the progression to epithelial dysplasia and gastric cancer[892].

7.13.7   Ovarian cancer

7.13.7.1   The genes BRCA1 and BRCA2 that predispose to breast cancer also increase risk of ovarian cancer (see section 7.2). The protective effects of parity and oral contraceptive use against ovarian cancer suggest that hormonal mechanisms are important and may involve pituitary and/or sex hormones[443].

8.   Other Metabolically Active Constituents of Plants

8.1   Introduction

8.1.1   Overall, the epidemiological evidence on the link between diet and cancer provides consistent evidence for an inverse association between risk of certain cancers and the consumption of fruit and vegetables (see Chapter 5). Fruits and vegetables are a rich source of micronutrients and other metabolically active substances. Many of the micronutrients appear to be good candidates for anticarcinogens because of their intimate involvement in physiological processes associated with cell proliferation and the maintenance of normal function[893]. Examples are folate, ascorbic acid (vitamin C), vitamin E and the carotenoids. However, although similar inverse associations between dietary intakes and serum levels of these micronutrients have also been observed, the few intervention trials which have been conducted to test these hypotheses have, so far, generally failed to demonstrate any benefit. It is possible that none of these trials were long enough to demonstrate a protective effect. If the antioxidant nutrients exert a protective effect at an early stage of the carcinogenic process, for example by protecting against free-radical induced genetic damage, trials lasting only 5 years would be unlikely to demonstrate any difference in cancer rates. Nevertheless, the evidence for a protective effect of fruits and vegetables is stronger than that for individual micronutrients and it is reasonable to hypothesise that other components of fruits and vegetables might also play a role.

8.1.2   There are a large number of metabolically active compounds that occur in fruits and vegetables and for which putative anti-carcinogenic mechanisms have been demonstrated at a cellular level, or at whole body level in experimental animals or humans. Many of these compounds have previously been regarded as natural toxicants but if their biological activity contributes to the probable protective effect of fruits and vegetables against cancer, a balance of risk and benefits must be considered.

8.1.3   There are a number of biologically plausible mechanisms of anti-carcinogenesis, as has been described in Chapter 7. However, most of the evidence for the anti-carcinogenic properties of different compounds has been obtained from *in vitro* techniques or using experimental animal models whose relevance to human carcinogenesis is highly questionable. In addition, much of the work has been done using isolated compounds, often at dose levels which exceed those likely to occur in normal diets, if this is known. Furthermore, there is little information on the bioavailability of these compounds. Nevertheless, there is some evidence that at least some of the mechanisms described might have nutritional relevance in humans. This chapter concentrates on compounds for which the evidence is more extensive; phenolic compounds, glucosinolates and their derivatives, compounds from allium species and chlorophyll and its derivatives.

8.2 Phenolic compounds

8.2.1 Phenolic compounds all possess an aromatic ring with one or more hydroxy groups. Phenols and polyphenols include flavonoids, phytoestrogens and tannins. They are widely distributed in plants and are responsible for many of the colour and flavour characteristics of vegetables, fruits and beverages. Human intakes vary enormously but diets rich in plant foods, tea and wine can provide more than a gram of phenolic compounds per day. However, there are many gaps in the data on the phenolic content of foods, particularly processed foods. In addition, little is known about the bioavailability of different phenolic compounds. The biological effects of phenolic compounds varies greatly, both in terms of potency and specificity. Dose relative to potency is therefore important in considering the effect of different substances. Most naturally occurring antioxidants are phenolic compounds.

8.2.2 *Flavonoids* Flavonoids include compounds such as quercetin, kaempferol, luteolin and catechins. In addition to their antioxidant properties, flavonoids can modify the expression of phase I and phase II enzymes and can therefore function as blocking agents (see 7.11.3). They have also been shown to inhibit the arachidonic cascade (see 7.12.4), inhibit PKC activity (see 7.12.3) and interfere with the expression of the mutated *Ras* oncogene and so could also function as suppressing agents (see 7.12.2). The wide range of effects, in addition to the relatively high intakes of flavonoids, have led to suggestions that phenolic compounds might potentially be the most important source of anti-carcinogenic activity in the diet[894]. However, no association between the intake of 5 major flavonoids and mortality from total cancer, lung cancer, colorectal cancer or stomach cancer was observed in an analysis of data from the Seven Countries Study after 25 years of follow-up[895] or with mortality from cancer at all sites in the Zutphen Elderly Study[896]. Therefore, despite plausible mechanisms, there is little observational evidence for a protective effect of flavonoids against cancer.

8.2.3 *Phytoestrogens*

8.2.3.1 An important class of phenolic compounds is the phytoestrogens. The principle compounds in this class are the isoflavones and lignans. Linseed is a rich source of lignans while soya protein products contain high concentrations of isoflavones[897]. Average intake of isoflavones in the UK is estimated to be less than 1mg/day[898] whereas average intakes in Asian countries is approximately 50mg/day[899].

8.2.3.2 Phytoestrogens are structurally similar to the mammalian oestrogen, oestradiol and possess weakly oestrogenic activity. Their oestrogenic activity ranges from 1/500 to 1/1000 of the activity of oestradiol and they produce typical oestrogenic responses when administered to animals[900]. Certain foods contain relatively large amounts of phytoestrogens however, so that urinary excretion and plasma concentrations may exceed levels of endogenous oestrogens by several orders of magnitude. Oestrogenic compounds can be agonistic or antagonistic to oestradiol when they act simultaneously at target tissues. Antagonistic compounds normally compete for oestradiol receptors but fail to stimulate the nucleus to respond fully[901]. In animal models and in *in vitro* experimental systems, the isoflavones appear to act as anti-oestrogens. Phytoestrogens are postulated to play a preventive role in hormone dependent cancers. The evidence for this is discussed in section 7.13.2.6.

8.2.3.3 *Conclusions* Despite plausible mechanisms, there is little observational evidence for a protective effect of flavonoids against cancer. There is insufficient evidence to draw conclusions on the effect of phytoestrogens on the risk of breast cancer.

8.3 Glucosinolates and their derivatives

8.3.1 Glucosinolates derive almost entirely from brassica vegetables (for example, broccoli, cabbage, cauliflower, Brussels sprouts, kale, mustard). About 120 compounds have been isolated. Average intakes in the UK are around 46mg/day[902]. Glucosinolates are broken down to a number of products including isothiocyanates and indolylic compounds which appear to be responsible for the bioactive properties of glucosinolates[903,904]. A summary of case-control studies found that vegetables with a high content of glucosinolates were associated with a lower risk of cancer, particularly colon cancer, which was independent of fibre[905].

8.3.2 There are plausible mechanisms whereby glucosinolates might exert a protective effect on carcinogenesis. Cell culture assays can be used to determine anticarcinogenesis potential, although the relevance of these assays to human carcinogenesis is questionable. One of the few dietary compounds which is positive in all assays is indole-3-carbinol, which is derived from indolylglucosinolates. Numerous studies have found that brassica vegetables and components of them induce phase II enzymes in a number of different organs in mice and rats[906,907]. Numerous other studies have found that cabbage, broccoli, Brussels sprouts and components of them reduce the formation of tumours in rats and mice where cancer is induced experimentally by the administration of a tumour inducer[908-914]. A review by Steinmetz and Potter[905] found that of 16 studies reviewed, 12 showed a reduction in a measure of cancer risk, e.g. number and size of tumours, DNA damage, urine mutagenicity or lipid peroxidation. Other studies have shown that cabbage and broccoli fed to rats one week after treatment with a mammary carcinogen reduced the number of tumours in the experimental group[908]. However, the relevance of these studies to human carcinogenesis is not clear. Most of the cancers were induced by carcinogens which are unlikely to be involved in human carcinogenesis and the dose of the test food or compound was higher than would be found in the human diet. Nevertheless, it is clear that under experimental conditions, many constituents of brassica vegetables can inhibit the induction of cancer through both blocking and suppressing mechanisms.

8.3.4 However, concerns about potential toxic effects have also been raised. For example, indole-3-carbinol has also been shown to induce phase I

186

enzymes[915] and to elevate colonic tumour production[916] and toxic effects have been observed in animal models when fed high levels of glucosinolates or their breakdown products. Low glucosinolate varieties of rapeseed were developed after concerns of antinutritional effects were ascribed to high intakes of glucosinolates.

8.3.5   There are few experimental studies in humans. Large amounts of broccoli (5 portions per day), Brussels sprouts (300g/day) and cabbage (200g/day) have been shown to induce cytochrome P450 levels after 10 days (a phase I enzyme)[917,918]. Three portions of Brussels sprouts/day increased plasma gluta-thione-S-transferase (GST) levels (a phase II enzyme)[919] and reduced DNA dam-age[920] in another study. There have been claims that endemic goitre in man is linked to eating cruciferous vegetables (a type of brassica) but this is generally considered unlikely, except where dietary iodine is deficient[937].

8.3.6   *Conclusions*   There is insufficient evidence to draw conclusions on the effect of glucosinolates and the risk of cancer. Plausible mechanisms whereby glucosinolates might protect against carcinogen activation have been proposed and there is some evidence of phase II enzyme induction and reduced DNA damage with high intakes of brassica vegetables and glucosinolates. There are also concerns about possible toxic effects from these or other components of brassica vegetables and more research is required to clarify their mechanisms of action.

8.4   Sulphur containing compounds from *Allium* species

8.4.1   Plants of the genus *Allium*, for example onions, garlic, leeks, are a major source of sulphur compounds in the diet. The metabolism of these compounds is complex and they undergo enzymically mediated reactions during processing and cooking. The end products of these reactions contribute to the smell, flavour and lachrymatory effects of onions and garlic[921]. The most important compounds are the sulphur substituted cysteine sulphoxides. A small number of case-control studies in a number of countries have found a lower risk of gastric cancer in those consuming relatively large amounts of *Allium* species[376,380,922].

8.4.2   There is some evidence that onions and garlic and compounds derived from them can exhibit blocking and suppressing activity (see 7.11.3) in animal models of carcinogenesis. The addition of deodorised garlic powder in the diets of rats treated with the carcinogen, DMBA, markedly reduced the formation of mammary tumours[923]. Other studies have shown that high levels of garlic powder can reduce the formation of DNA adducts by DMBA[924] and by N-nitroso compounds[925], compounds which might be involved in the aetiology of gastric cancer in humans (see 7.13.6). The authors suggested that constituents of garlic might modify the formation, activation or denitrosation of N-nitroso compounds.

8.4.3   *Conclusions*   The experimental studies described above involve the use of animal carcinogens and levels of exposure to the putative protective factors which are of doubtful relevance to human disease. Nevertheless, the existence of some epidemiological evidence suggesting a possible protective effect combined with experimental evidence for antimutagenic effects of the sulphur compounds of onions and garlic suggests that further research on these constituents is warranted.

8.5 Chlorophyll and its derivatives

8.5.1   Chlorophyll is ubiquitous in green plants and is the plant pigment capable of photosynthesis. It contains the metal ion, magnesium. Much of the information relating to chlorophyll has been obtained using the Ames *Salmonella* microsome test system. This *in vitro* approach is limited and cannot establish activity *in vivo*. An inverse relationship between mutagenic activity and the chlorophyll component of extracts has been observed and a purified derivative of chlorophyll was effective at similar concentrations[926–928]. There is evidence that chlorophyll binds carcinogens by forming reversible complexes and thereby prevents DNA damage[929,930]. Chlorophyll derivatives have also been shown to reduce the frequency of chromosome damage by a range of clastogenic compounds in a dose dependent manner[931]. However, it has also been shown that the anti-carcinogenic activity of plants and plant extracts does not always correspond to their chlorophyll content[931].

8.5.2   *Conclusions*   The relevance of the antimutagenic and anticlastogenic effects of chlorophyll seen in experimental systems to cancer induction in humans is unclear.

8.6 Conclusions

There is good evidence that plant foods contain metabolically active components that can inhibit carcinogenesis under experimental conditions. Further research is necessary to evaluate whether these processes are of any importance to human health. In addition, a high proportion of these compounds could also be classified as potential carcinogens as they have also been shown to be genotoxic *in vitro*. The relevance of these *in vitro* tests to human carcinogenesis is unclear and the activity might depend, in part, on the dose. This highlights the need for caution when considering the possibility of increasing the concentration of particular constituents of fruits and vegetables either by selective breeding or by genetic manipulation. The possibility that some of the putative protective factors might also show toxic effects, or that other toxic constituents might be synthesised by the same metabolic pathway or that the balance between different components might be particularly important should be considered.

9. Conclusions and Recommendations

9.1 Introduction

9.1.1   Section 1.5 describes the principles used by the Working Group to evaluate the body of evidence relating aspects of the diet to the development of cancers. Section 5.1.4 describes how the Working Group drew their conclusions on the consistency of the epidemiological evidence. This chapter considers both the epidemiological evidence and the evidence from mechanistic studies and assesses how likely the observed associations are to be causal relationships. Finally, a judgement must be made on the basis of usually incomplete data as to whether the evidence in total warrants the making of recommendations, taking into account the overall balance of possible benefits and adverse effects.

9.1.2   In the light of the widespread assumption that there are specific dietary characteristics which are known to influence the risk of development of cancer, it is worth noting that in no case did the Working Group consider the evidence sufficient to conclude that a causal link had been established, for instance compared to the link between smoking and lung cancer, though in some cases the evidence was more persuasive than in others. Equally, the evidence was generally insufficient to exclude with confidence a plausible causal connection (see 1.5), and there is no reason to challenge the estimates of others that about one third of cancers might be attributable to dietary and nutritional factors. The Working Group has made recommendations on the basis of the best evidence currently available, though the evidence falls short of absolute proof. Such absolute certainty, unlikely ever to be found in relation to human health, is unnecessarily stringent in the context of public health recommendations and where the evidence is sufficient, we have made recommendations on the balance of the evidence.

9.1.3   *Public health implications*   The public health importance of any individual diet/cancer relationship depends not only on the size of the relative risk for a given difference in consumption but also on the incidence of the cancer in question; in other words, the public health implications of a small increase in risk of a common cancer may be greater than a large risk from a relatively rare one (see section 4.1.7). The recommendations arising out of this review of the relationship between diet and cancer take into account these factors against the background of uncertainty regarding the causality of the associations.

9.1.4   *Recommendations*   The recommendations arising out of this review of diet and cancer need to be made in the light of existing recommendations. Therefore, in addition to considering the strength of a relationship between a constituent of the diet and a particular cancer, it is also necessary to take into

189

account whether any recommendation might have effects on health, particularly adverse effects, other than in relation to cancer; and if so, whether it is sufficiently strong and of sufficient public health importance to warrant a change to existing recommendations. Judgements need to be made about the potential consequences, both beneficial and adverse, and the expected net benefit, of any recommended change in consumption. Recommendations to the general population which, though reducing risk of some cancers, might have a net adverse effect would be unhelpful. The recommendations arising out of this review are therefore made in the context of COMA's existing recommendations. They are generally directed at the population as a whole. Better characterization of individual susceptibilities to various cancers, and other diseases, might eventually allow more targeted recommendations to particular at risk groups or people. Such precision in targeting recommendations, though desirable in principle is not yet possible in the state of current knowledge.

9.1.5 *Format* The following paragraphs combine the relevant conclusions for each cancer and the particular food or nutrient groups. A common format was adopted: for each cancer an assessment first of epidemiological evidence; then of the evidence for plausible mechanisms; then a conclusion. Finally conclusions and sometimes recommendations are made following an assessment of the overall impact of particular nutritional factors on cancer.

9.1.6 The epidemiological associations are described in terms of their consistency (strongly, moderately, weakly, inconsistent or insufficient); the evidence for mechanisms is described in terms of the extent of its existence (no/little/some/substantial, exists in animals/in vitro, operates in humans) and in terms of its strength (convincing, equivocal, unconvincing, lacking/no evidence); and the overall conclusion in terms of the strength of evidence (strong, moderate, weak, not enough) (see Annex 2). The overall conclusion might differ from that in relation to, say, the epidemiology alone, for instance, because of a lack of evidence for mechanisms.

9.2 Fruit(s) and vegetables

9.2.1 The term "fruit(s) and vegetables" is used in most studies in a dietetic, rather than botanical, sense, and covers a wide variety of plants and parts of plants. Botanically, they are not mutually exclusive and in many studies it is often not clear which are included or excluded in the analysis. The Working Group followed the original studies' definitions of fruits and vegetables to include variously all fresh, canned, frozen and dried fruits and vegetables *except* potatoes and pulses. These latter are generally regarded as starchy foods, having a different place in the diet. Some studies distinguish between cruciferous, salad and green or green yellow vegetables and between citrus and non-citrus fruits. However, most studies refer only to fruit or vegetable consumption (or both) in general.

9.2.2 *Fruits and vegetables and breast cancer*

- The evidence from case-control studies is weakly consistent that higher intakes of fruits and moderately consistent that higher intakes of vegetables are associated with lower risk of breast cancer. There are few cohort studies on the association of fruit and vegetable consumption with risk of breast cancer. Such evidence as there is, is weakly consistent that higher intakes of fruits and moderately consistent that higher intakes of total and green/yellow vegetables are associated with lower risk of breast cancer (see section 5.2.5).

- Mechanisms have been postulated to explain how fruits and vegetables might protect against breast cancer. There are components present in fruits and vegetables which might account for the observed association. One such component, dietary fibre, was found in pre-menopausal women to produce a significant reduction in one or more oestrogen fractions but not in post-menopausal women (see 7.13.2).

- *Overall, the evidence to conclude that higher intakes of fruits and vegetables would reduce the risk of breast cancer is weak.*

9.2.3 *Fruits and vegetables and lung cancer*

- The overwhelming risk for lung cancer remains cigarette smoking (see section 5.3.1) There is moderately consistent evidence that higher consumption of fruits and weakly consistent evidence that higher consumption of vegetables are associated with a lower risk of lung cancer (see section 5.3.2).

- Many studies have failed adequately to characterise the lifetime exposure to tobacco smoking and it is not possible to exclude confounding.

- The suggestion that the mechanism for a possible protective effect of fruits and vegetables is through the antioxidant capacity of components of fruits and vegetables in protecting against free-radical induced DNA damage remains plausible. However, β-carotene and α-tocopherol appear unlikely to be the mediators of any effect. Although higher intakes and blood levels of β-carotene and α-tocopherol have generally been associated with a lower risk of lung cancer, supplementation with β-carotene and α- tocopherol supplements did not reduce lung cancer rates in three intervention trials after up to 12 years. Nevertheless, if these nutrients have an effect at an early stage in the carcinogenic process, these trials might not be capable of demonstrating a protective effect.

- *Overall, there is not enough evidence to conclude that higher fruit and vegetable consumption would mitigate the overwhelming effect of smoking in increasing the risk of lung cancer.*

191

9.2.4 Fruits and vegetables and colorectal cancer

- There is moderately consistent evidence from case-control studies, especially higher scoring studies, that higher consumption of vegetables is associated with a lower risk of colon cancer, but the evidence from cohort studies is only weakly consistent (see section 5.4.4). There is only limited and inconsistent evidence of an effect of fruit consumption.

- There are a number of plausible mechanisms postulated to explain why vegetables might reduce the risk of colorectal cancer, and there is some evidence that some might operate in humans (see 7.13.4 and 8.2, 8.3, 8.4 and 8.5).

- *Overall, there is moderate evidence to conclude that higher intakes of vegetables would reduce the risk of colorectal cancer.*

9.2.5 Fruits and vegetables and gastric cancer

- There is moderately consistent evidence that higher intakes of fruits and vegetables are associated with lower risk of gastric cancer (see 5.7.3). Although it is possible that confounding by *Helicobacter pylori* infection may partly account for these findings, the strength and consistency and dose response relationship argue against this.

- Although a plausible mechanism via vitamin C has been proposed (see section 7.13.6), the evidence that it operates in human gastric carcinogenesis is equivocal. Hypotheses relating diet to gastric cancer have generally not taken account of the aetiological importance of infection with *H. pylori* (see 7.13.6).

- *Overall, there is moderate evidence to conclude that higher fruit and vegetable consumption would reduce risk of gastric cancer.*

9.2.6 Fruits and vegetables and oesophageal cancer

- The evidence that higher consumption of fruits and vegetables reduces the risk of oesophageal cancer is strongly consistent, but what prospective data exist cannot directly be extrapolated to the UK (see 5.12.3). Smoking, a risk factor for oesophageal cancer, may cause confounding.

- Plausible mechanisms have been postulated, and higher dietary intakes of antioxidant nutrients, β-carotene, vitamin C and vitamin E, are associated with lower risk of oesophageal cancer in case-control studies, but intervention trials using supplements of various combinations of vitamins and minerals have not found any effect on the appearance of precancerous lesions, oesophageal cancer incidence or mortality (see 5.12.4).

- *Overall there is not enough evidence to conclude that consumption of fruits and vegetables influences risk of oesophageal cancer in the UK.*

9.2.7 *Fruits and vegetables and other cancers*

● There are few studies of fruit and vegetable consumption and risk of prostate cancer, cervical cancer, pancreatic cancer or bladder cancer. The limited data for all four cancers are moderately or strongly consistent for reduced risk with higher fruit and vegetable consumption, although the data are too limited to draw firm conclusions.

9.2.8 *Fruits and vegetables and cancer*

9.2.8.1   Overall, there is moderate evidence that higher vegetable consumption would reduce the risk of colorectal cancer, and that higher fruit and vegetable consumption would reduce the risk of gastric cancer. There is weak evidence, based on fewer data, that higher fruit and vegetable consumption would reduce the risk of breast cancer. These cancers combined represent about 18% of the cancer burden in men and about 39% of the cancer burden in women in the UK. Even a small reduction in relative risk would have important public health benefits in terms of the reduction in the absolute numbers of people affected. In addition, the data are generally consistent with a graded reduction in risk for higher fruit and vegetable consumption and no cancer consistently shows a higher risk with higher fruit and vegetable consumption. The overall picture, therefore, is consistent and supports the hypothesis that the consumption of fruits and vegetables protects against the development of some cancers. **The Working Group recommends that fruit and vegetable consumption in the UK should increase.**

9.2.8.2   There is insufficient evidence to quantify the optimum level of fruit and vegetable consumption associated with the lowest cancer risk. There is some suggestion from observational studies that there might be a level of consumption above which no further benefit is seen, but this is well above the current average consumption in the UK. Advice from the COMA Working Group on Nutritional Aspects of Cardiovascular Disease[2] to increase fruit and vegetable consumption by 50%, to at least 5 portions per person per day on average, is a potentially achievable goal and is likely to be conducive to better health in general and a lower risk of cancer in particular. The Working Group considers that any increase in fruit and vegetable consumption would be expected to confer benefit.

9.2.8.3   There is insufficient evidence to recommend particular types of fruits or vegetables. Dietary advice to eat more fruits and vegetables should emphasise the advantages of variety rather than focusing on particular types. Though the lack of demonstrable effect of vitamins C, E and β-carotene may be due to methodological problems with the intervention trials used to assess their effects, the evidence that they are responsible for a protective effect of fruits and vegetables is at best equivocal (see sections 9.6). It is likely that a range of compounds, including non-starch polysaccharides and the essential nutrients, is involved. There are many potentially protective chemical constituents in foods, and a variety of mechanisms through which they might act, and current knowledge does not suggest that any one should be singled out as of paramount importance. Although the evidence for a protective effect of components of fruits and vegetables such as non-starch polysaccharides, folates, antioxidant nutrients and other metabolically active compounds, is not conclusive and is insufficient to recommend an increase in their intake specifically, an increase in fruit and vegetable consumption would, *inter alia,* lead to an increase in the intake of these substances.

9.2.8.4   Some studies have observed adverse outcomes associated with supplements of β-carotene in doses of the same order as might conceivably be obtained from ordinary foods (see section 5.3.3). However, it is unlikely that ordinary unsupplemented diets would have similar adverse effects attributable to β-carotene. Firstly, achieving similar habitual intakes, though theoretically possible, is unlikely. Secondly, the balance of various carotenoids and nutrients is markedly different. Thirdly, blood levels of β-carotene achieved through supplementation are many times higher than those achieved through ordinary diets even for equivalent intakes. An increase in intakes of β-carotene consequent on raising consumption of a variety of vegetables would not therefore be expected to carry adverse effects.

9.2.8.5   Our conclusions are more cautious than some other commentators. The results of the intervention trials reported so far do not support the notion that either vitamin supplements or fortified foods provide an equivalent alternative to increasing the consumption of fruit and vegetables. In addition, efforts to increase the concentration of particular chemical constituents of fruit and vegetables for instance by selective breeding or genetic manipulation should be done cautiously with careful evaluation of the possible risks and benefits.

9.3   Meat and fish

9.3.1   The term "meat", which includes "meat products", in epidemiological studies encompasses a wide variety of foods which are all complex mixtures of different substances. Not all studies define what is meant by meat and where definitions are offered, they are not always the same or comparable from study to study. Some studies include poultry and fish in the definition of meat and others differentiate between "red meat", poultry, processed meat and meat products and fish. In general red meat refers to beef, lamb and pork in main dishes and processed meat refers to sausages, hamburgers, smoked, cured and salted meat, and canned meats.

9.3.2   *Meat and fish and breast cancer*

●   There is moderately consistent epidemiological evidence that higher meat consumption, particularly red or fried/browned meat, is associated with a higher risk of breast cancer. The evidence is largely in the direction of higher risks with higher frequency of consumption, which in the diets of British adults is strongly correlated with the amount consumed (see 3.2.4.2). Nevertheless, half the higher scoring prospective studies have failed to find statistically significant relative risks. There are insufficient data on poultry or fish consumption and the risk of breast cancer to draw any conclusions (see section 5.2.2).

194

- A number of plausible mechanisms has been proposed, but evidence that they operate in humans is lacking (see 7.13.2). In one prospective study consumption of meat in childhood was associated with 6 months earlier menarche (see 7.13.2.8)

- Although most studies have tried to allow for the effects of other differences in diet or lifestyle associated with meat consumption, it is difficult to exclude the effect of confounding completely.

- *Overall, the evidence to conclude that lower meat consumption in adult life would reduce the risk of breast cancer is weak.*

9.3.3   *Meat and fish and lung cancer*

- The evidence that higher total meat consumption is associated with a higher risk of lung cancer is weakly consistent (see section 5.3.5), and most studies do not achieve statistical significance. This suggests that any increase in risk is small if one exists at all. Alternatively these findings might be accounted for by confounding by other diet or lifestyle factors, for example cigarette smoking and social class. There is no evidence for a protective effect of consuming higher amounts of fish.

- No specific mechanism has been proposed for a role of meat in causing lung cancer.

- *Overall, the evidence to conclude that lower intakes of meat would reduce the risk of lung cancer is weak.*

9.3.4   *Meat and fish and colorectal cancer*

- There is inconsistent epidemiological evidence of an effect of total meat consumption on risk of colorectal cancer. There is moderately consistent evidence from cohort studies of a positive association between the consumption of red or processed meat and the risk of colorectal cancer with relative risks between 1 and 2 (see section 5.4.2). No prospective study has found a significantly lower risk of colorectal cancer with higher intakes of red meat or processed meat. There is moderately consistent evidence that poultry (white meat) and fish consumption are not associated with risk of colorectal cancer (see section 5.4.2). Confounding by other diet or lifestyle factors might have influenced these findings.

- A number of plausible mechanisms has been proposed to explain these observations (see 7.13.4). The importance in human cancer of nitrogenous residues, e.g. ammonia and N-nitrosocompounds from meat and other protein containing foods, and heterocyclic aromatic amines from cooked meats, is uncertain and there is no direct evidence that they are involved in human colorectal carcinogenesis.

- *Overall, there is moderate evidence to conclude that lower red meat and processed meat consumption would reduce the risk of colorectal cancer.*

9.3.5 Meat and fish and prostate cancer

- There is weakly consistent evidence that total meat and moderately consistent evidence that red meat consumption are associated with higher risk of prostate cancer. Although the evidence is largely in the direction of higher risk with higher meat consumption, in the majority of studies, it does not reach statistical significance (see 5.5.2). The data relating to poultry, fish or processed meat consumption on risk of prostate cancer are insufficient to draw conclusions (see 5.5.2).

- No specific mechanisms have been proposed for the role of meat in causing prostate cancer.

- *Overall, the evidence to conclude that lower intakes of meat would reduce the risk of prostate cancer is weak.*

9.3.6 Meat and fish and gastric cancer

- The epidemiological evidence for meat and fish and gastric cancer is generally related to salted or preserved meat and fish. The few prospective studies identified showed moderately consistent evidence that high intakes of salted meat and fish are associated with higher risk of gastric cancer, although such foods do not generally relate to foods commonly consumed in the UK (see 5.7.2). Furthermore the epidemiological studies did not take account of *Helicobacter pylori* infection which is an important potential confounder (see below).

- One mechanism proposed to explain these observations is that components of preserved meats and fish, such as salt, initiated the process of chronic injury and repair postulated as the precursor of gastric carcinogenesis. However, it is now thought that infection with the bacterium *Helicobacter pylori* is the major causative agent in the development of gastric cancer. Whether preserved meats and fish might influence this process has not been demonstrated (see section 7.13.6).

- *Overall, the evidence is not enough to conclude that lower consumption of preserved meats eaten in the UK would reduce the risk of gastric cancer.*

9.3.7 Meat and fish and pancreatic cancer

- Though based on limited data, the evidence is moderately consistent that higher total meat and red meat (beef and pork) consumption is associated with higher risk of pancreatic cancer. The evidence that consumption of poultry, fish and processed meat are associated with risk of pancreatic cancer is inconsistent (see section 5.11.2). Smoking increases risk of pancreatic cancer, which may have caused confounding.

- There is no evidence for any mechanism operating in humans.

- *Overall, the evidence to conclude that lower consumption of total meat and red meat would result in a lower risk of pancreatic cancer is weak.*

9.3.8 Meat and fish and other cancers

9.3.8.1 The evidence relating meat consumption to oesophageal cancer is inconsistent. Furthermore, the relevance of the evidence to meat as commonly eaten in the UK is limited. There is insufficient evidence for an association between meat consumption and bladder, cervical, ovarian, testicular, oral, pharyngeal and laryngeal cancers. Although most studies have tried to allow for the effects of other differences in diet or lifestyle associated with meat consumption such as smoking, it is difficult to exclude the effect of confounding completely.

9.3.9 Meat and meat products and cancer

9.3.9.1 There is moderate evidence for a relationship between red and processed meat consumption and colorectal cancer. Colorectal cancers represent about 12% of all cancers. The evidence indicates that the risk of colorectal cancer is greatest in people with the highest intakes of red and processed meat. Overall, therefore, there is moderate evidence that lower red meat or processed meat consumption would reduce the risk of colorectal cancer. The overall evidence that lower meat consumption would reduce risk of breast cancer, lung cancer, prostate cancer and pancreatic cancer is weak. There is insufficient evidence that lower consumption of preserved meat as eaten in the UK would reduce the risk of gastric cancer. The nature and mechanisms of the observed associations between meat consumption and the risk of cancers, should be the subject of research. It is feasible that the observed associations between meat consumption and the risk of various cancers could be explained by confounding due to other dietary or lifestyle factors, for example low fruit and vegetable consumption, and such confounding is difficult to disentangle.

9.3.9.2 Besides any potential effect meat and meat products have on cancers, they are a valuable source of a number of nutrients, including iron, whose average intake in some sectors of the population is low. Total meat consumption, as measured by the National Food Survey has been falling since 1980. Within this trend, however, consumption of poultry and meat products has risen whilst consumption of carcase (red) meats has fallen. **The Working Group concluded that lower consumption of red and processed meat would probably reduce the risk of colorectal cancer**. However, the Working Group are aware of the possible associated adverse implications of a reduction in meat consumption on other aspects of health, particularly iron status, and **recommend that this should be the subject of review**. The Working Group was concerned that any general recommendations regarding red or processed meat should not compromise those for whom an intake of red meat, in moderation, is making an important contribution to micronutrient status. **The Working Group recommend for adults that individuals' consumption of red and processed meat should not rise; that higher consumers should consider a reduction; and as a consequence of** this the population average will fall. **Adults with intakes of red and processed meats greater than the current average, especially those in the upper reaches of the distrubtion of intakes where the scientific data are more robust, might benefit from, and should consider, a reduction in intake. It is not recommended that adults with intakes below the current average, should reduce their intakes. The wider nutritional implications of any reduction should be assessed**. As a guide to help identify where people's patterns of consumption lie in the distribution of intakes, the current average consumption of red and processed meats in the UK is around 90g/day cooked weight (8–10 portions per week), and consumers in the upper reaches of the distribution of intakes above 140g/day cooked weight (12–14 portions per week). This latter figure represents one standard deviation above the mean. 15% of consumers eat more than this amount. **These recommendations should be followed in the context of COMA's wider recommendations for a balanced diet rich in cereals, fruits and vegetables**. There is insufficient evidence to make recommendations on the consumption of white meat or fish or on different cooking methods in relation to cancer risk.

9.4 Energy and obesity

9.4.1 *Energy, obesity and breast cancer*

- There is no evidence of a relationship between energy intake and risk of pre- or post-menopausal breast cancer (see section 6.2.1). The evidence for a relationship between risk of pre-menopausal breast cancer and BMI is inconsistent (see 6.2.2) and there is no clear association with height (see 6.2.6). There is strongly consistent evidence for a positive association between BMI and post-menopausal breast cancer although the relative risks are between 1 and 2 (see 6.2.3). There is increasing evidence that central obesity and weight gain in adult life are associated with higher risks of post-menopausal breast cancer (see 6.2.4). There is also evidence that taller women are at greater risk of post-menopausal breast cancer (see 6.2.6).

- The evidence for a mechanism proposed to explain increased risk of post-menopausal breast cancer associated with obesity is convincing. High levels of total and available oestradiol have been associated with higher risk of post-menopausal breast cancer in a number of prospective studies (see section 7.13.2).

- *Overall, there is not enough evidence to conclude that energy intake or body size or composition influence the risk of pre-menopausal breast cancer. There is strong evidence that greater, particularly central, adiposity, and greater weight gain in adulthood, increase risk of post-menopausal breast cancer.*

9.4.2 *Energy, obesity and colorectal cancer*

- There is no evidence for a significant association between energy intake and risk of colorectal cancer (see section 6.3.1). The evidence for a positive association between body weight and BMI and risk of

198

colon cancer is moderately consistent in men (see section 6.3.2) and weakly consistent in women (see section 6.3.3).

- There are no well established mechanisms to explain the different relationships observed between obesity and colorectal cancer in men and women. There is no evidence that increasing body fatness protects against colorectal cancer.

- *Overall, the evidence to conclude that energy intake, body weight or adiposity influence the risk of colorectal cancer is weak.*

9.4.3 *Energy, obesity and endometrial cancer*

- There is moderately consistent evidence from epidemiological studies that higher energy intakes are associated with an increased risk of endometrial cancer (see section 6.5). There is strongly consistent evidence that higher body weight and higher BMI are associated with higher risk of endometrial cancer.

- The higher levels of available oestradiol associated with increasing body fatness could explain the increased risk of endometrial cancer associated with obesity as oestrogens stimulate the proliferation of endometrial tissue (see section 7.12.5).

- *Overall, there is strong evidence to conclude that greater adiposity increases risk of endometrial cancer.*

9.4.4 *Energy, obesity and other cancers*

- There are too few studies to draw conclusions on the risk of prostatic, ovarian, pancreatic and testicular cancers associated with obesity. Studies of gastric cancer and lung cancer tend to find a lower risk with increasing body weight or BMI but this is more likely to be a consequence of the disease or due to confounding, for example by smoking, than a causal factor (see section 6.6.1).

9.4.5 *Energy, obesity and cancer*

Overall, there is moderate to strong evidence that maintaining a healthy weight would reduce the risk of post-menopausal breast cancer and endometrial cancer. There is weak evidence that it would reduce the risk of colon cancer. There is no evidence that increasing obesity protects against cancers. Breast cancer is the most common cancer in women in the UK, accounting for about 25% of the cancer burden in women. England and Wales have one of the highest rates of breast cancer in the world. Endometrial cancer accounts for about 3% of cancers in women. **The Working Group therefore endorsed current advice to maintain a healthy body weight, in the BMI range of 20–25, and to prevent weight gain with age, through regular physical activity and eating appropriate amounts of food conforming to COMA dietary recommendations.**

9.5 Total fat

9.5.1 Total fat and breast cancer

● Within the range found in Western populations and after correcting for any confounding by BMI, the evidence from case-control studies for an association between higher total fat and saturated fatty acid intakes and risk of breast cancer is weakly consistent. The evidence from prospective studies alone is moderately consistent that no such association exists (see section 5.2.4). It remains possible that dietary fat intake during childhood and adolescence may affect breast cancer risk several decades later. The evidence for a lack of association between intakes of mono- and polyunsaturated fatty acids and the risk of breast cancer is moderately consistent.

● A number of plausible mechanisms by which fat could be involved in the aetiology of breast cancer have been postulated, but while there is moderately consistent evidence that circulating levels of free and albumin bound oestradiol, the most bioavailable form of oestrogen, are associated with a higher future risk of post-menopausal breast cancer (see section 7.13.2), the evidence that low fat diets lead to a reduction in total and free oestradiol in either pre- or post-menopausal women is weak and inconsistent. The possibility that an increased risk of breast cancer through earlier menarche might be caused by higher fat intake leading to higher body fat has not been sufficiently investigated.

● *Overall, there is moderate evidence to conclude that total fat intake in adult life does not influence the risk of breast cancer independently of BMI.*

9.5.2 Total fat and colorectal cancer

● There is weakly consistent epidemiological evidence that higher total fat intakes are associated with a higher risk of colorectal cancer. Although the majority of studies are in the direction of higher risks with higher fat consumption, most do not reach conventional levels of statistical significance (see section 5.4.3).

● Though possible mechanisms have been suggested, for example through the action of secondary bile acids (see section 7.13.4), the evidence is equivocal that these mechanisms operate in humans.

● *Overall, the evidence to conclude that total fat intake influences risk of colorectal cancer is weak.*

9.5.3 Total fat and prostate cancer

● The limited epidemiological data are weakly consistent that higher total fat intakes are associated with higher risks of prostate cancer (see section 5.5.3).

- No plausible mechanisms to explain this observation have been proposed.

- *Overall, there is not enough evidence to conclude that total fat intake influences risk of prostate cancer.*

9.5.4 Total fat and other cancers

- There is insufficient evidence to conclude that total fat intakes are associated with risk of cancers such as lung cancer, gastric cancer, cervical cancer, pancreatic cancer or oesophageal cancer (see sections 5.3, 5.7, 5.8, 5.11, 5.12).

9.5.5 Total fat and cancer

Overall, therefore, the evidence to conclude that higher total fat intakes in adult life result in higher risks of colorectal cancer is weak. There is insufficient evidence to conclude that total fat intakes influence risk of prostate cancer; and moderate evidence to conclude that they do not influence risk of breast cancer. **The Working Group made no specific recommendations on total fat intake.** Current dietary advice to reduce the proportion of energy from fat would not be expected to influence the risk of cancer, though it might reduce the likelihood of obesity.

9.6 Vitamins A, C, E and β-carotene

9.6.1 Vitamins A, C and E and breast cancer

- There is weakly consistent epidemiological evidence that higher intakes of vitamin A, either total, pre-formed retinol or carotenoids, are associated with a reduced risk of breast cancer. There is a suggestion that among women with the lowest dietary intakes of vitamin A, the use of supplements of vitamin A reduces the risk of breast cancer, but vitamin A supplements are unlikely to influence the risk of breast cancer among women whose dietary intake of vitamin A is not low. There is insufficient evidence to draw conclusions on vitamins C and E and risk of breast cancer (see section 5.2.7).

- There is no evidence for a specific mechanism.

- *Overall, there is not enough evidence to conclude that intakes of vitamins A, C and E modulate the risk of breast cancer.*

9.6.2 Vitamins A, C and E and β-carotene and lung cancer

- Although there is strongly consistent evidence from case-control studies that higher vitamin A and/or β-carotene intakes are associated with a lower risk of lung cancer, the evidence from prospective studies is only weakly consistent and this has not been confirmed in three intervention trials lasting up to 12 years. There is strongly consistent evidence that higher plasma levels of β-carotene are associated with lower risk of developing lung cancer. It is possible that the associations seen in the observational studies were due to confounding, for example by smoking or by other nutrients associated with β-carotene; or that any protective effect of β-carotene is seen at an earlier stage in the development of lung cancer. Two intervention trials in smokers have found increases in the incidence of lung cancer in those taking β-carotene supplements which emphasises the need to consider the possibility of adverse effects of high doses of single nutrients (see section 5.3.3).

● The evidence for an association of intakes of vitamin C with risk of lung cancer is inconsistent. The limited epidemiological evidence for an association between serum vitamin E and lung cancer is inconsistent (see section 5.3.4).

● Plausible mechanisms have been postulated for a role of antioxidants in general in reducing risk of cancers, but evidence that any effect in humans resides in these particular nutrients, or operates in human lung cancer, is lacking (see section 7.6.4).

● *Overall, data from intervention trials provide moderate evidence that β-carotene supplements do not mitigate risk of lung cancer, for which the major risk is smoking, and emphasise the need to consider the possibility of adverse effects due to moderate to high biologically active doses of nutrient supplements in general, and of β-carotene in particular. There is not enough evidence to draw conclusions specifically on vitamin E in relation to risk of lung cancer.*

9.6.3   Vitamins A, C, E and β-carotene and colorectal cancer

● There is inconsistent epidemiological evidence that the vitamins C and E and β-carotene are associated with risk of colorectal cancer and insufficient evidence that vitamin A (retinol) is associated with risk of colorectal cancer. Intervention trials in people with FAP or adenomatous polyps have generally failed to find a protective effect of supplements of vitamin C, E and β-carotene on polyp recurrence. Although such interventions are not conclusive, the evidence that higher intakes of these vitamins would reduce the risk of colorectal cancer is not compelling. The findings of increased risk of large adenomas in two intervention studies cautions against the widespread use of β-carotene supplements (see section 5.4.6).

● Though there are mechanisms hypothesised for a potential role for antioxidants in general in reducing risk of cancers (see section 7.6.4), evidence that such an effect in humans either resides in these particular nutrients, or exists at all, is lacking.

● *Overall, there is not enough evidence to conclude that higher intakes of these vitamins would reduce the risk of colorectal cancer.*

9.6.4 Vitamins A, C, E and β-carotene and prostate cancer

- The evidence that intakes of vitamin A, C and E and β-carotene are associated with a lower risk of prostate cancer is inconsistent (see section 5.5.5).

- Though there are mechanisms hypothesised for a potential role for antioxidants in general in reducing risk of cancers (see section 7.6.4), evidence that such an effect in humans either resides in these particular nutrients, or exists at all, is lacking.

- *Overall, there is not enough evidence to conclude that vitamins A, C and E and β-carotene influence risk of prostate cancer.*

9.6.5 Vitamins C, E and β-carotene and gastric cancer

- There are few studies reporting dietary intake and blood levels of vitamin C, β-carotene and vitamin E. From these there is strongly consistent evidence that higher levels of vitamin C and moderately consistent evidence that higher intakes of carotenoids reduce the risk of gastric cancer. The evidence for vitamin E is inconsistent. Evidence from intervention studies suggests that reduced risk of gastric cancer with a multisupplement of β-carotene, α-tocopherol and selenium may be limited to those with low intakes of these nutrients (see section 5.7.4).

- Mechanisms have been proposed for a possible role of antioxidants in prevention of gastric cancer, but their plausibility needs re-evaluation in the light of the recently established role of *Helicobacter pylori* (see 7.13.6).

- *Overall, there is not enough evidence to conclude that vitamins C, E and β-carotene influence risk of gastric cancer.*

9.6.6 Vitamins A, C, E and β-carotene and cervical cancer

- There are few studies, especially cohort studies, which have examined the relationship between antioxidant vitamins and cervical cancer. Evidence for dietary vitamin A and /or carotenoids and blood carotenoids are weakly consistent and for dietary vitamin C are moderately consistent for a reduced risk of developing cervical cancer with higher intakes. The very limited evidence for dietary and blood levels of vitamin E are moderately consistent for a reduced risk of developing cervical cancer with higher intakes but insufficient to draw firm conclusions (see section 5.8.3).

- Though there are mechanisms hypothesised for a potential role for antioxidants in general in reducing risk of cancers, evidence that such an effect in humans either resides in these particular nutrients, or exists at all, is lacking.

203

- *Overall, there is not enough evidence to draw conclusions on vitamins A, C, E and β-carotene intake in relation to risk of cervical cancer.*

9.6.7   *Vitamins C, E and β-carotene and oesophageal cancer*

- Although higher dietary intakes of antioxidant nutrients, β-carotene, vitamin C and vitamin E, are associated with a lower risk of oesophageal cancer in case-control studies, the results from intervention trials have not demonstrated any effect on either the prevalence of pre-cancerous lesions or on the incidence and mortality of oesophageal cancer. The evidence is, therefore, inconsistent (see section 5.12.4). It is possible that the apparent effect observed in epidemiological studies is due to confounding by other factors, for example smoking.

- There is no evidence that the plausible mechanisms proposed operate in human oesophageal cancer (see 7.6.4).

- *Overall, there is not enough evidence to conclude that vitamins C and E or β-carotene influence risk of oesophageal cancer.*

9.6.8   *Vitamins A, C, E and β-carotene and cancer*

9.6.8.1   Overall, therefore, there is not enough evidence to conclude that vitamins A, C, E or β-carotene protect against the development of various cancers. Higher intakes of the antioxidant vitamins, β-carotene, vitamin C and vitamin E have been variously associated with lower risks of breast cancer, colorectal cancer, lung cancer, gastric cancer and cervical cancer in case-control and prospective studies. Most of the intervention trials that have been carried out so far with supplements of these vitamins have failed to confirm a hypothesised protective effect of these vitamins on cancer. The lack of effect in the intervention trials raises questions about the capability of such (relatively) short term trials to demonstrate a protective effect. If these vitamins exert a protective effect at an early stage of the carcinogenic process, for example by protecting against free-radical induced DNA damage (see section 7.6.4), the relatively short-term trials reported so far would be unable to demonstrate a protective effect even if one existed. Alternatively, the observed associations may relate to a substance or mixture of substances in the diet for which intakes of these nutrients are acting as a marker.

9.6.8.2   The intervention studies also highlight the lack of information on the long term safety of sustained intakes of moderate to high doses of micronutrient supplements. In particular, the unexpected finding of an increased incidence of lung cancer in those taking β-carotene supplements in two intervention trials in people at high risk raises the possibility that a change in the usual balance of carotenoids in the diet (for instance by high dose purified supplements) might lead to potentially adverse perturbations in their absorption, metabolism or function. Such findings caution against the widespread use of moderate to high dose micronutrient supplements, which cannot be assumed to be without adverse effects.

9.7 Non-starch polysaccharides (dietary fibre)

The definition and analyses of dietary fibre is not clear in most studies, but non-starch polysaccharides (NSP) is the common factor.

9.7.1 Non-starch polysaccharides (dietary fibre) and breast cancer

- The epidemiological evidence that higher intakes of dietary fibre are associated with a lower risk of breast cancer is inconsistent. Whilst most case-control studies show a significantly reduced risk of breast cancer with higher intakes of fibre in post-menopausal women, three out of four prospective studies have failed to find an association between dietary fibre intake and breast cancer (see section 5.2.6).

- Plausible mechanisms have been proposed whereby higher intakes of dietary fibre might reduce the risk of breast cancer. Several studies have found that high NSP diets, with or without low fat, lead to a reduction in total and free oestradiol, a risk factor for breast cancer (see 7.13.2.5). However, as weight loss was also seen in some of these studies, the results are difficult to interpret.

- *Overall, there is not enough evidence to draw conclusions about the relationship between NSP (dietary fibre) and the risk of breast cancer.*

9.7.2 Non-starch polysaccharides (dietary fibre) and colorectal cancer

- There is moderately consistent evidence that higher intakes of dietary fibre are associated with a lower risk of colon cancer. Although the majority of studies have not found significantly lower risks, the evidence is largely in the direction of lower risk with higher intake. This may indicate a protective effect of diets characterised by high consumption of plant foods (in particular cereals, vegetables and fruits) and low consumption of meats and fat or it might indicate a protective effect of dietary fibre through one of the physiological effects or fermentation products (see section 5.4.5).

- Plausible mechanisms through colonic fermentation and increasing stool weight have been suggested, and there is some direct evidence that they operate in humans (see section 7.13.4).

- *Overall, there is moderate evidence to conclude that diets rich in NSP (dietary fibre) would reduce the risk of colorectal cancer.*

9.7.3 Non-starch polysaccharides (dietary fibre) and other cancers
There is insufficient evidence to associate NSP (dietary fibre) with other cancers except pancreatic cancer where there is moderately consistent evidence that higher intakes of dietary fibre are associated with lower risk of pancreatic cancer.

9.7.4 Non-starch polysaccharides (dietary fibre) and cancer
The definition and analyses of dietary fibre is not clear in most studies, but NSP is the common

factor. Overall, therefore, there is moderate evidence that higher intakes of NSP from a variety of food sources would reduce the risk of colorectal cancer, and possibly pancreatic cancer. **The Working Group therefore recommends an increase in intakes of non-starch polysaccharides from a variety of food sources.** The COMA Panel on Dietary Reference Values recommended an increase in average intake of NSP in the adult population from 12 g/day to 18 g/day and the Working Group endorse this recommendation.

9.8 Other nutrients (starch, sugars, folates, selenium, calcium, iron and zinc)

9.8.1 These nutrients have variously been proposed to be involved in the causation or prevention of some cancers. However, there is not enough evidence to reach conclusions for any specific links.

9.9 Diet, nutrition and cancer

9.9.1 There is a large body of evidence pertaining to the relationships between diet, nutritional factors and the development of human cancers. However, partly because of poor quality of many studies, and partly because of a lack of data on mechanisms postulated to act in humans, the value of the data is limited. No causal links between diet and cancers were established with confidence. These uncertain conclusions do not challenge the estimates of others that about one third of cancers might be attributable to dietary or nutritional factors. A lack of understanding of the potential molecular mechanisms underlying any impact of diet on cancer has hampered the development of knowledge. In addition the data are limited almost exclusively to adults. Nevertheless, we considered that there was sufficient evidence relating dietary patterns or the consumption of broad categories of food or nutritional status with various cancers to justify making recommendations. The Working Group did not consider the evidence in respect of any specific nutrient or constituent of food other than NSP to be sufficient to make recommendations.

9.9.2 **The Working Group made its recommendations in the light of existing COMA recommendations. The following summaries are derived from and are cross-referenced to the paragraphs containing the Working Group's more detailed recommendations with any quantified guidance:**

- **to maintain a healthy body weight within the BMI range 20–25 and not to increase it during adult life (9.4.5);**

- **to increase intakes of a wide variety of fruits and vegetables (9.2.8.1 and 9.2.8.2);**

- **to increase intakes of non-starch polysaccharides (dietary fibre) from a variety of food sources (9.7.4);**

- **for adults, individuals' consumption of red and processed meat should not rise; higher consumers should consider a reduction; and as a consequence of this the population average will fall (9.3.9.2);**

- these recommendations should be followed in the context of COMA's wider recommendations for a balanced diet rich in cereals, fruits and vegetables (9.3.9.2).

Adoption of dietary patterns conforming to these recommendations would be expected to reduce the burden resulting from some of the commonest cancers in the UK significantly.

In addition the Working Group recommended:

- the avoidance of β-carotene supplements as a means of protecting against cancer (9.6.8.2);

- the need to exercise caution in the use of high doses of purified supplements of other micronutrients as they cannot be assumed to be without risk (9.6.8.2).

9.9.3   Varying degrees of certainty surround our conclusions which reflect the current evidence. We have made recommendations where the evidence is clearly sufficient. Further data are already accumulating in this rapidly evolving field. It is therefore likely that firmer conclusions in at least some aspects of our review will be possible in a few years. **We therefore recommend that this topic be the subject of further review in the future.**

10. Research Recommendations

10.1 Introduction

10.1.1   Research into cancer and into the role that diet might play in the development of cancer is challenging for a number of reasons. Firstly, there is a long latent period in the development of most cancers, making it difficult to combine intervention at early stages with clinically relevant end-points in a single study. Secondly, it is difficult to measure accurately exposure to diet (especially over the long period of development of most cancers). Together, these considerations make the study of factors involved in the early development of cancer particularly demanding. There are, as yet, few intermediate markers of risk which have been shown to be part of the causal pathway. Although the development of cardiovascular disease shows features common with that of cancer, the identification of such markers of risk, for example serum cholesterol levels and blood pressure, has enabled research into the role of diet in the development of cardiovascular disease to progress further.

10.1.2   The inconclusive nature of much of the existing research into diet and cancer highlights the need for better methodologies and new research strategies. The Working Group agreed that further case-control studies of the common cancers would not improve the identification of potentially important dietary factors, and the inclusion of markers of dietary exposure would not provide clearer answers to the questions posed. They might, paradoxically, give unwarranted credence to false positive findings, in particular because of the bias inherent in this study design. They agreed that prospective studies of cancers which incorporated the use of biomarkers of exposure and intermediate markers of risk, including nested case-control studies, might help elucidate the role of diet in their development. However, prospective studies have tended to be conducted amongst homogeneous population groups and have used methods of dietary assessment with large measurement error, which leads to underestimation of risk from diet. Not all have included repeat measures of diet during follow-up, and possible relationships between early diet and later cancer at some sites has not usually been assessed. In many prospective studies, biological samples have not been collected, so that the interplay between dietary, metabolic and genetic factors could not be investigated.

10.1.3   Given the large and diverse nature of research into diet and cancer, the Working Group have put forward general recommendations for the direction of further research into diet and cancer rather than more specific research recommendations. The challenge for the research community is to close the gap between the 30% of cancer deaths thought to be attributable to diet, and the relatively few more or less firm links established by this review.

10.2 Future research directions

10.2.1 The development of meaningful markers both of risk and of exposure would help research into human carcinogenesis. Such markers could reduce measurement errors in estimates of exposure, and reduce the time for human studies to achieve relevant end points. Intervention trials in "at risk" groups, for example those with a genetic predisposition or with precursor lesions, would also be expected to render meaningful results more practicably than in unselected groups.

10.2.2 The elucidation of the possible "reciprocal relationship" between meat consumption and fruit and vegetable consumption, for example, by designing studies which control for one of the two variables whilst studying the other variable are required. In addition, more precise definition of meats and fruits and vegetables in all epidemiological studies is recommended.

10.2.3 More intervention trials of dietary change are in principle desirable, though there are practical problems (see 4.1.6). Prospective studies should involve appropriate storage of biological samples, which would allow the later development and testing of specific hypotheses.

10.2.4 The elucidation of both cellular and physiological mechanisms of cancer development, for example by the use of transgenic animals with defects in cancer susceptibility genes, would contribute to the understanding of the potential for nutritional involvement in the process.

10.2.5 Better clarification of the interaction between diet and genetic predisposition in determining susceptibility to cancer will help the understanding of differences in rates of cancer between different groups and, possibly, to enable appropriate advice to be targeted to particular groups of the population. For example, the links between central adiposity, insulin resistance, sex hormone binding globulin (SHBG) synthesis and increased oestrogen availability in relation to breast cancer should be studied.

10.2.6 The better specification of potentially important dietary factors in influencing cancer risk, of their interactions and of their metabolic handling, is essential to understanding any role of diet in cancer development. The most consistent associations are with dietary patterns rather than with individual nutrients and, it is possible that, there are important interactions between the many nutrients in foods that are not seen with single nutrient supplements. In particular, possible mechanisms relating to the association between meat consumption and colorectal cancer, including preparation and cooking methods, should be investigated.

10.2.7 The long timescale involved in the development of cancer means that factors occurring early in life might have consequences for cancer development in later life. For instance, the growth of the fetus and the role of diet in infancy and childhood, including the nutritional influences on the timing of puberty and menarche, and the consequent risk of later cancers should be studied.

10.2.8   Investigations into the relationship between physical activity levels and cancer incidence are warranted and more research based on a systematic review of the literature.

10.2.9   The population risk benefit needs to be considered in the light of the recommendations made in this report on a disaggregated basis (i.e. individual risks against individual genetic and metabolic background). In addition better specification of the factors that operate at individual level is required.

11. References

[1] Department of Health. *Dietary Reference Values for Food Energy and Nutrients for the United Kingdom.* London: HMSO, 1991. (Report on Health and Social Subjects; No. 41).

[2] Department of Health. *Nutritional Aspects of Cardiovascular Disease.* London: HMSO, 1994. (Report on Health and Social Subjects; No. 46).

[3] Department of Health. *The Health of the Nation. A strategy for health in England.* London: HMSO, 1992.

[4] Doll R, Peto R. The causes of cancer: quantitative estimates of avoidable risks of cancer in the United States today. *J Natl Cancer Inst* 1981; **66**: 1191-1308.

[5] Riboli E. Background and Rationale of EPIC. *Annals of Oncology,* 1992; **3**: 783-791.

[6] Willett WC. Diet, nutrition, and avoidable cancer. *Enviro Health Perspect* 1995; **103(Suppl 8)**: 165-170.

[7] Committees on Toxicity, Mutagenicity, Carcinogenecity of Chemicals in Food, Consumer Products and the Environment. *Annual Report 1995.* London: HMSO, 1996.

[8] Hill AB. The environment and disease: association or causation. *Proc Roy Soc Med* 1965; **58**: 295-300.

[9] Rothman KJ. *Modern epidemiology.* Little Brown & Co., Boston; 1986.

[10] International Agency for Research on Cancer. Some naturally occurring substances: food items and constituents, heterocyclic aromatic amines and mycotoxins. *IARC Monographs on the Evaluation of Carcinogenic Risks of Chemicals to Humans* 1993; **56**. IARC: Lyon, France.

[11] Segi M. *Cancer Mortality for Selected Sites in 24 Countries (1950-1957).* Sendai, Tohoku: University School of Medicine; 1960.

[12] Parkin DM, Muir CS, Whelan SL, Gao Y-T, Ferlay J, Powell J.(ed). *Cancer Incidence in Five Continents Volume VI.* IARC Scientific Publications No **120** 1992. International Agency for Research on Cancer. Lyon, France.

[13] Office of Population Censuses & Surveys. *Cancer Statistics. Registrations 1989. England & Wales.* Series MB1; No.**22**. London: HMSO, 1994.

[14] Sharp LS, Black RJ, Harkness EF, Finlayson A, Muir CS. *Cancer Registration Statistics Scotland 1981-1990.* Edinburgh: Information and Statistics Division, 1993.

[15] *Scottish Health Statistics 1993.* Edinburgh: Information and Statistics Division, 1995.

[16] WHO. *International Statistical Classification of Diseases, Injuries, and Causes of Death.* 9th Revision. Geneva: WHO, 1977.

[17] Tominaga S, Aoki K, Fujimoto I, Kurihara M. *Cancer Mortality and Morbidity Statistics. Japan and the World - 1994.* Gann Monograph on Cancer Research No. **41**. Tokyo: Japan Scientific Societies Press, 1994.

[18] Coleman MP, Estève J, Damiecki P, Arslan A, Renard H. *Trends in Cancer Incidence and Mortality.* IARC Scientific Publication No **121**, 1993. International Agency for Research on Cancer. Lyon, France.

[19] Welsh Office. *Cancer Registration in Wales 1984-1988.* Cardiff: Welsh Office, 1994.

[20] Office of Population, Census and Surveys. *Cancer Statistics. Registrations 1984. England & Wales.* Series MB1 No. **16**. London: HMSO, 1988.

[21] Carstairs V, Morris R. *Deprivation and Health in Scotland.* Aberdeen: Aberdeen University Press, 1991.

[22] Muir CS, Choi NW, Schifflers E. Time trends in cancer mortality in some countries - their possible causes and significance. *Proceedings of Skandia International Symposium.* Stockholm: Almqvist and Wiksell; 1981: 269-309.

[23] Ministry of Agriculture, Fisheries and Food. *Household Food Consumption and Expenditure 1995.* London: HMSO, 1996.

[24] Gregory J, Foster K, Tyler H, Wiseman M. *The Dietary and Nutritional Survey of British Adults.* London: HMSO, 1990.

[25] Gregory JR, Collins DL, Davies PSW, Hughes JM, Clarke PC. *National Diet and Nutrition Survey: Children aged 1½ to 4½ years. Volume 1: Report of the Diet and Nutrition Survey.* London: HMSO, 1995.

[26] Department of Health. *The Diets of British Schoolchildren.* London: HMSO, 1989. (Report on Health and Social Subjects; No. 36)

[27] Ministry of Agriculture, Fisheries and Food. *The British Diet: Finding the Facts 1989-1993.* London: HMSO, 1994: 56-60.

[28] Ministry of Agriculture, Fisheries and Food. *Food Surveillance Information Sheet, July 1994;* No. **34** London: MAFF.

[29] Armstrong B, Doll R. Environmental factors and cancer incidence in different countries with special reference to dietary practices. *Int J Cancer* 1975; **15**: 617-631.

[30] McMichael AJ, Potter JD, Hetzel BS. Time trends in colorectal cancer mortality in relation to food and alcohol consumption. *Int J Epidemiol* 1979; **8**: 295-303.

[31] Office of Population, Census and Surveys. *Registrations of cancer diagnosed in 1990, England and Wales.* OPCS Monitor. Series MB1 **95/1**. London: HMSO, 1995.

[32] Giovannucci E, Stampfer MJ, Colditz GA, Manson JAE, Rosner BA, Longnecker M, Speizer FE, Willett WC. A comparison of prospective and retrospective assessment of diet in the study of breast cancer. *Am J Epidemiol* 1993; **137**: 502-511.

[33] Friedenreich CM, Howe GR, Miller AB. The effect of recall bias on the association of calorie providing nutrients and breast cancer. *Epidemiology* 1991; **2**: 424-429.

[34] Trichopoulos D, Lipworth L. Is cancer causation simpler than we thought, but more intractable? *Epidemiology* 1995; **6**: 347-349.

[35] Tibblin G, Eriksson M, Cnattingius S, Ekbom A. High birth weight as a predictor of prostate cancer risk. *Epidemiology* 1995; **6**: 423-424.

[36] Michels KB, Trichopoulos D, Robins JM, Rosner BA, Manson JE, Hunter DJ, Colditz GA, Hankinson SE, Speizer FE, Willett WC. Birthweight as a risk factor for breast cancer. *Lancet* 1996; **348**: 1542-1546.

[37] Barker DPJ, Winter PD, Osmond C, Phillips DIW, Sultan HY. Weight gain in infancy and cancer of the ovary. *Lancet* 1995; **345**: 1087-1088.

[38] Beaglehole R, Bonita R, Kjellström T. *Basic Epidemiology.* WHO: Geneva, 1993.

[39] Friedenreich CM, Slimani N, Riboli E. Measurement of past diet: Review of previous and proposed methods. *Epidemiol Rev* 1992; **14**: 177-196.

[40] Willett WC. *Nutritional epidemiology.* New York: Oxford University Press, 1990.

[41] Bingham S. The dietary assessment of individuals: methods, accuracy, new techniques and recommendations. *Nut Abs Revs* 1987; **57**: 705-742.

[42] Gaard M, Tretli S, Loken EB. Dietary fat and the risk of breast cancer: A prospective study of 25,892 Norwegian women. *Int J Cancer* 1995; **63**: 13-17.

[43] Isaksson B. Urinary nitrogen output as a validity test in dietary surveys. *Am J Clin Nutr* 1980; **33**: 4-6.

[44] Steen B, Isaksson B, Svanborg A. Intake of energy and nutrients and meal habits in 70 year old males and females in Gothenburg, Sweden: a population study. *Acta Med Scand* 1977; **Suppl 611**: 39-86.

[45] Prentice AM, Coward WA, Davies HL, Murgatroyd PR, Black AE, Goldberg GR, Ashford J, Sawyer M, Whitehead RG. Unexpectedly low levels of energy expenditure in healthy women. *Lancet* 1985; **i**: 1419-1422.

[46] Prentice AM, Black AE, Coward WA, Davies HL, Goldberg GR, Murgatroyd PE, Ashford J, Sawyer M, Whitehead RG. High levels of energy expenditure in obese women. *BMJ* 1986; **292**: 983-987.

[47] Livingstone MBE, Prentice AM, Strain JJ, Coward WA, Black AE, Barker ME, McKenna PG, Whitehead RG. Accuracy of weighed dietary records in studies of diet and health. *BMJ* 1990; **300**: 708-712.

[48] Heitman BL, Lissner L. Dietary underreporting by obese individuals - is it specific or non-specific? *BMJ* 1995; **311**: 986-989.

[49] Visser M, de Groot LCPG, Deurenburg P, van Staverren WJA. Validation of dietary history method in a group of elderly women using measurements of total energy expenditure. *Br J Nutr* 1995; **74**: 775-785.

[50] Bingham SA, Cassidy A, Cole T, Welch A, Runswick S, Black AE, Thurnham D, Bates CE, Khaw KT, Day NE. Validation of weighed records and other methods of dietary assessment using the 24h urine technique and other biological markers. *Br J Nutr* 1995; **73**: 531-50.

[51] Black AE, Prentice AM, Goldberg GR, Jebb SA, Bingham SA, Livingstone MBE, Coward WA. Measurements of total energy expenditure provide insights into the validity of dietary measurements of energy intake. *J Am Diet Ass* 1993; **93**: 572-579.

[52] Bingham SA. Methodological problems in nutritional epidemiology. *Acta Cardiol* 1993; **48**: 433.

[53] Bingham SA, Day NE. Use of biomarkers to validate dietary assessments and the effect of energy adjustment. *Am J Clin Nutr* 1997; **65**: 1130-1137S.

[54] Ursin G, Ziegler RG, Subar AF, Graubard BI, Haile RW, Hoover R. Dietary patterns associated with a low fat diet in the national health examination follow-up study: identification of potential confounders for epidemiologic analyses. *Am J Epidemiol* 1993; **137**: 916-927.

[55] Willett WC, Hunter DJ, Stampfer MJ, *et al*. Dietary fat and fibre in relation to risk of breast cancer. An eight year follow up. *J Am Med Ass* 1992; **268**: 2037-2044.

[56] Gapstur SM, Potter JD, Sellers TA, Folsom AR. Increased risk of breast cancer with alcohol consumption in post menopausal women. *Am J Epidemiol* 1992; **136**: 1221-1231.

[57] Porrini M, Gentile MG, Fidanza F. Biochemical validation of a self administered FFQ. *Br J Nutr* 1995; **74**: 323-333.

[58] Yong LC, Forman M, Beecher GR, Graubard BI, Campbell WS, Reichman ME, Taylor PR, Lanza E, Holden JM, Judd JT. Relationship between dietary intake and plasma concentration of carotenoids in pre-menopausal women. *Am J Clin Nutr* 1994; **60**: 223-230.

[59] Rothenberg E. Validation of the FFQ with the 4 day record method and analysis of 24h urinary nitrogen. *Eur J Clin Nutr* 1994; **48**: 725-35.

[60] O'Donnell MG, Nelson M, Wise P, Walker D. A computerised diet questionnaire for use in health education. *Br J Nutr* 1991; **66**: 3-15.

[61] Quian G, Ross K, Yu M, Yuan J, Gao Y, Henderson B, Wogan G, Groopman J. A follow-up study of urinary markers of aflatoxin exposure and liver cancer risk in Shangai, People's Republic of China. *Cancer Epid, Biomarkers Prev* 1994; **3**: 3-10.

[62] The Nutrition Society (Nutrition Epidemiology Group). *Diet and Cancer: A review of the epidemiological literature.* London: Nut Soc, 1993.

[63] Margetts B, Thompson Rl, Key T, Duffy S, Nelson M, Bingham S, Wiseman M. Development of a scoring system to judge the scientific quality of information from case-control and cohort studies of nutrition and disease. *Nutr Cancer* 1995; **24**: 231-239

[64] Goodwin PJ, Boyd NF. Critical appraisal of the evidence that dietary fat intake is related to breast cancer in humans. *J Natl Cancer Inst*, 1987; **79**: 473-485.

[65] Schatzkin A, Piantadosi S, Miccozzi M, Bartee D. Alcohol consumption and breast cancer: A cross-national correlation study. *Int J Epidemiol* 1989; **18**: 28-31.

[66] Hankin JH. Role of nutrition in women's health: Diet and breast cancer. *J Am Diet Ass* 1993; **93**: 994-999.

[67] United Kingdom National Case-Control Study Group. Breastfeeding and risk of breast cancer in young women. *BMJ* 1993; **307**: 17-20.

[68] Taioli E, Nicolosi A, Wynder EL. Dietary habits and breast cancer. A comparative study of United States and Italian data. *Nutr Cancer* 1991; **16**: 259-265.

[69] Hems G. Associations between breast-cancer mortality rates, child-bearing and diet in the UK. *Br J Cancer* 1980; **41**: 429-437.

[70] Ingram DM. Trends in diet and breast cancer mortality in England and Wales 1928-1977. *Nutr Cancer* 1981; **3**: 75-80.

[71] Kato I, Tominaga S, Kuroishi T. Relationship between westernization of dietary habits and mortality from breast and ovarian cancers in Japan. *Jpn J Cancer Res* 1987; **78**: 349-357.

[72] Kodama M, Kodama T, Miura S, Yoshida M. Nutrition and breast cancer risk in Japan. *Anticancer Res* 1991; **11**: 745-754.

[73] Key TJ, Darby SC, Pike MC. Trends in breast cancer mortality and diet in England and Wales from 1911-1980. *Nutr Cancer* 1987; **10**: 1-9.

[74] Michels KB, Willett WC, Rosner BA, Manson JE, Hunter DJ, Colditz GA, Hankinson SE, Speizer FE. Prospective assessment of breastfeeding and breast cancer incidence among 89,887 women. *Lancet* 1996; **347**: 431-436.

[75] Brinton LA, Potischman NA, Swanson CA, Schoenberg JB, Coates RJ, Gammon MD, Malone KE, Stanford JL, Daling JR. Breastfeeding and breast cancer risk. *Cancer Causes Control* 1995; **6**: 199-208.

[76] Ewertz M, Gill C. Dietary factors and breast cancer risk in Denmark. *Int J Cancer* 1990; **46**: 779-784.

[77] Goodman MT, Nomura AMY, Wilkens LR, Hankin J. The association of diet, obesity, and breast cancer in Hawaii. *Cancer Epid, Biomarkers Prev* 1992; **1**: 269-275.

[78] Matos EL, Thomas DB, Sobel N, Vuoto D. Breast cancer in Argentina: case-control study with special reference to meat eating habits. *Neoplasm* 1991; **38**: 357-366.

[79] Richardson S, Gerber M, Cenee S. The role of fat, animal protein and some vitamin consumption in breast cancer: A case control study in southern France. *Int J Cancer* 1991; **48**: 1-9.

214

[80] Talamini R, La Vecchia C, Decarli A, Franceschi S, Grattoni E, Grigoletto E, Liberati A, Tognono G. Social factors, diet and breast cancer in a northern Italian population. *Br J Cancer* 1984; **49**: 723-9.

[81] Toniolo P, Riboli E, Protta F, Charrel M, Cappa APM. Calorie-providing nutrients and the risk of breast cancer. *J Natl Cancer Inst* 1989; **81**: 278-286.

[82] Kato I, Miura S, Kasumi F, Iwase T, Tashiro H, Fujita Y, Koyama H, Ikedo T, Fujiwara K, Sootome K, Asaishi K, Abe R, Nihei M, Ishida T, Yokoe T, Tamamoto H, Morata M. A case-control study of breast cancer among Japanese women: with special reference to family history and reproductive and dietary factors. *Breast Cancer Res Treat* 1992; **24**: 51-59.

[83] Katsouyanni K, Trichopoulou A, Boyle P, et al. Diet and breast cancer: A case control study in Greece. *Int J Cancer* 1986; **38**: 815-820.

[84] Hislop TG, Coldman AJ, Elwood JM, Brauer G, Kan L. Childhood and recent eating patterns and risk of breast cancer. *Cancer Detect Prev* 1986; **9**: 47-58.

[85] Holmberg L, Ohlander EM, Byers T, *et al.* Diet and breast cancer risk: results from a population-based, case- control study in Sweden. *Arch Int Med* 1994; **154**: 1805-1811.

[86] Ingram DM, Nottage E, Roberts T. The role of diet in the development of breast cancer: A case control study of patients with breast cancer, benign epithelial hyperplasia and fibrocystis disease of the breast. *Br J Cancer* 1991; **64**: 187-191.

[87] Iscovich JM, Iscovich RB, Howe GR, Shiboski S, Kaldor JM. A case-control study of diet and breast cancer in Argentina. *Int J Cancer* 1989; **44**: 770-776.

[88] Landa MC, Frago N, Tres A. Diet and the risk of breast cancer in Spain. *Eur J Cancer Prev* 1994; **3**: 313-320.

[89] La Vecchia C, Decarli A, Franceschi S, Gentile A, Negri E, Parazzini F. Dietary factors and the risk of breast cancer. *Nutr Cancer* 1987; **10**: 205-214.

[90] Lee HP, Courley L, Duffy SW, Esteve J, Lee J, Day NE. Risk factors for breast cancer by age and menopausal status: a case-control study in Singapore, *Cancer Causes Control* 1992; **3**: 313-322.

[91] Levi F, La Vecchia C, Gulie C, Negri E. Dietary factors and breast cancer risk in Vaud, Switzerland. *Nutr Cancer* 1993; **19**: 327-335.

[92] Lubin JH, Burns PE, Blot WJ, Ziegler RG, Lees AW, Fraumeni JFJ. Dietary factors and breast cancer risk. *Int J Cancer* 1981; **28**: 685-689.

[93] Qi XY, Zhang A, Wu G, Pang W. The association between breast cancer and diet and other factors. *Asia Pac J Public Health* 1994; **7**: 98-104.

[94] Ronco A, De Stefani E, Mendilaharsu M, Deneo-Pellegrini H. Meat, fat and risk of breast cancer: A case-control study from Uruguay. *Int J Cancer* 1996; **65**: 328-331.

[95] van't Veer P, Kok FJ, Brants HAM, Ockhuizen T, Sturmans F, Hermus RJJ. Dietary fat and the risk of breast cancer. *Int J Epidemiol* 1990; **19**: 12-18.

[96] Toniolo P, Riboli E, Shore RE, Pasternack BS. Consumption of meat, animal products, protein, and fat and risk of breast cancer: A prospective cohort study in New York. *Epidemiology* 1994; **5**: 391-397.

[97] Vatten LJ, Kvinnsland S. Body height and risk of breast cancer. A prospective study of 23,831 Norwegian women. *Br J Cancer* 1990; **61**: 881-885.

[98] Hirayama T. Lifestyle and mortality: a large-scale census-based cohort study in Japan. Basel, Switzerland: Karger, 1990.

[99] Knekt P, Steineck G, Jarvinen R, Hakulinen T, Aromaa A. Intake of fried meat and risk of cancer: a follow-up study in Finland. *Int J Cancer* 1994; **59**: 756-760.

[100] Nomura AMY, Henderson BE, Lee J. Breast cancer and diet among the Japanese in Hawaii. *Am J Clin Nutr* 1978; **31**: 2020-2025.

[101] van den Brandt PA, van't Veer P, Goldbohm RA, *et al*. A prospective cohort study on dietary fat and risk of post menopausal breast cancer. *Cancer Res* 1993; **53**: 75-82.

[102] Mills PK, Beeson WL, Phillips RL, Fraser GE. Dietary habits and breast cancer incidence among seventh day adventists. *Cancer* 1989; **64**: 582-590.

[103] Hunter DJ, Willett WC. Diet, body size, and breast cancer. *Epidemiol Rev* 1993; **15**: 110-132.

[104] Boyd NF, Martin LJ, Noffel M, Lockwood GA, Tritchler DL. A meta-analysis of studies of dietary fat and breast cancer risk. *Br J Cancer* 1993; **68**: 627-636.

[105] Knekt P, Järvinen R, Seppänen R, Pukkala E, Aromaa A. Intake of dairy products and risk of breast cancer. *Br J Cancer* 1996; **73**: 687-691.

[106] Mills PK, Beeson WL, Abbey DE, Fraser GE, Phillips RL. Dietary habits and past medical history as related to fatal pancreas cancer risk among adventists. *Cancer* 1988; **61**: 2578-2585.

[107] Ursin G, Bjelke E, Heuch I, *et al*. Milk consumption and cancer incidence. A Norweigen prospective study. *Br J Cancer* 1990; **61**: 454-459.

[108] Cooper JA, Rohan TE, Cant ELMCK Horsfall DJ, Tilley WD. Risk factors for breast cancer by oestrogen receptor status: a population-based case-control study. *Br J Cancer* 1989; **59**: 119-125

[109] Hirohata T, Nomura AMY, Hankin JH, Kolonel LN, Lee J. An epidemiological study on the association between diet and breast cancer. *J Natl Cancer Inst* 1987; **78**: 595-600.

[110] Miller AB, Kelly A, Choi NW, *et al*. A study of diet and breast cancer. *Am J Epidemiol* 1978; **107**: 499-509.

[111] Shun-Zhang Y, Rui-Fang L, Da-Dao X, Howe GR. A case-control study of dietary and nondietary risk factors for breast cancer in Shanghai. *Cancer Res* 1990; **50**: 5017-5021.

[112] Yuan J, Wang Q, Ross RK, Henderson BE, Yu MC. Diet and breast cancer in Shanghai and Tianjin, China. *Br J Cancer* 1995; **71**: 1353-1358.

[113] Graham S, Hellmann R, Marshall J, *et al*. Nutritional epidemiology of postmenopausal breast cancer in Western New York. *Am J Epidemiol* 1991; **134**: 552-566.

[114] Katsouyanni K, Trichopoulous A, Stuver S, *et al*. The association of fat and other macronutrients with breast cancer: a case-control study from Greece. *Br J Cancer* 1994; **70**: 537-541.

[115] Lee HP, Gourley L, Duffy SW, Estève J, Lee J, Day NE. Dietary effects on breast-cancer risk in Singapore. *Lancet* 1991; **337**: 1197-1200.

[116] Martin-Moreno JM. Dietary fat, olive oil intake and breast cancer risk. *Int J Cancer* 1994; **58**: 774-780.

[117] Pryor M, Slattery ML, Robinson LM, Egger M. Adolescent diet and breast cancer in Utah. *Cancer Res* 1989; **49**: 2161-2167.

[118] Rohan TE, McMichael AJ, Baghurst PA. A population-based case-control study of diet and breast cancer in Australia. *Am J Epidemiol* 1988; **128**: 478-489.

[119] Franceschi S, Favero A, Decarli A, Negri E, La Vecchia C, Ferraroni M, Russo A, Salvini S, Amadori D, Conti E, Montella M, Giacosa A. Intake of macronutrients and risk of breast cancer. *Lancet* 1996; **347**: 1351-1356.

[120] Howe GR, Hirohata T, Hislop TG, *et al*. Dietary factors and risk of breast cancer: combined analysis of 12 case-control studies. *J Natl Cancer Inst* 1990; **82**: 561-569.

[121] Graham S, Zielezny M, Marshall J, *et al*. Diet in the epidemiology of post menopausal breast cancer in New York state cohort. *Am J Epidemiol* 1992; **136**: 1327-1337.

[122] Knekt P, Albanes D, Seppanen A, *et al.* Dietary fat and risk of breast cancer. *Am J Clin Nutr* 1990; **52**: 903-908.

[123] Willett WC, Stampfer MJ, Colditz GA, Rosner BA, Hennekens CH, Speizer FE. Dietary fat and risk of breast cancer. *New Engl J Med* 1987; **316**: 22-28.

[124] Ballard-Barbash R, Schatzkin A, Taylor PR, Kahle LL. Association of change in body mass with breast cancer. *Cancer Res* 1990; **50**: 2152-2155.

[125] Howe GR, Friedenreich CM, Jain M, Miller AB. A cohort study of fat intake and risk of breast cancer. *J Natl Cancer Inst* 1991; **83**: 336-340.

[126] Kushi LH, Sellers TA, Potter JD, *et al.* Dietary fat and post menopausal breast cancer. *J Natl Cancer Inst* 1992; **84**: 1092-1099.

[127] Hunter DJ, Spigelman D, Adami HO, Beeson L, van den Brandt PA, *et al.* Cohort studies of fat intake and the risk of breast cancer - a pooled analysis. *New Engl J Med* 1996; **334**: 356-361.

[128] Zaridze D, Lifanova Y, Maximovitch D, Day NE, Duffey SW. Diet, alcohol consumption and reproductive factors in a case-control study of breast cancer in Moscow. *Int J Cancer* 1991; **48**: 493-501.

[129] Gerber M, Richardson S, Crastes de Paulet P, Pujol H, Crastes de Paulet A. Relationship between vitamin E and polyunsaturated fatty acids in breast cancer. Nutritional and metabolic aspects. *Cancer* 1989; **64**: 2347-2353.

[130] Trichopoulos A, Katsouyanni K, Stuver S, *et al.* Consumption of olive oil and specific food groups in relation to breast cancer risk in Greece. *J Natl Cancer Inst* 1995; **87**: 110-116.

[131] van't Veer P, Kolb CM, Verhoef P, *et al.* Dietary fiber, beta carotene and breast cancer: results from a case-control study. *Int J Cancer* 1990; **45**: 825-828.

[132] Freudenheim JL, Marshall JR, Vena JE, Laughlin R, Brasure JR, Swanson MK, Nemoto T, Graham S. Premenopausal breast cancer risk and intake of vegetables, fruit and related nutrients. *J Natl Cancer Inst* 1996; **88**: 340-348.

[133] Negri E, La Vecchia C, Franceschi S, D'Avanzo B, Parazzini F. Vegetable and fruit consumption and cancer risk. *Int J Cancer* 1991; **48**: 350-354.

[134] Rohan TE, Howe GR, Friedenreich CM, Jain M, Miller AB. Dietary fiber, vitamins A, C, and E, and risk of breast cancer: a cohort study. *Cancer Causes Control* 1993; **4**: 29-37.

[135] Pawlega J. Breast cancer and smoking, vodka drinking and dietary habits. *Acta Oncologica* 1992; **31**: 387-392.

[136] Young TB. A case control study of breast cancer and alcohol consumption habits. *Cancer* 1989; **64**: 552-558.

[137] Graham S, Marshall J, Mettlin C, Rzepka T, Nemoto T, Byers T. Diet in the epidemiology of breast cancer. *Am J Epidemiol* 1982; **116**: 68-75.

[138] Marubini E, Decarli A, Costa A, *et al.* The relationship of dietary intake and serum levels of retinol and beta-carotene with breast cancer. Results of a case-control study. *Cancer* 1988; **61**: 173-180.

[139] Potischman N, McCulloch CE, Byers T, *et al.* Breast cancer and dietary and plasma concentrations of carotenoids and vitamin A. *Am J Clin Nutr* 1990; **52**: 909-915.

[140] Katsouyanni K, Willett W, Trichopoulos D, *et al.* Risk of breast cancer among Greek women in relation to nutrient intake. *Cancer* 1988; **61**: 181-185.

[141] Paganini-Hill GM, Chao AA, Ross RK, Henderson BE. Vitamin A, β-carotene and risk of cancer: A prospective study. *J Natl Cancer Inst* 1987; **79**: 443-448.

217

[142] Comstock GW, Helzlsouer KJ, Bush TL. Prediagnostic serum levels of carotenoids and vitamin E as related to subsequent cancer in Washington County, Maryland. *Am J Clin Nutr* 1991; **53**: 260S-264S.

[143] Wald NJ, Boreham J, Hayward JL, Bulbrook RD. Plasma retinol, β-carotene and vitamin E in relation to the future risk of breast cancer. *Br J Cancer* 1984; **49**: 321-324.

[144] Adlercreutz H, Fotsis T, Heikkinen R, Dwyer JT, Goldin BR, Gorbach SL, Lawson AM, Setchell KDR. Diet and urinary excretion of lignans in female subjects. *Med Biol* 1981; **59**: 259-261.

[145] Adlercreutz H, Fotsis T, Heikkinen R, Dwyer JT, Woods M, Goldin BR, Gorbach SL. Excretion of the lignans enterolactone and enterdiol and of equol in omnivorous and vegetarian post-meno-pausal women and in women with breast cancer. *Lancet* 1982; **2**: 1295-1299.

[146] Adlercreutz H, Fotsis T, Bannwart C, Wahala K, Makela T, Brunow G, Hase T. Determination of urinary lignans and phytoestrogen metabolites, potential antiestrogens and anticarcinogens, in the urine of women of various habitual diets. *J Steroid Biochem* 1986; **25**: 791-797.

[147] Adlercreutz H, Fotsis T, Bannwart C, Wahala K, Brunow G, Hase T. Isotope dilution gas chroma-tographic-mass spectrometric method for the determination of lignans and isoflavonoids in human urine, including the identification of genistein. *Clinica Chimica Acta* 1991; **199**: 263-278.

[148] Adlercreutz H, Honjo H, Higashi A, Fotsis T, Hamamainen E, Hasegawa T, Okada H. Urinary excretion of lignans and isoflavonoid phytoestrogens in Japanese men and women consuming a traditional Japanese diet. *Am J Clin Nutr* 1991; **54**: 1093-1100.

[149] Adlercreutz H, Hamalainen E, Gorbach S, Goldin B. Dietary phytoestrogens and the menopause in Japan. *Lancet* 1992; **339**: 1233.

[150] Adlercreutz H, Fotsis T, Lampe J, Wahala K, Makela T, Brunow G, Hase T. Quantitative determi-nation of lignans and isoflavonoids in plasma of omnivorous and vegetarian women by isotope dilution gas chromatography-mass spectrometry. *Scand J Clin Lab Invest* 1993; **53(Suppl 215)**: 5-18.

[151] Cassidy A, Bingham S, Setchell K, Watson D. Plant oestrogen excretion in a group of post-meno-pausal women. *Proc Nut Soc* 1990; **50**: 105A.

[152] Cassidy A, Bingham S, Setchell K. Biological effects of isoflavones in young women - import-ance of the chemical composition of soya products. *Br J Nutr* 1995; **74**: 587-601.

[153] Frentzel-Beyme R, Chang-Claude J, Eilber U. Mortality among German vegetarians: first results after five years follow-up. *Nutr Cancer* 1988; **11**: 117-126

[154] Adlercreutz H, Fotsis T, Kurzer MS, Wahala K, Makela T, Hase T. Isotope dilution gas chromato-graphic-mass spectrometric method for the determination of unconjugated lignans and isoflavo-noids in human faeces, with preliminary results in omnivorous and vegetarian women. *Anal Biochem* 1995; **225**: 101-108.

[155] Hirohata T, Shigematsu T, Nomura AM, Nomura Y, Horie A, Hirohata I. Occurrence of breast cancer in relation to diet and reproductive history: A case-control study in Fukuoka, Japan. *Nat Cancer Inst Monogr* 1985; **69**: 187-190.

[156] Hirayama T. A large scale cohort study on cancer risks by diet with special reference to the risk reducing effects of green-yellow vegetable consumption. In: Hayashi Y, *et al.* eds. *Diet, nutrition and cancer.* Tokyo: Sci. Soc. Press. 1986; 41-53.

[157] CNERNA-CNRS. Alimentation et Cancer. Évaluation des Données Scientifiques. Coordinnateurs: Riboli E, Decloître F, Dollet-Ribbing C. London, New York & Paris: TEC & DOC Lavoisier, 1996.

[158] Chow WH, Schuman LM, McLaughlin JK, *et al.* A cohort study of tobacco use, diet, occupation, and lung cancer mortality. *Cancer Causes Control* 1992; **3**: 247-254.

[159] Wynder EL. Amount and type of fat /fibre in nutritional carcinogenesis. *Prev Med* 1987; **16**: 451-459.

218

[160] Xie J, Lesaffe E, Kesteloot H. The relationship between animal fat intake, cigarette smoking, and lung cancer. *Cancer Causes Control* 1991; **2**: 79-83.

[161] Kodama M, Kodama T. Interrelations between Western type cancers and non Western type cancers as regards their risk variations in time and space. II Nutrition and cancer risk. *Anticancer Res* 1990; **10**: 1043-1049.

[162] Maruchi N, Aoki S, Tsuda K, Tanaka Y, Toyokawa H. Relation of food consumption to cancer mortality in Japan with special reference to international figures. *Gann* 1977; **68**: 1-13.

[163] Hursting SD, Thornquist M, Henderson MM. Types of dietary fat and the incidence of cancer at 5 sites. *Prev Med* 1990; **19**: 242-253.

[164] Schrauzer GN, White DA, Schneider CJ. Cancer mortality studies - III: Statistical associations with dietary selenium intakes. *Bioinorg Chem* 1977; **7**: 23-34.

[165] Cheng KK, Day NE, Duffy SW, Lam TH, Fok M, Wong J. Pickled vegetables in the aetiology of oesophageal cancer in Hong Kong Chinese. *Lancet* 1992; **339**: 1314-1318.

[166] Decarli A, La Vecchia C. Environmental factors and cancer mortality in Italy: Correlation exercise. *Oncology* 1986; **43**: 116-126.

[167] Taioli E, Nicolosi A, Wynder EL. Possible role of diet as a host factor in the aetiology of tobacco induced lung cancer. An ecological study in Southern and Northern Italy. *Int J Epidemiol* 1991; **20**: 611-614.

[168] Axelsson G, Liljeqvist T, Andersson L, Bergamn B, Rylander R. Dietary factors and lung cancer among men in West Sweden. *Int J Eidemiol* 1996; **25**: 32-39.

[169] Candelora EC, Stockwell HG, Armstrong AW, Pinkham PA. Dietary intake and risk of lung cancer in women who never smoked. *Cancer* 1992; **17**: 263-270.

[170] Dorgan JF, Ziegler RG, Schoenberg JB, *et al*. Race and sex differences in associations of vegetables, fruits, and carotenoids with lung cancer risk in New Jersey (United States). *Cancer Causes Control* 1993; **4**: 273-281.

[171] Fontham ETH, Pickle LW, Haenszel W, Correa P, Lin Y, Falk RT. Dietary vitamins A and C and lung cancer risk in Louisiana. *Cancer* 1988; **62**: 2267-2273.

[172] Forman MR, Yao SX, Graubard BI, *et al*. The effect of dietary intake of fruits and vegetables on the odds ratio of lung cancer among Yunnan tin miners. *Int J Epidemiol* 1992; **21**: 437-441.

[173] Goodman MT, Kolonel LN, Wilkens LR, Yoshizawa CN, LeMarchand L, Hankin JH. Dietary factors in lung cancer prognosis. *Eur J Cancer*, 1992; **28**: 495-501.

[174] Jain M, Burch JD, Howe GR, Risch HA, Miller AB. Dietary factors and risk of lung cancer: results from a case-control study Toronto, 1981-1985. *Int J Cancer* 1990; **45**: 287-293.

[175] Lei Y, Cai W, Chen Y, Du Y. Some lifestyle factors in human lung cancer: a case-control study of 792 lung cancer cases. *Lung Cancer* 1996; **14**: S121-S136.

[176] Le Marchand L, Yoshizawa CN, Kolonel LN, Hankin JH, Goodman MT. Vegetable consumption and lung cancer risk: A population-based case-control study in Hawaii. *J Natl Cancer Inst* 1989; **81**: 1158-1164.

[177] Mayne ST, Janerich DT, Greenwald P, *et al*. Dietary Beta Carotene and lung cancer risk in US nonsmokers. *J Natl Cancer Inst* 1994; **86**: 33-38.

[178] MacLennan R, Da-Costa J, Day NE, Law CH, Ng YK, Shanmugaratnam K. Risk factors for lung cancer in Singapore Chinese, a population with high female incidence rates. *Int J Cancer* 1977; **20**: 854-860.

[179] Ziegler RG. Epidemiologic studies of vitamins and cancer of the lung, oesophagus and cervix. *Adv Exp Med Biol* 1986; **206**: 11-26.

219

[180] Alavanja MCR, Brown CC, Swanson C, Brownson RC. Saturated fat intake and lung cancer risk among nonsmoking women in Missouri. *J Natl Cancer Inst* 1993; **85**: 1906-1916.

[181] Kalandidi A, Katsouyanni K, Voropoulou N, Bastas G, Saracci R, Trichopoulos D. Passive smoking and diet in the etiology of lung cancer and among non-smokers. *Cancer Causes Control* 1990; **1**: 15-21.

[182] Steinmetz KA, Potter JD, Folsom AR. Vegetables, fruit, and lung cancer in the Iowa Women's Health Study. *Cancer Res* 1993; **53**: 536-543.

[183] Kvale G, Bjelke E, Gart JJ. Dietary habits and lung cancer risk. *Cancer* 1983; **31**: 397-405.

[184] Shibata A, Paganini-Hill RK, Henderson R, Henderson BE. Intake of vegetables, fruit, beta-carotene, vitamin C, supplements and cancer among the elderly: a prospective study. *Br J Cancer* 1992; **66**: 673-679.

[185] Knekt P, Jarvinen R, Seppanen R, *et al*. Dietary antioxidants and risk of lung cancer. *Am J Epidemiol* 1991; **134**: 471-479.

[186] Dorant E, van den Brandt PA, Goldbohm RA, Sturmans F. Consumption of onions and a reduced risk of stomach carcinoma. *Gastroent* 1996; **110**: 12-20.

[187] Koo LC. Dietary habits and lung cancer risk among Chinese females in Hong Kong who never smoked. *Nutr Cancer* 1988; **11**: 155-172.

[188] Axelsson G, Liljeqvist T, Andersson L, Bergamn B, Rylander R. Dietary factors and lung cancer among men in West Sweden. *Int J Eidemiol* 1996; **25**: 32-39.

[189] Wu-Williams AH, Dai XD, Blot WJ, *et al*. Lung cancer among women in North-East China. *Br J Cancer* 1990; **62**: 982-987.

[190] Swanson CA, Mao BL, Li JY, *et al*. Dietary determinants of lung cancer risk: results from a case-control study in Yunnan province China. *Int J Cancer* 1992; **50**: 876-880.

[191] de Long W, Cuyler Hammond E. Lung cancer fruit, green salad and vitamin pills. *Chin Med J* 1985; **98**: 206-210.

[192] Fraser GE, Beeson WL, Phillips RL. Diet and lung cancer in California Seventh-day Adventists. *Am J Epidemiol* 1991; **133**: 683-693.

[193] Kromhout D. Essential micronutrients in relation to carcinogenesis. *Am J Clin Nutr* 1987; **45**: 1361-1367.

[194] Byers TE, Graham S, Haughey BP, Marshall JR, Swanson MK. Diet and lung cancer risk findings from the Western New York Diet Study. *Am J Epidemiol* 1987; **125**: 351-363.

[195] Dartigues JF, Dabis F, Gros N, *et al*. Dietary vitamin A, beta carotene and risk of epidermoid lung cancer in south western France. *Eur J Epid* 1990; **6**: 261-265.

[196] Hinds MW, Kolonel LN, Hankin JH, Lee J. Dietary vitamin A, carotene, vitamin C and risk of lung cancer in Hawaii. *Am J Epidemiol* 1984; **119**: 227-237.

[197] Gregor A, Lee PN, Roe FJC, Wilson MJ, Melton A. Comparison of dietary histories in lung cancer cases and controls with special reference to vitamin A. *Nutr Cancer* 1980; **2**: 93-97.

[198] Harris RWC, Key TJA, Silcocks PB, Bull D, Wald NJ. A case-control study of dietary carotene in men with lung cancer and in men with other epithelial cancers. *Nutr Cancer* 1991; **15**: 63-68.

[199] Mettlin C, Selenskasn S, Natarajan N, Huben R. Beta-carotene and animal fats and their relationship to prostate cancer risk. *Cancer* 1989; **64**: 605-612.

[200] Samet JM, Skipper BJ, Humble CG, Pathak DR. Lung cancer risk and vitamin A consumption in New Mexico. *Am Rev Resp Dis* 1985; **131**: 198-202.

[201] Wu AH, Hendersen BE, Pike MC, Yu MC. Smoking and other risk factors for lung cancer in women. *J Natl Cancer Inst* 1985; **74**: 747-751.

[202] Ziegler RG, Mason TJ, Stemhagen A, *et al*. Dietary carotene and vitamin A and risk of lung cancer among white men in New Jersey. *J Natl Cancer Inst* 1984; **73**: 1429-1435.

[203] Bjelke E. Dietary vitamin A and human lung cancer. *Int J Cancer* 1975; **15**: 561-565.

[204] Bond GG, Flores GH, Shellenberger RJ, Cartmill JB, Fishbeck WA, Cook RR. Nested case-control study of lung cancer among chemical workers. *Am J Epidemiol* 1986; **124**: 53-66.

[205] Bond GG, Thompson FE, Cook RR. Dietary vitamin A and lung cancer: results of a case-control study among chemical workers. *Nutr Cancer* 1987; **9**: 109-121.

[206] Connett JE, Kuller LH, Kjelsberg MO, *et al*. Relationship between carotenoids and cancer. The multiple risk factor intention trial (MRFIT) study. *Cancer* 1989; **64**: 126-134.

[207] Knekt P, Aromaa A, Maatela J, *et al*. Serum vitamin A and subsequent risk of cancer: cancer incidence follow up of the Finnish mobile clinic health examination survey. *Am J Epidemiol* 1990; **132**: 857-870.

[208] Nomura AMY, Stemmermann GN, Heilbrun LK, Salkeld RM, Vuilleumier JP. Serum vitamin levels and the risk of cancer at specific sites in men of Japanese ancestry in Hawaii. *Cancer Res* 1985; **45**: 2369-2372.

[209] Stahelin HB, Rosel F, Buess E, Brubacher G. Cancer vitamins and plasma lipids: Prospective Basel study. *J Natl Cancer Inst* 1984; **73**: 1463-1468.

[210] Wald NJ, Thompson SG, Densem JW, Boreham J, Bailey A. Serum beta-carotene and subsequent risk of cancer: Results from the BUPA study. *Br J Cancer* 1988; **57**: 428-433.

[211] van Poppel G, Kok FJ, Hermus RJJ. Beta-carotene supplementation in smokers reduces the frequency of micronuclei in sputum. *Br J Cancer* 1992; **66**: 1164-1168.

[212] Alpha-Tocopherol, Beta-Carotene Cancer Prevention Study Group (ATBC). The effect of vitamin E and beta-carotene on the incidence of lung cancer and other cancers in male smokers. *New Engl J Med* 1994; **330**: 1029-1035.

[213] Omenn GS, Goodman GE, Thornquist MD, *et al*. Effects of a combination of beta-carotene and vitamin A on lung cancer and cardiovascular disease. *New Engl J Med* 1996; **334**: 1150-1155.

[214] Hennekens CH, Buring JE, Mason JE, Stampfer M. Lack of effect of long-term supplementation with beta-carotene on the incidence of malignant neoplasms and cardiovascular disease. *New Engl J Med* 1996; **334**: 145-149.

[215] Knekt P, Aromaa A, Maatela J, *et al*. Serum vitamin E and the risk of cancer among Finnish men during a 10-year follow up. *Am J Epidemiol* 1988; **127**: 28-41.

[216] Knekt P, Aromaa A, Maatela J, *et al*. Serum selenium and subsequent risk of cancer among Finnish men and women. *J Natl Cancer Inst* 1990; **82**: 864-868.

[217] Salonen JT, Salonen R, Lappetelainen R, Maenpaa PH, Alfthan G, Puska P. Risk of cancer in relation to serum concentrations of selenium and vitamins A and E : Matched case-control analysis of prospective data. *BMJ* 1985; **290**: 417-420.

[218] van den Brandt PA, Goldbohm RA, van't Veer P, *et al*. Toenail selenium levels and the risk of breast cancer. *Am J Epidemiol* 1994; **140**: 120-126.

[219] Willett WC, Morris JS, Pressel S, *et al*. Prediagnostic serum selenium and risk of cancer. *Lancet* 1983; **ii**: 130-134.

[220] Coates RJ, Weiss NS, Daling JR, Morris JS, Labbe RF. Serum levels of selenium and retinol and subsequent risk of cancer. *Am J Epidemiol* 1988; **128**: 515-523.

[221] Kok FJ, van Duyn CM, Hofman A, Vermeeren R, de Bruyn AM, Valkenburg HA. Micronutrients and the risk of lung cancer. *New Engl J Med* 1987; **316**: 1916.

[222] Virtamo J, Valkeila E, Alfthan G, Punsar S, Huttunen JK, Karvonen MJ. Serum selenium and risk of cancer. A prospective follow-up of nine years. *Cancer* 1987; **60**: 145-148.

221

[223] Ringstad J, Jacobsen BK, Tretli S, Thomassen Y. Serum selenium concentration associated with risk of cancer. *J Clin Pathol* 1988; **41**: 454-457.

[224] Peleg I, Morris S, Hames CG. Is serum selenium a risk factor for cancer? *Med Oncol Tumor Pharmacother* 1985; **2**: 157-163.

[225] Menkes MS, Comstock GW, Vuilleumier JP, Helsing KJ, Rider AA, Brookmeyer R. Serum beta-carotene, vitamins A and E, selenium, and the risk of lung cancer. *New Engl J Med* 1986; **315**: 1250-1254.

[226] Nomura Y, Tashiro H, Hamada Y, Shigematsu T. Relationship between estrogen receptors and risk factors of breast cancer in Japanese pre- and post-menopausal patients. *Breast Cancer Res Treat* 1984; **4**: 37-43.

[227] Heimburger DC, Alexander CB, Birch R, Butterworth CE, Bailey WC, Krumdieck CL. Improvement in bronchial squamous metaplasia in smokers treated with folate and vitamin B12. *J Am Med Ass* 1988; **259**: 1525-1530.

[228] Sankaranarayanan R, Varghese C, Duffy SW, Padmakumary G, Day NE, Nair MK. A case-control study of diet and lung cancer in Kerala, South India. *Int J Cancer* 1994; **58**: 644-649.

[229] Pisani P, Berrino F, Macaluso M, Pastorino U, Crosignani P, Baldasseroni A. Carrots, green vegetables and lung cancer: A case-control study. *Int J Epidemiol* 1986; **15**: 463-468.

[230] Knekt P, Seppanen R, Jarvinen R, *et al*. Dietary cholesterol, fatty acids, and the risk of lung cancer among men. *Nutr Cancer* 1991; **16**: 267-275.

[231] Shekelle RB, Rossof AH, Stamler J. Dietary cholesterol and incidence of lung cancer: The Western Electric study. *Am J Epidemiol* 1991; **134**: 480-484.

[232] Muir C, Waterhouse J, Mack T, Powell J, Whenal S eds. *Cancer incidence in five continents vol 5*. Lyon: International Agency for Research on Cancer, 1987.

[233] Cannon-Albright LA, Skolnick MH, Bishop DT, Lee RG, Burt RW. Common inheritance of susceptibility to colonic adenomatous polyps and associated colorectal cancers. *N Engl J Med* 1988; **319**: 533-537.

[234] Houlston RS, Collins A, Slack J, Morton NE. Dominant genes for colorectal cancer are not rare. *Ann Hum Genetics* 1992; **56**: 99-103.

[235] Kinzler KW, Volgelstein B. Lessons from hereditary colorectal cancer. *Cell* 1996; **87**: 159-170.

[236] Haenszel W, Berg JW, Segi M, *et al*. Large bowel cancer in Hawaiian Japanese. *J Natl Can Inst* 1973; **51**: 1765-1779.

[237] McMichael AJ, McCall MG, Hartshorne JM, Woodings TL. Patterns of gastro intestinal cancer in European migrants to Australia: the role of dietary change. *Int J Cancer* 1980; **25**: 431-437.

[238] Minowa M, Bingham S, Cummings JH. Dietary fibre intake in Japan. *Human Nut:Applied Nut* 1983; **37A**: 113-119.

[239] Kuratsune M, Honda T, Englyst H, Cummings JH. Dietary fibre in the Japanese diet. *Jap J Cancer Res* 1986; **77**: 736-738.

[240] Powles J, Williams DRRR. Trends in bowel cancer in selected countries in relation to wartime changes in flour milling. *Nutr Cancer* 1984; **6** :40-48.

[241] Drasar BS, Irving D. Environmental factors and cancer of the colon and breast. *Br J Cancer* 1973; **27**: 167-172.

[242] Thind I. Diet and cancer: an international study. *Int J Epidemiol* 1986; **15**: 160-63.

[243] Howell M. Diet as an etiologic factor in the development of cancers of the colon and rectum. *J Chron Dis* 1975; **28**: 67-80.

[244] Bingham S. Diet and large bowel cancer. *J Roy Soc Med* 1990; **83**: 420-422.

[245] Trock B, Lanza E, Greenwald P. Dietary fiber, vegetables and colon cancer: critical review and meta analysis of the epidemiological evidence. *J Natl Cancer Inst* 1990; **82**: 650-661.

[246] Potter JD, Slattery ML. Bostick RM, Gapstur SM. Colon cancer: a review of the epidemiology. *Epidemiol Revs* 1994; **15**: 489-545.

[247] Bostick RM, Potter JD, Kushi LH, Sellers TA, Steinmetz KA, McKenzie DR, Gapstur SM, Folsom AR. Sugar, meat and fat intake and non-dietary risk factors for colon cancer incidence in Iowa women (US). *Cancer Causes Control* 1994; **5**: 38-52.

[248] Giovannucci E, Rimm EB, Stampfer MJ, Colditz GA, Ascherio A, Willett WC. Intake of fat, meat, and fiber in relation to risk of colon cancer in men. *Cancer Res* 1994; **54**: 2390-2397.

[249] Goldbohm RA, Van den Brandt PA, van't Veer P, *et al*. A prospective cohort study on the relation between meat consumption and the risk of colon cancer. *Cancer Res* 1994; **54**: 718-723.

[250] Heilbrun LK, Nomura A, Hankin JH, Stemmermann GN. Diet and colorectal cancer with special reference to fiber intake. *Int J Cancer* 1989; **44**: 1-6.

[251] Phillips RL, Snowdon DA. Dietary relationships with fatal colorectal cancer among Seventh Day Adventists. *J Natl Cancer Inst* 1985; **74**: 307-317.

[252] Thun MJ, Calle EE, Namboodiri MM, *et al*. Risk factors for fatal colon cancer in a large prospective study. *J Natl Cancer Inst* 1992; **84**: 1491-1500.

[253] Willett WC, Stampfer MJ, Colditz GA, Rosner BA, Speizer FE. Relation of meat, fat and fiber intake to the risk of colon cancer in a prospective study among women. *New Engl J Med* 1990; **323**: 1664-1672.

[254] Schofield PF, Jones DJ. Colorectal neoplasia I: benign colonic tumours. *BMJ* 1992; **304**: 1498-1500.

[255] Lofti AM, Spencer RJ, Ilstrup D, Melton J. Colorectal polyps and risk of subsequent carcinoma. *Mayo Clin Proc* 1986; **61**: 337-343.

[256] Roberts-Thompson IC, Ryan P, Khoo KK, Hart WJ, McMichael AJ, Butler RN. Diet, acetylator phenotype, and risk of colorectal neoplasia. *The Lancet* 1996; **347**: 1372-74.

[257] Giovannucci E, Stampfer MJ, Colditz G, Rimm EB, Willett WC. Relationship of diet to risk of colorectal adenoma in men. *J Natl Cancer Inst* 1992; **84**: 91-98.

[258] Stemmermann GN, Heilbrun LK, Nomura AMY. Association of diet and other factors with adenomatous polyps of the large bowel: A prospective autopsy study. *Am J Clin Nutr* 1988; **47**: 312-317.

[259] Potter JD. Nutrition and colorectal cancer. *Cancer Causes and Control* 1996; **7**: 127-146.

[260] Garland C, Shekelle RB, Barrett-Connor E, Criqui MH, Rossof AH, Paul O. Dietary Vitamin D and calcium and risk of colorectal cancer: 19-year prospective study in men. *Lancet* 1985; 307-309.

[261] Olsen J, Kronbor O, Lynggaard J, Ewertz M. Dietary risk factors for cancer and adenomas of the large intestine. A case-control study within a screening trial in Denmark. *Eur J Cancer* 1994; **30A**: 53-60.

[262] Stemmermann GN, Nomura AMY, Heilbrun LK. Dietary fat and the risk of colorectal cancer. *Cancer Res* 1984; **44**: 4633-4637.

[263] MacLennan R, Macrae F, Bain C, *et al*. Randomized trial of intake of fat, fiber, and beta-carotene to prevent colorectal adenomas. *J Natl Cancer Inst* 1995; **87**: 1760-1766.

[264] McKeown-Eyssen G. Review: Triglycerides, glucose and colorectal cancer. *Cancer Epid, Biomarkers Prev* 1994; **3**: 687-695.

[265] Johansson GK. Effects of a shift from a mixed diet to a lactovegetarian diet: influence on some cancer associated intestinal bacterial enzyme activities. *Nutr Cancer* 1990; **14**: 239-246.

[266] Frentzel-Beyme R, Chang-Claude J. Vegetarian diets and colon cancer - the German experience. *Am J Clin Nutr* 1994; **59**: 1143S-1152S.

[267] Bingham S, Williams DRR, Cole TJ, James WPT. Dietary fibre and regional large-bowel cancer mortality in Britain. *Br J Cancer* 1979; **40**: 456-463.

[268] Potter JD, Slattery M, Bostick RM, Gapstur SM. Colon cancer: A review of the Epidemiology. *Epidemiol Rev* 1993; **15(2)**: 499-545.

[269] Phillips RL. Role of lifestyle and dietary habits in risk of cancer among seventh day adventists. *Cancer Res* 1975; **35**: 3513-3522.

[270] Steinmetz KA, Kushi LH, Bostick RM, Folsom AR, Potter JD. Vegetables, fruit, and colon cancer in the Iowa women's Health Study. *Am J Epidemiol* 1994; **139**: 1-15.

[271] Hirayama T. A large-scale cohort study on the relationship between diet and selected cancers of the digestive organs. In: Bruce WR, Correa P, Lipkins M, Tannenbaum SR, Wilkins TD, eds. *Gastrointestinal cancer: endogenous factors.* New York: Cold Springs Harbor, Banbury report, 1981; 409-429.

[272] Trowell H. Definition of fibre. *Lancet* 1974; **i**: 503.

[273] McKeown-Eyssen GE, Bright-See E. Dietary factors in colon cancer: International relationships. An update. *Nutr Cancer* 1985; **7**: 251-253.

[274] Bingham S, Williams DRR, Cummings JH. Dietary fibre consumption in Britain: new estimates and their relation to large bowel cancer mortality. *Br J Cancer* 1985; **52**:399-402.

[275] International Agency for Research on Cancer. Large Bowel Cancer Group. Second international collaborative study on diet and cancer in Denmark and Finland. *Nutr Cancer* 1982; **4**: 3-79.

[276] Boing H, Martinez L, Frentzel-Beyme R, Oltersdorf U. Regional nutritional pattern and cancer mortality in the Federal Republic of Germany. *Nutr Cancer* 1985; **7**: 121-130.

[277] Kaaks R, Riboli E. Colorectal cancer and intake of dietary fibre. A summary of the epidemiological evidence. *Eur J Clin Nut* 1995; **49**: S10-S17.

[278] Bingham SA. Mechanisms and experimental and epidemiological evidence relating dietary fibre (non starch polysaccharides) and starch to protection against large bowel cancer. *Proc Nut Soc* 1990; **49**: 153-171.

[279] Howe GR, Benito E, Castello R, *et al.* Dietary intake of fibre and decreased risk of cancers of the colon and rectum: evidence from the combined analysis of 13 case-control studies. *J Natl Cancer Inst* 1992; **84**: 1887-96.

[280] Slattery ML, Sorensen AW, Mahoney AW, French TK, Kritchevsky D, Street JC. Diet and colon cancer: assessment of risk of fibre type and food source. *J Natl Cancer Inst* 1988; **80**: 1474-1480.

[281] Morgan JW, Fraser GE, Phillips RL, Andress MH. Dietary factors and colon cancer incidence among seven-day adventists. *Am J Epidemiol* 1988; **128**: 918A

[282] Freudenheim JL, Graham S, Marshall JR, Haughey BP, Wilkinson G. A case-control study of diet and rectal cancer in Western New York. *Am J Epidemiol* 1990; **131**: 612-621.

[283] Freudenheim JL, Graham S, Norvath J, Marshall JR, Haughey BP, Wilkinson G. Risks associated with source of fibre and fibre components in cancer of the colon and rectum. *Cancer Res* 1990; **50**: 3259-3300.

[284] DeCosse JJ, Miller HH, Lesser ML. Effect of wheat fiber and vitamins C and E on rectal polyps in patients with Familial Adenomatous Polyposis. *J Natl Cancer Inst* 1989; **81**: 1290-1297.

[285] MacLennan R, Ward W, Macrae F, *et al.* Effect of fat, fiber and betacarotene on occurrence of colorectal adenomas, after 24 months. *Gastroent* 1991; **100**: A382.

[286] Tuyns AJ, Haelterman M, Kaaks R. Colorectal cancer and the intake of nutrients: Oligosaccharides are a risk factor, fats are not. A case-control study in Belgium. *Nutr Cancer* 1987; **10**: 181-196.

[287] Zaridze D, Filipchenko V, Kustov V, Serdyuk V, Duffy S. Diet and colorectal cancer: Results of two case-control studies in Russia. *Eur J Cancer* 1993; **29A**: 112-115.

[288] Longnecker MP, Moreno JMM, Knekt P, Nomura AMY, Schober SM, Stahelin HB, Wald NJ, Gey F, Willett W. Serum alpha tocopherol concentration in relation to subsequent colorectal cancer: pooled data from five cohorts. *J Natl Cancer Inst* 1992; **84**: 430-435.

[289] Bostick RM, Potter JD, McKenzie DR, *et al*. Reduced risk of colon cancer with high intake of vitamin E: the Iowa Women's Health Study. *Cancer Res* 1993; **53**: 4230-4237.

[290] Stahelin HB, Gey KF, Eichholzer M, *et al*. Plasma antioxidant vitamins and subsequent cancer mortality in a 12 y follow-up of the prospective Basel study. *Am J Epidemiol* 1991; **133**: 766-775.

[291] Paganelli GM, Biasco G, Brandi G, Santucci R, Gizzi G, Villani V, Migiolo M, Barbara L. Effect of vitamins A, C, and E on rectal cell proliferation in patients with colorectal adenomas. *J Natl Cancer Inst*, 1992; **84**: 47-51.

[292] McKeown-Eyssen GE, Holloway C, Jazmaji V, Bright-See E, Dion P, Bruce WR. A randomized trial of vitamin C and E in the prevention or recurrence of colorectal polyps. *Cancer Res* 1988; **48**: 4701-4705.

[293] Greenberg ER, Baron JA, Tosteson TD, *et al*. A clinical trial of antioxidant vitamins to prevent colorectal adenoma. *New Engl J Med* 1994; **33**: 141-147.

[294] Lashner BA, Heidenriech PA, Su GL, Kane SV, Hanauer SB. Effect of folate supplementation on the incidence of dysplasia and cancer in ulcerative colitis. *Gastroent* 1989; **97**: 255-259.

[295] Lashner BA. Red cell folate is associated with the development of dysplasia and cancer in ulcerative colitis. *J Can Res Clin Oncol* 1993; **119**: 549-554.

[296] Giovannucci E, Stampfer MJ, Colditz GA, *et al*. Folate, methionine, and alcohol intake and risk of colorectal adenoma. *J Natl Cancer Inst* 1993; **85**: 875-884.

[297] Giovannucci E, Rimm EB, Ascherio A, Stampfer MJ, Colditz GA, Willett WC. Alcohol, low-methionine low-folate diets, and risk of colon cancer in men. *J Natl Cancer Inst* 1995; **87**: 265-273.

[298] Wu AH, Paganini-Hill A, Ross RK, Henderson BE. Alcohol, physical activity and other risks of colorectal cancer: A prospective study. *Br J Cancer* 1987; **55**: 687-694.

[299] Stemmermann GN, Nomura AMY, Chyou PH, Yoshizawa C. Prospective study of alcohol intake and large bowel cancer. *Dig Dis Sci* 1990; **35**:1414-1420.

[300] Slob ICM, Lambregts LMC, Schuit AJ, Kok FJ. Calcium intake and 28 year GI cancer mortality in Dutch civil servants. *Int J Cancer* 1993; **54** :20-25.

[301] Kampman E, van't Veer P, Hiddink GJ, Van Aken-Schneijder P, Kok FJ. Fermented dairy products, dietary calcium and colon cancer a case-study in the Netherlands. *Int J Cancer* 1994; **59**: 170-176.

[302] Cats A, Kleibeuker JH, van der Meer R, *et al*. Randomised, double-blinded placebo-controlled intervention study with supplemental calcium in families with hereditary nonpolyposis colorectal cancer. *J Natl Can Inst* 1995; **87**: 598-603.

[303] Garland CF, Helsing KJ, Garland FC, Comstock GW, Shaw EK, Gorham ED. Serum 25 hydroxy-vitamin D and colon cancer: eight-year prospective study. *Lancet* 1989; 1176-1178.

[304] Hoff G, Moen K, Trygg K, Frolich W, Vatn M, Gjone E, Larson S. Epidemiology of polyps of the rectum and sigmoid colon. *Scand J Gastroen* 1986; **21**: 199-204.

225

[305] Nelson RL, Davis FG, Sutter E, Sobin LH, Kikendall JW, Bowen P. Body iron stores and risk of colonic neoplasia. *J Natl Cancer Inst* 1994; **86**: 455-460.

[306] Stevens RG, Graubard BI, Micozzi M, Nershi K, Blumberg BS. Moderate elevation of body iron level and increased risk of cancer occurrence and death. *Int J Cancer* 1994; **56**: 364-369.

[307] Knekt P, Reunanen A, Takkunene H, Aromaa A, Heliovaara M, Hakulinene T. Body iron stores and risk of cancer. *Int J Cancer* 1994; **56**: 379-382.

[308] Rose DP, Boyar AP, Wynder EL. International comparisons of mortality rates for cancer of the breast, ovary, prostate, and colon and per capita food consumption. *Cancer* 1986; **58**: 2363-2371.

[309] Hirayama T. Cancer epidemiology in Japan. *Envir Health Perspect* 1979; **32**: 11-15.

[310] McMichael AJ, Giles GG. Cancer in migrants to Australia: extending the descriptive epidemiological data. *Cancer Res* 1988; **48**: 751-756.

[311] Kolonel LN, Hankin JH, Lee J, Chu SY, Nomura AMY, Hinds MW. Nutrient intakes in relation to cancer incidence in Hawaii. *Br J Cancer* 1981; **44**: 332-339.

[312] Bravo MP, Castellanos E, del Rey Calero J. Dietary factors and prostatic cancer. *Urol Int* 1991; **46**: 163-166.

[313] Ewings P, Bowie C. A case-control study of cancer of the prostate in Somerset and east Devon. *Br. J Cancer* 1996; **74**: 661-666.

[314] Ross RK, Shimizu H, Paganini-Hill A, Honda G, Henderson BE. Case-control studies of prostate cancer in blacks and whites in Southern California. *J Natl Cancer Inst* 1987; **78**: 869-874.

[315] Walker ARP, Walker BF, Tsotetsi NG, Sebitso C, Siwedo D, Walker AJ. Case-control study of prostate cancer in black patients in Soweto, South Africa. *Br J Cancer* 1992; **65**: 438-441.

[316] Graham S, Haughey B, Marshall, *et al*. Diet in the epidemiology of carcinoma of the prostate gland. *J Natl Cancer Inst* 1983; **70**: 687-692.

[317] Talamini R, Franceschi S, LaVecchia C, Serraino D, Barra S, Negri E. Diet and prostatic cancer: A case-control study in Northern Italy. *Nutr Cancer* 1992; **18**: 277-286.

[318] Giovannucci E, Rimm EB, Colditz GA, *et al*. A prospective study of dietary fat and risk of prostate cancer. *J Natl Cancer Inst* 1993; **85**: 1571-1579.

[319] Mills PK, Beeson L, Phillips RL, Fraser GE. Cohort study of the diet, lifestyle and prostate cancer in Adventist men. *Cancer* 1989; **64**: 598-604.

[320] Le Marchand L, Kolonel LN, Wilkens LR, Myers BC, Hirohata T. Animal fat consumption and prostate cancer: A prospective study in Hawaii. *Epidemiol* 1994; **5**: 276-282.

[321] Snowdon DA, Phillips RL, Choi W. Diet, obesity and risk of fatal prostate cancer. *Am J Epidemiol* 1984; **120**: 244-250.

[322] Severson RK, Nomura AMY, Grove JS, Stemmermann GN. A prospective study of demographics, diet and prostate cancer among men of Japanese ancestry in Hawaii. *Cancer Res* 1989; **49**: 1857-1860.

[323] Hsing AW, McLaughlin JK, Schuman LM, *et al*. Diet, tobacco use and fatal prostate cancer: Results from the Lutheran Brotherhood cohort study. *Cancer Res* 1990; **50**: 6836-6840.

[324] Key T. Risk factors for prostate cancer. *Cancer Surveys* 1995; **23**: 63-77.

[325] West DW, Slattery ML, Robison LR, French TK, Mahoney AW. Adult dietary intake and prostate cancer risk in Utah: A case-control study with special emphasis on aggressive tumors. *Cancer Causes Control* 1991; **2**: 85-94.

[326] Whittemore AS, Kolonel LN, Wu AH, *et al*. Prostate cancer in relation to diet, physical activity, and body size in blacks, Whites, and Asians in the United States and Canada. *J Natl Cancer Inst* 1995; **87**: 652-661.

226

[327] Kolonel LN, Yoshizawa CN, Hankin JH. Diet and prostatic cancer: a case-control study in Hawaii. *Am J Epidemiol* 1988; **127**: 999-1012.

[328] Ohno Y, Yoshida O, Oishi K, Okada K, Yamabe H, Schroeder FH. Dietary β-carotene and cancer of the prostate : A case-control study in Kyoto Japan. *Cancer Res* 1988; **48**: 1331-1336.

[329] Kaul L, Heshmat MY, Kovi J, *et al.* The role of diet in prostate cancer. *Nutr Cancer* 1987; **9**: 123-128.

[330] Neugut AI, Grabowski GC, Lee WC, Murray T, Nieves JW, Forde KA, Treat MR, Waye JD, Fenogliopreiser C. Dietary risk factors for the incidence and recurrence of colorectal adenomatous polyps. A case control study. *Ann Int Med* 1993; **118**: 91-95.

[331] Fincham SM, Hill GB, Hanson J, Wijayasinghe C. Epidemiology of prostatic cancer. A case-control study. *Prostate* 1990; **17**: 189-206.

[332] Le Marchand L, Hankin JH, Kolonel LN, Wilkens LR. Vegetable and fruit consumption in relation to prostate cancer risk in Hawaii: A re-evaluation of the effect of dietary beta carotene. *Am J Epidemiol* 1991; **133**: 215-219.

[333] Giovannucci E, Ascherio A, Rimm EB, Stampfer MJ, Colditz GA, Willett WC. Intake of carotenoids and retinol in relation to risk of prostate cancer. *J Natl Cancer Inst* 1995; **87**: 1767-1776.

[334] Oishi K, Okada K, Yoshida O, *et al.* A case-control study of prostatic cancer with reference to dietary habits. *Prostate* 1988; **12**: 179-190.

[335] Heshmat MY, Kaul L, Kovi J, *et al.* Nutrition and prostate cancer : A case-control study. *Prostate* 1985; **6**: 7-17.

[336] Middleton B, Byess T, Marshall J, Graham S. Dietary vitamin A and cancer - a multi case-control study. *Nutr Cancer* 1986; **8**: 107-116.

[337] Kolonel LN, Hankin JH, Yoshizawa CN. Vitamin A and prostate cancer in elderly men: enhancement of risk. *Cancer Res* 1987; **47**: 2982-2985.

[338] Rohan TE, Howe GR, Burch JD, Jain M. Dietary factors and risk of prostate cancer: a case-control study in Ontario, Canada. *Cancer Causes Control* 1995; **6**: 145-154.

[339] Hsing AW, Comstock GW, Abbey H, Polk BF. Serologic precursors of cancer. Retinol, carotenoids and tocopherol and risk of prostate cancer. *J Natl Cancer Inst* 1990; **82**: 941-946.

[340] Reichman ME, Hayes RB, Ziegler RG, *et al.* Serum vitamin A and the subsequent development of prostate cancer in the first National Health and Nutrition Examination Survey epidemiologic follow-up study. *Cancer Res* 1990; **50**: 2311-2315.

[341] La Vecchia C, Negri E. Nutrition and bladder cancer. *Cancer Causes Control* 1996; **7**: 95-100.

[342] Riboli E, Gonzalez CA, Lopez-Abente G, *et al.* Diet and bladder cancer in Spain: a multi-centre case-control study. *Int J Cancer* 1991; **49**: 214-219.

[343] Steineck G, Hagman U, Gerhardsson M, Norell SE. Vitamin A supplements, fried foods, fat and urothelial cancer. A case reference study in Stockholm - 1985-87. *Int J Cancer* 1990; **45**: 1008-1011.

[344] Steineck G, Norell SE, Feychting M. Diet, tobacco and urothelial cancer. A 14 year follow-up of 16,477 subjects. *Acta Oncologica* 1988; **27**: 323-327.

[345] La Vecchia C, Negri E, Decarli A, D'Avanzo B, Liberati C, Franceschi S. Dietary factors in the risk of bladder cancer. *Nutr Cancer* 1989; **12**: 93-101.

[346] Claude J, Kunze E, Frentzel-Beyme R, Paczkowski K, Schneider J, Schubert H. Life-style and occupational risk factors in cancer of the lower urinary tract. *Am. J. Epidemiol* 1986; **124**: 578-589.

[347] Mettlin C, Graham S. Dietary risk factors in human bladder cancer. *Am J Epidemiol* 1979; **110**: 255-263.

227

[348] Nomura AM, Kolonel LN, Hankin JH, Yoshizawa CN. Dietary factors in cancer of the lower urinary tract. *Int J Cancer* 1991; **48**: 199-205.

[349] Ohno Y, Aoki K, Obata K, Morrison AS. Case-control study on urinary bladder cancer in Metropolitan, Nagoya. *Natl Cancer Inst Monogr* 1985; **69**: 229-234.

[350] Momas I, Daures JP, Festy B, *et al.* Relative importance of risk factors in bladder carcinogenesis: some new results about Mediterranean habits. *Cancer Causes Control* 1994; **5**: 326-332.

[351] Mills PK, Beeson L, Phillips RL, Fraser GE. Bladder cancer in a low risk population: results from the Adventists health study. *Am J Epidemiol* 1991; **133**: 230-239.

[352] Kolonel LN, Hinds MW, Nomura AW, Hankin JH, Lee J. Relationship of dietary vitamin A and ascorbic acid intake to the risk for cancers of the lung, bladder and prostate in Hawaii. *Natl Cancer Inst Monogr* 1985; **69**: 137-142.

[353] Knekt P, Aromaa A, Maatela J, Alfthan G, Aaran RK, Nikkari T, Hakama M, Hakulinen, Teppo L. Serum micronutrients and risk of cancers of low incidence in Finland. *Am J Epidemiol* 1991; **134**(4): 356-361.

[354] Department of Health. *Public Health Common Data Set, England, Volume 1.* Surrey: National Institute of Epidemiology, 1996.

[355] Pujolar-Escolar A, Gonzalez CA, Lopez-Abente G, *et al.* Bladder cancer and coffee consumption in smokers and non-smokers in Spain. *Int J Epidemiol* 1993; **22**: 38-44.

[356] International Agency for Research on Cancer. Coffee, Tea, Mate, Methylxanthines and Methylglyoxal. *IARC Monographs on the Evaluation of Carcinogenic Risks of Chemicals to Humans* 1991; **51**: 207-271. IARC: Lyon, France.

[357] Heilbrun LK, Nomura A, Stemmermann GN. Black tea consumption and cancer risk: A prospective study. *Br J Cancer* 1986; **54**: 677-683.

[358] International Agency for Research on Cancer. Liver flukes and *Helicobacter pylori*. *IARC Monographs on the Evaluation of Carcinogenic Risk of Chemicals to Humans* 1994; **61**; 177-240. IARC: Lyon, France.

[359] Kato I, Tominaga S, Matsumoto K. A prospective study of stomach cancer among a rural Japanese population. A 6 year survey. *Jpn J Cancer Res* 1992; **83**: 568-575.

[360] Kono S, Hirohata T. Nutrition and stomach cancer. *Cancer Causes Control* 1996; **7**: 41-55.

[361] Haenszel W, Kurihara M. Studies of Japanese migrants. I. Mortality from cancer and other diseases among Japanese in the United States. *J Nat Cancer Inst* 1968; **40**: 43-68.

[362] Office of Population, Census and Surveys. *Occupational mortality 1979-80, 1982-83.* Decennial supplement, England and Wales. London: HMSO, 1986.

[363] Franceschi S, Levi F, La Vecchia C. Epidemiology of gastric cancer in Europe. *Eur J Cancer* 1994; **3(suppl 2)**: 5-10.

[364] Hakama M, Saxen EA. Cereal consumption and gastric cancer. *Int J Cancer* 1967; **2**: 265-268.

[365] Thouez JP, Ghadirian P, Petitclerc C, Hamelin P. International comparisons of nutrition and mortality from cancers of the oesophagus, stomach and pancreas. *Geogr Med* 1990; **20**: 39-50.

[366] Tominaga S, Ogawa H, Kuroishi T. Usefulness of correlation analysis in the epidemiology of stomach cancer. *Nat Cancer Inst Monogr* 1982; **62**: 135-140.

[367] Nagai M, Hashimoto T, Yanagawa H, Yokoyama H, Minowa M. Relationship of diet to the incidence of oesophageal and stomach cancer in Japan. *Nutr Cancer* 1982; **3**: 257-268.

[368] Benito E, Cabeza E, Moreno V, Obrador A, Bosch FX. Diet and colorectal adenomas: a case-control study in Majorca. *Int J Cancer* 1993; **55**: 213-219.

228

[369] Lu JB, Qin YM. Correlation between high salt intake and mortality rates for oesophageal and gastric cancers in Henan Province China. *Int J Epidemiol* 1987; **16**: 171-176.

[370] Chen J, Geissler C, Parpia B, Li J, Campbell TC. Antioxidant status and cancer mortality in China. *Int J Epidemiol* 1992; **21**: 625-635.

[371] Zaldivar R. Epidemiology of gastric and colorectal cancer in the United States and Chile with particular reference to the role of dietary and nutritional variables, nitrate fertilizer pollution and N-nitroso compounds. *Zentralb Bacteriol* 1977; **164**: 193-217.

[372] Hirayama T. Epidemiology of cancer of the stomach with special reference to its decrease in Japan. *Cancer Res* 1975; **35**: 3460-63.

[373] Jedrychowski W, Wahrendorf J, Popiela T, Rachtan J. A case-control study of dietary factors and stomach cancer risk in Poland. *Int J Cancer* 1986; **37**: 837-842.

[374] MacDonald WC. Gastric cancer among the Japanese of British Columbia: dietary studies. *Can Cancer Conf* 1966; **6**: 451-459.

[375] Boeing H, Frentzel-Beyme R, Berger M, *et al*. Case-control study on diet and stomach cancer in Germany. *Int J Cancer* 1991; **47**: 858-864.

[376] Buiatti E, Palli D, Decarli A, *et al*. A case-control study of gastric cancer and diet in Italy. *Int J Cancer* 1989; **44**: 611-616.

[377] Coggon D, Barker DJP, Cole RB, Nelson M. Stomach cancer and food storage. *J Natl Cancer Inst* 1989; **81**: 1178-1182.

[378] Gonzalez CA, Sanz JM, Marcos G, *et al*. Dietary factors and stomach cancer in Spain: A multicentre case-control study. *Int J Cancer*, 1991; **49**: 513-519.

[379] Graham S, Haughey B, Marshall J, *et al*. Diet in the epidemiology of gastric cancer. *Nutr Cancer* 1990; **13**: 19-34.

[380] Haenszel W, Kurihara M, Segi M, Lee RKC. Stomach cancer among Japanese in Hawaii. *J Natl Cancer Inst*, 1972; **49**: 969-988.

[381] Haenszel W, Kurihara M, Locke FB, Shimuzu K, Segi M. Stomach cancer in Japan. *J Natl Cancer Inst*, 1976; **56**: 265-274.

[382] La Vecchia C, Negri E, Decarli A, Avanzo B, Franceschi S. A case-control study of diet and gastric cancer in Northern Italy. *Int J Cancer* 1987; **40**: 484-489.

[383] Kono S, Ikeda M, Tokudome S, Kuratsune M. A case-control study of gastric cancer and diet in Northern Kyushu, Japan. *Jpn J Cancer Res* 1988; **79**: 1067-1074.

[384] Lee J, Park B, Yoo K, Ahn Y. Dietary factors and stomach cancer: A case-control study in Korea. *Int J Epidemiol* 1995; **24**: 33-41.

[385] Nazario CM, Szklo M, Diamond E, Roman-Franco A, Climent C, Suarez E, Conde JG. Salt and gastric cancer: a case-control study in Puerto Rico. *Int J Epidemiol* 1993; **22**: 790-797.

[386] Ramón JM, Serra L, Cerdó C, Oromi J. Dietary factors and gastric cancer risk: a case-control study in Spain. *Cancer* 1993; **71**: 1731-1735.

[387] Tuyns AJ. Salt and gastrointestinal cancer. *Nutr Cancer* 1988; **11**: 229-232.

[388] Yu GP, Hsieh CC. Risk factors for stomach cancer: a population based case-control study in Shanghai. *Cancer Causes Control* 1991; **2**: 169-174.

[389] You WC, Blot WJ, Chang YS, *et al*. Diet and high risk of stomach cancer in Shandong, China. *Cancer Res* 1988; **48**: 3518-3523.

[390] Hansson LE, Nyrén O, Bergström R, *et al*. Diet and risk of gastric cancer. A population-based case-control study in Sweden. *Int J Cancer* 1993; **55**:181-189.

[391] Boeing H, Jedrychowski W, Wahrendorf J, Popiela T, Tobiasz-Adamczy KB, Kulig A. Dietary risk factors in intestinal and diffuse types of stomach cancer: a multicentre case-control study in Poland. *Cancer Causes Control* 1991; **2**: 227-233.

[392] Risch HA, Jain M, Choi NW, *et al*. Dietary factors and the incidence of cancer of the stomach. *Am J Epidemiol* 1985; **122**: 947-959.

[393] Hirohata T. A case-control study of stomach cancer (in Japanese). *Proceedings of the 21st General Congress of Japan Medical Association* 1983; 953-955.

[394] Nomura A, Grove JS, Stemmermann GN, Severson RK. A prospective study of stomach cancer and its relation to diet, cigarettes, and alcohol consumption. *Cancer Res* 1990; **50**: 627-631.

[395] Kneller RW, McLaughlin JK, Bjelke E, *et al*. A cohort study of stomach cancer in a high-risk American population. *Cancer* 1991; **68**: 672-678.

[396] Caygill CPJ (ECP-EURONUT IM Study Group). ECP-EURONUT Intestinal metaplasia study: gastric juice and urine analyses. *Eur J Cancer Prev* 1994; **3(suppl 2)**: 89-92

[397] Johnson BJ (ECP-EURONUT IM Study Group). The prevalence of *Helicobacter pylori* infection in patients with intestinal metaplasia and in controls: a serological and histological study in four UK centres. *Eur J Cancer Prev*, 1994; **3(suppl 2)**: 69-73.

[398] Buiatti E, Palli D, Bianchi S, *et al*. A case-control study of gastric cancer and diet in Italy III. Risk patterns by histologic type. *Int J Cancer* 1991; **48**: 369-74.

[399] Cornee J, Pobel D, Riboli E, Guyader M, Hemon B. A case-control study of gastric cancer and nutritional factors in Marseille, France. *Eur J Epid* 1995; **11**: 55-65.

[400] Correa P, Fontham E, Williams-Pickle L, Chen V, Lin YP, Haenszel W. Dietary determinants of gastric cancer in South Louisiana inhabitants. *J Natl Cancer Inst* 1985; **75**: 645-654.

[401] Demirer T, Icli F, Uzunalimoglu O, Kucuk O. Diet and stomach cancer incidence. A case-control study in Turkey. *Cancer* 1990; **65**: 2344-2348.

[402] De Stefani E, Correa P, Fierro L, Carzoglio J, Deneo-Pellegrini H, Zavala D. Alcohol drinking and tobacco smoking in gastric cancer. A case-control study. *Rev Epidemiol Sante Pub* 1990; **38**: 297-307.

[403] Hansson LE, Nyrén O, Bergström R, *et al*. Nutrients and gastric cancer risk. A population-based case-control study in Sweden. *Int J Cancer* 1994; **57**: 638-644.

[404] Hoey J, Montvernay C, Lambert R. Wine and tobacco: risk factors for gastric cancer in France. *Am J Epidemiol* 1981; **113**: 668-674.

[405] Inoue M, Tajima K, Hirose K, Kuroishi T, Gao CM, Kitoh T. Lifestyle and subsite of gastric cancer - Joint effect of smoking and drinking habits. *Int J Cancer* 1994; **56**: 494-499.

[406] Jedrychowski W, Maugeri U, Jedrychowski I, Tobiasz-Adamczk B, Gomola K. The analytic epidemiologic study on occupational factors and stomach cancer occurrence. *G Ital Med Lav* 1990; **12**: 3-8.

[407] Modan B, Cuckle H, Lubin F. A note on the role of dietary retinol and carotene in human gastro-intestinal cancer. *Int J Cancer* 1981; **28**: 421-424.

[408] Sanchez-Diez A, Hernandez-Mejia R, Cueto-Espinar A. Study of the relationship between diet and gastric cancer in a rural area of the province of Leon, Spain. *Eur J Epid* 1992; **8**: 233-237.

[409] Trichopoulos D, Ouranos G, Day NE, *et al*. Diet and cancer of the stomach: a case-control study in Greece. *Int J Cancer* 1985; **36**: 291-297.

[410] Tuyns AJ, Kaaks R, Haelterman M, Riboli E. Diet and gastric cancer. A case-control study in Belgium. *Int J Cancer* 1992; **51**: 1-6.

[411] Hirayama T. Actions suggested by gastric cancer epidemiological studies in Japan. In: Reed PI and Hill MJ eds. *Gastric carcinogenesis*. Amsterdam, Exerpta Medica: 1988, pp 209-227.

[412] Nomura AMY, Stemmermann GN, Chyou PH. Gastric cancer among the Japanese in Hawaii. *Jpn J Cancer Res* 1995; **86**: 916-923.

[413] Chyou PH, Nomura AMY, Hankin JH, Stemmermann GN. A case-cohort study of diet and stomach cancer. *Cancer Res* 1990; **50**: 7501-7504.

[414] Paganini-Hill GH, Ross RK, Gray GE, Henderson BE. Vitamin A and cancer incidence in a retirement community. *Nat Cancer Inst Monogr* 1985; **69**: 133-135.

[415] Guo W, Blot WJ, Li J, *et al*. A nested case-control study of oesophageal and stomach cancers in the Linxian Nutrition Intervention trial. *Int J Epidemiol* 1994; **23**: 444-450.

[416] Kono S, Ikeda M, Ogata M. Salt and geographical mortality of gastric cancer and stroke in Japan. *J Epidemiol* 1983; **37**: 43-46.

[417] Enstrom JE, Kanim LE, Klein MA. Vitamin C intake and mortality among a sample of the United States population. *Epidemiology* 1992; **3**: 194-202.

[418] Knekt P, Aromaa A, Maatela J, *et al*. Serum vitamin E, serum selenium and risk of gastro intestinal cancer. *Int J Cancer* 1988; **42**: 846-850.

[419] Blot WJ, Li JY, Taylor PR, *et al*. Nutrition intervention trial in Linxian, China: supplementation with specific vitamin/mineral combinations, cancer incidence, and disease-specific mortality in the general population. *J Natl Cancer Inst* 1993; **85**: 1483-1492.

[420] Potischman N, Brinton LA. Nutrition and cervical neoplasia. *Cancer Causes Control* 1996; **7**: 113-126.

[421] de Vet HCW, Knipschild PG, Grol ME, Schouten HJA, Sturmans F. The role of beta-carotene and other dietary factors in the aetiology of cervical dysplasia: results of a case-control study. *Int J Epidemiol* 1991; **20**: 603-610.

[422] La Vecchia C, Decarli A, Fasoli M, *et al*. Dietary vitamin A and the risk of epithelial and invasive cervical neoplasia. *Gynecol Oncol* 1988; **30**: 187-195.

[423] Verreault R, Chu J, Mandelson M, Shy K. A case-control study of diet and invasive cervical cancer. *Int J Cancer* 1989; **43**: 1050-1054.

[424] Ziegler RG, Jones CJ, Brinton LA, *et al*. Diet and the risk of in situ cervical cancer among white women in the United States. *Cancer Causes Control* 1992; **2**: 17-29.

[425] Herrero R, Potischman N, Brinton LA, *et al*. A case-control study of nutrient status and invasive cervical cancer. *Am J Epidemiol* 1991; **134**: 1335-1346.

[426] Peng HQ, Liu SL, Mann V, Rohan T, Rawls W. Human papillomavirus types 16 and 33, herpes simplex virus type 2 and other risk factors for cervical cancer in Sichuan province, China. *Int J Cancer* 1991; **47**: 711-716.

[427] Marshall JR, Graham S, Byerss T, Swanson M, Brasure J. Diet and smoking in the epidemiology of cancer of the cervix. *J Natl Cancer Inst* 1983; **70**: 847-851.

[428] Romney SL, Palan PR, Duttagupta C, *et al*. Retinoids and the prevention of cervical dysplasias. *Am J Obstet Gynecol* 1981; **141**: 890-894.

[429] VanEenwyk J, Davis FG, Bowen PE. Dietary and serum carotenoids and cervical intraepithelial neoplasia. *Int J Cancer* 1991; **48**: 34-38.

[430] Wylie-Rosett JA, Romney SL, Slagle NS, *et al*. Influence of vitamin A on cervical dysplasia and carcinoma in situ. *Nutr Cancer* 1984; **6**: 49-57.

[431] Brock KE, Berry G, Mock PA, MacLennan R, Truswell AS, Brinton LA. Nutrients in diet and plasma and risk of in situ cervical cancer. *J Natl Cancer Inst* 1988; **80**: 580-585.

[432] MacQuart-Moulin G, Riboli E, Cornée J, Kaaks R, Berthezène P. Colorectal polyps and diet: a case-control study in Marseilles. *Int J Cancer* 1987; **40**: 179-188.

231

[433] Buckley DI, McPherson RS, North CQ, Becker TM. Dietary micronutrients and cervical dysplasia in south western American Indian women. *Nutr Cancer* 1992; **17**: 179-185.

[434] Slattery ML, Abbott TM, Overall JC, *et al*. Dietary vitamins A, C, and E and selenium as risk factors for cervical cancer. *Epidemiol* 1990; **1**: 8-15.

[435] VanEenwyk J, Davis FG, Colman N. Folate, vitamin C and cervical intraepithelial neoplasia. *Cancer Epid Biomarkers Prev* 1992; **1**: 119-124.

[436] Cuzick J, De Stavola BL, Russell MJ, Thomas BS. Vitamin A, vitamin E and the risk of cervical intraepithelial neoplasia. *Br J Cancer* 1990; **62**: 651-652.

[437] Knekt P. Serum Vitamin E level and risk of female cancers. *Int J Epidemiol* 1988; **17**: 281-286.

[438] Batieha AM, Armenian HK, Norkus EP, Morris JS, Spate VE, Comstock GW. Serum micronutrients and the subsequent risk of cervical cancer in the population based nested case-control study. *Cancer Epid Biomarkers Prev* 1993; **2**: 335-339.

[439] Potischman N, Herrero R, Brinton LA, *et al*. A case-control study of nutrient status and invasive cervical cancer: II. Serological indicators. *Am J Epidemiol* 1991; **134**: 1347-55.

[440] Butterworth CE, Hatch KD, Macaluso M, *et al*. Folate deficiency and cervical dysplasia. *J Am Med Ass* 1992; **267**: 528-533.

[441] Butterworth CE, Hatch KD, Soong SJ, *et al*. Oral folic acid supplementation for cervical dysplasia: A clinical intervention study. *Am J Obstet Gynecol* 1992; **166**: 803-809.

[442] Butterworth CE, Hatch KD, Gore H, Mueller H, Krumdieck CL. Improvement in cervical dysplasia associated with folic acid therapy in users of oral contraceptives. *Am J Clin Nutr* 1982; **35**: 73-82.

[443] Parazzini F, Franceschi S, La Vecchia C, Fasoli M. Review. The epidemiology of ovarian cancer. *Gynaecol Oncol* 1991; **43**: 9-23.

[444] Serra-Majem L, La Vecchia C, Ribas-Barba L, Prieto-Ramos F, Lucchini F, Ramon JM, Salleras L. Changes in diet and mortality from selected cancers in southern Mediterranean countries. *Eur J Clin Nutr* 1993; **47(suppl 1)**: S25-S34.

[445] Phillips RL, Garfinkel L, Kuzma JW, Beeson WL, Lotz T, Brin B. Mortality among California Seventh-Day adventists for selected cancer sites. *J Natl Cancer Inst* 1980; **65**: 1097-1107.

[446] Kinlen LJ. Meat and fat consumption and cancer mortality: A study of strict religious orders in Britain. *Lancet* 1982; **1**: 946-949.

[447] Lyon JL, Gardner JW, West DW. Cancer risk and life-style: Cancer among Mormons from 1967-1975 In: Cairns J, Lyon JL, Skolnick M, eds. *Cancer incidence in defined populations*. New York: Cold Springs Harbor, Banbury Report no 4, 1980; 3-31.

[448] Risch HA, Jain M, Marrett LD, Howe GR. Dietary fat intake and risk of epithelial ovarian cancer. *J Natl Cancer Inst* 1994; **86**: 1409-1415.

[449] La Vecchia C, Decarli A, Negri E, Parazzini F, Gentile A, Cecchetti G, Fasoli M, Franceschi S. Dietary factors and the risk of epithelial ovarian cancer. *J Natl Cancer Inst* 1987; **75**; 663-669.

[450] Shu XO, Gao JM. Dietary factors and epithelial ovarian cancer. *Br J Cancer* 1989; **59**: 92-96.

[451] Tzonou A, Hsief CC, Polychronopoulou A, Kaprinis G, Toupadaki N, Trichopoulou A, Karakatsani A, Trichopoulos D. Diet and ovarian cancer: a case-control study in Greece. *Int J Cancer* 1993; **55**: 411-414.

[452] Engle A, Muscat JE, Harris RE. Nutritional risk factors and ovarian cancer. *Nutr Cancer* 1991; **15**: 239-247.

[453] Slattery ML, Schuman KL, West DW, French TK, Robinson LM. Nutrient intake and ovarian cancer. *Am J Epidemiol* 1989; **130**: 497-502.

454 Harlow BL, Cramer DW, Geller J, Willett WC, Bell DA, Welch WR. The influence of lactose consumption on the association of oral contraceptive use and ovarian cancer risk. *Am J Epidemiol* 1991; **134**: 445-453.

455 Sandler RS, Lyles CM, Peipins LA, McAuliffe CA, Woosley JT, Kupper LL. Diet and risk of colorectal adenomas - macronutrients, cholesterol and fiber. *J Natl Cancer Inst* 1993; **85**: 884-891.

456 Barbone F, Austin H, Partridge EE. Diet and endometrial cancer: a case-control study. *Am J Epidemiol* 1993; **137**: 393-403.

457 Levi F, Franceschi S, Negri E, La Vecchia C. Dietary factors and the risk of endometrial cancer. *Cancer* 1993; **71**: 3575-3581.

458 Shu XO, Zheng W, Potischman N, Brinton LA, Hatch MC, Gao Y-T, Fraumeni JF. A population based case-control study of dietary factors and endometrial cancer in Shanghai, People's Republic of China. *Am J Epidemiol* 1993; **137**: 155-165.

459 Ghadirian P, Simard A, Baillargeon G, Maisonneuve P, Boyle P. Nutritional factors and pancreatic cancer in the Francophore community in Montreal, Canada. *Int J Cancer* 1991; **47**: 1-6.

460 Hirayama T. Epidemiology of pancreatic cancer in Japan. *Jpn J Clin Oncol* 1989; **19**: 208-215.

461 Bueno de Mesquita HB, Maisonneuve P, Runia S, Moerman CJ. Intake of foods and nutrients and cancer of the exocrine pancreas: a population-based case-control in the Netherlands. *Int J Cancer* 1991; **48**: 540-549.

462 Falk RT, Williams-Pickle L, Fontham ET, Correa P, Fraumeni JFJ. Life-style risk factors for pancreatic cancer in Louisiana: A case- control study. *Am J Epidemiol* 1988; **128**: 324-336.

463 Farrow DC, Davis S. Diet and the risk of pancreatic cancer in men. *Am J Epidemiol* 1990; **132**: 423-431.

464 Fernandez E, La Vecchia C, Decarli A. Attributable risks for pancreatic cancer in Northern Italy. *Cancer Epid Biomarker Prev* 1996; **5**: 23-27.

465 La Vecchia C, Negri E, D'Avanzo B, *et al*. Medical history, diet and pancreatic cancer. *Oncology* 1990; **47**: 463-466.

466 Mack TM, Yu MC, Hanisch R, Henderson BE. Pancreas cancer and smoking, beverage consumption and past medical history. *J Natl Cancer Inst* 1986; **76**: 49-60.

467 Olsen GW, Mandel JS, Gibson RW, Wattenberg LW, Schuman LM. A case-control study of pancreatic cancer and cigarettes, alcohol, coffee and diet. *Am J Public Health* 1989; **79**: 1016-1019.

468 Norell SE, Ahlbom A, Erwald R, *et al*. Diet and pancreatic cancer : a case-control study. *Am J Epidemiol* 1986; **124**: 894-902.

469 Baghurst PA, McMichael AJ, Slavotinek AH, Baghurst KI, Boyle P, Walker AM. A case-control study of diet and cancer of the pancreas. *Am J Epidemiol* 1991; **134**: 167-179.

470 Friedman GD, van den Eeden SK. Risk factors for pancreatic cancer: an exploratory study. *Int J Epidemiol* 1993; **22**: 30-37.

471 Durbec JP, Chevillotte G, Bidart JM, Berthezene P, Sarles H. Diet, alcohol, tobacco and risk of cancer of the pancreas: a case-control study. *Br J Cancer* 1983; **47**: 463-470.

472 Bueno de Mesquita HB, Moerman CJ, Runia S, Maisonneuve P. Are energy and energy-providing nutrients related to exocrine carcinoma of the pancreas? *Int J Cancer* 1990; **46**: 435-444.

473 Howe GR, Jain M, Miller AB. Dietary factors and risk of pancreatic cancer: results of a Canadian population-based case-control. *Int J Cancer* 1990; **45**: 604-608.

474 Kalaphothaki V, Tzonou A, Hsieh C-c, *et al*. Nutrient intake and cancer of the pancreas: a case-control study in Athens, Greece. *Cancer Causes Control* 1993; **4**: 383-389.

233

[475] Zatonski W, Przewozniak K, Howe GR, Maisonneuve P, Walker AM, Boyle P. Nutritional factors and pancreatic cancer: A case-control study from South West Poland. *Int J Cancer* 1991; **48**: 390-394.

[476] Howe GR, Ghadirian P, Bueno de Mesquita HB, *et al*. A collaborative case-control study of nutrient intake and pancreatic cancer within the Search Programme. *Int J Cancer* 1992; **51**: 365-372.

[477] Knekt P, Heliovaara M, Rissanen A, Aromaa A, Seppanen R, Teppo L, Pukkala E. Leanness and lung cancer risk. *Int J Cancer* 1991; **49(2)**: 208-213.

[478] Gold EB, Gordis L, Diener MD, *et al*. Diet and other risk factors for cancer of the pancreas. *Cancer* 1985; **55**: 460-467.

[479] Shibata A, Mack TM, Paganini-Hill A, Ross RK, Henderson BE. A prospective study of pancreatic cancer in the elderly. *Int J Cancer* 1994; **58**: 46-49.

[480] Burney PGJ, Comstock GW, Morris JS. Serologic precursors of cancer: Serum micronutrients and the subsequent risk of pancreatic cancer. *Am J Clin Nutr* 1989; **49**: 895-900.

[481] Schottenfeld D. Epidemiology of cancer of the esophagus. *Semin Oncol* 1984; **11**: 92-100.

[482] Pera M, Cardesa A, Pera C, Mohr U. Nutritional aspects in oesophageal carcinogenesis. *Anticancer Res* 1987; **7**: 301-308.

[483] Ghadirian P, Vobecky J, Vobecky JS. Factors associated with cancer of the oesophagus: An overview. *Cancer Detect Prev* 1988; **11**: 225-234.

[484] Yang CS, Miao J, Huang M, *et al*. Diet and vitamin nutrition of the high esophageal cancer risk population in Linxian, China. *Nutr Cancer* 1982; **4**: 154-164.

[485] Homozdiari H, Day NE, Aramesh B, Mahboubi E. Dietary factors and esophageal cancer in the Caspin Littoral of Iran. *Cancer Res* 1975; **35**: 3493-3498.

[486] Joint Iran IARC. Esophageal cancer studies in the Caspian littoral of Iran: results of population studies - a prodrome. *J Natl Inst Cancer* 1977; **59**: 1127-1138.

[487] Mahboubi EO, Aramesh B. Epidemiology of esophageal cancer in Iran with special reference to nutritional and cultural aspects. *Prev Med* 1980; **9**: 613-621.

[488] Ghadirian P. Thermal irritation and esophageal cancer in Northern Iran. *Cancer* 1987; **60**: 1909-1914.

[489] Jaskiewicz K, Marasas WF, Lazarus C, Beyers AD, Van-Helden PD. Association of esophageal cytological abnormalities with vitamin and lipotrophe deficiencies in populations at risk for esophageal cancer. *Anticancer Res* 1988; **8**: 711-715.

[490] Jaskiewicz K. Oesophageal carcinoma: cytopathology and nutritional aspects in aetiology. *Anticancer Res* 1989; **9**: 1847-1852.

[491] Adelstein AM, Staszewski J, Muir CS. Cancer mortality in 1970-1972 among Polish born migrants to England and Wales. *Br J Nutr* 1979; **40**: 464-475.

[492] Cheng KK, Day NE. Nutrition and esophageal cancer. *Cancer Causes Control* 1996; **7**: 33-40.

[493] Brown LM, Blot WJ, Schuman SH, *et al*. Environmental factors and high risk of esophageal cancer among men in coastal South Carolina. *J Natl Cancer Inst* 1988; **80**: 1620-1625.

[494] Brown LM, Swanson CA, Gridley G, *et al*. Adenocarcinoma of the Esophagus: role of obesity and diet. *J Natl Cancer Inst* 1995; **87**: 104-109.

[495] Decarli A, Liati P, Negri E, Franceschi S, La Vecchia C. Vitamin A and other dietary factors in the etiology of esophageal cancer. *Nutr Cancer* 1987; **10**: 29-37.

[496] De Stefani E, Munoz N, Estève J, Vasallo A, Victora CG, Teuchmann S. Mate, drinking alcohol, tobacco, diet and esophageal cancer in Uruguay. *Cancer Res* 1990; **50**: 426-431.

234

[497] Gao YT, McLaughlin JK, Gridley G, et al. Risk factors for esophageal cancer in Shanghai, China. II Role of diet and nutrients. *Int J Cancer* 1994; **58**: 197-202.

[498] Hu J, Nyren O, Wolk A, et al. Risk factors for oesophageal cancer in northeast China. *Int J Cancer* 1994; **57**: 38-46.

[499] Li JY, Ershow AG, Chen ZJ, et al. A case-control study of cancer of the esophagus and gastric cardia in Linxian. *Int J Cancer* 1989; **43**: 755-761.

[500] Nakachi K, Imai K, Hoshiyama Y, Sasaba T. The joint effects of two factors in the aetiology of oesophageal cancer in Japan. *J Epid Com Hlth* 1988; **42**: 355-364.

[501] Notani PN, Jayant K. Role of diet in upper aerodigestive tract cancers. *Nutr Cancer* 1987; **10**: 103-113.

[502] Tavani A, Negri E, Franceschi S, La Vecchia C. Risk factors for esophageal cancer in women in northern Italy. *Cancer* 1993; **72**: 2531-2536.

[503] Ziegler RG, Morris LE, Blot WJ, Pottern LM, Hoover R, Fraumeni JFJ. Esophageal cancer among black men in Washington, D.C. II. Role of nutrition. *J Natl Cancer Inst* 1981; **67**: 1199-1206.

[504] Victoria CG, Munoz N, Day NE, Barcelos LB, Peccin DA, Braga NM. Hot beverages and oesophageal cancer in Southern Brazil: A case-control study. *Int J Cancer* 1987; **39**: 710-716.

[505] Castelletto R, Castellsague X, Muñoz N, Iscovich J, Chopita N, Jmelnitsky A. Alcohol, tobacco, diet, Mate drinking, and esophageal cancer in Argentina. *Cancer Epid Biomarkers Prev* 1994; **3**: 557-564.

[506] Cook-Mozaffari PJ, Azordegan F, Day NE, Ressicaud A, Sabai C, Aramesh B. Oesophageal cancer studies in the Caspian Littoral of Iran: Results of a case-control study. *Br J Cancer* 1979; **39**: 293-308.

[507] Tuyns AJ, Riboli E, Doornbos G, Peguinot G. Diet and esophageal cancer in Calvados (France). *Nutr Cancer* 1987; **9**: 81-92.

[508] Yu Y, Taylor PR, Li JY, et al. Retrospective cohort study of risk-factors for esophageal cancer in Linxian, People's Republic of China. *Cancer Causes Control* 1993; **4**: 195-202.

[509] Wang YP, Han XY, Su W, et al. Esophageal cancer in Shanxi Province, People's Republic of China: a case-control study in high and moderate risk areas. *Cancer Causes Control* 1992; **3**: 107-113.

[510] Barone J, Taioli E, Hebert JR, Wynder EL. Vitamin supplement use and risk for oral and esophageal cancer. *Nutr Cancer* 1992; **18**: 31-41.

[511] Mettlin C, Graham S, Priore R, Marshall J, Swanson M. Diet and cancer of the esophagus. *Nutr Cancer* 1981; **2**: 143-147.

[512] Valsecchia MG. Modelling the relative risk of esophageal cancer in a case-control study. *J Clin Epid* 1992; **45**: 347-355.

[513] Graham S, Marshall J, Haughey B, et al. Nutritional epidemiology of cancer of the esophagus. *Am J Epidemiol* 1990; **131**: 454-467.

[514] Yu MC, Ho JH, Henderson BE, Armstrong RW. Epidemiology of nasopharyngeal carcinoma in Malaysia and Hong Kong. *Natl Cancer Inst Monogr* 1985; **69**: 203-207.

[515] Prasad MPR, Krishna TP, Pasricha S, Krishnaswamy K, Quereshi MA. Esophageal cancer and diet - A case-control study. *Nutr Cancer* 1992; **18**: 85-93.

[516] Li JY, Taylor PR, Li B, et al. Nutrition intervention trials in Linxian, China: multiple vitamin/mineral supplementation, cancer incidence, and disease-specific mortality among adults with esophageal dysplasia. *J Natl Cancer Inst* 1993; **85**: 1492-1498.

235

[517] Wang L. Effect of added dietary calcium on human esophageal precancerous lesions in a high risk area for oesophageal cancer-A randomised double-blind intervention trial. *Chung Hua Liu Hsing Ping Hsueh Tsa Chih* 1990; **12**: 332-335.

[518] Munoz N, Wahrendorf J, Jian Bang L, *et al.* No effect of riboflavin, retinol, and zinc on prevalence of precancerous lesions of oesophagus. *Lancet* 1985;111-114.

[519] Munoz N, Hayashi M, Jian Bang L, Wahrendorf J, Crespi M, Bosch X. Effect of riboflavin, retinol, and zinc on micronuclei of buccal mucosa and of esophagus: a randomized double-blind intervention study. *J Natl Cancer Inst* 1987; **79**: 687-691.

[520] Wahrendorf J, Munoz N, Jian-Bang L, Thurnham DI, Crespi M, Bosch FX. Blood, retinol and zinc riboflavin status in relation to precancerous lesions of the esophagus: findings from a vitamin intervention trial in the People's Republic of China. *Cancer Res* 1988; **48**: 2280-2283.

[521] Yu MC, Garabrant DH, Peters JM, Mack TM. Tobacco, alcohol, diet, occupation and carcinoma of the esophagus. *Cancer Res* 1988; **48**: 3843-3848.

[522] de Jong UW, Breslow N, Goh-Ewe-Hong J, Sridharan M, Shanmugaratnam K. Aetiological factors in oesophageal cancer in Singapore Chinese. *Int J Cancer* 1974; **13**: 291-303.

[523] Kirkpatrick CS, White E, Lee JAH. Case-control study of malignant melanoma in Washington State. II. Diet, alcohol and obesity. *Am J Epidemiol* 1994; **139**: 869-880.

[524] Bain C, Green A, Siskind V, Alexander J, Harvey P. Diet and melanoma: An exploratory case-control study. *Ann of Epidemiol* 1993; **3**: 235-238.

[525] Riboli E, Kaaks R, Estève J. Nutrition and laryngeal cancer. *Cancer Causes Control* 1996; **7**: 147-156.

[526] De Stefani, Correa P, Oreggia F, *et al.* Risk factors for laryngeal cancer. *Cancer* 1987; **60**: 3087-3091.

[527] La Vecchia C, Negri E, D'Avanzo B, Franceschi S, Decarli A, Boyle P. Dietary indicators of laryngeal cancer risk. *Cancer Res* 1990; **50**: 4497-4500.

[528] Estève J, Riboli E, Péquignot G, *et al.* Diet and cancers of the larynx and hypopharynx: The IARC multi-center study in south-western Europe. *Cancer Causes Control* 1996; **7**: 240-252.

[529] Zheng W, Blot WJ, Shu X, *et al.* Diet and other risk factors for laryngeal cancer in Shaghai, China. *Am J Epidemiol* 1992; **136**: 178-191.

[530] Winn D. Diet and nutrition in the etiology of oral cancer. *Am J Clin Nutr* 1995; **61(suppl)**: 437S-445S.

[531] Boyle P, Zaridze DG. Risk factor for prostate and testicular cancer. *Eur J Cancer* 1993; **29A**: 1048-1055.

[532] Davies TW, Prener A, Engholm G. Body size and cancer of the testis. *Acta Oncol* 1990: **3**: 287-290.

[533] Muir C, Waterhouse J, Mack T, Powell J, Whenal S eds. Cancer incidence in five continents. *International Agency for Research on Cancer*: Lyon, France; 1987.

[534] Davies TW, Palmer CR, Ruja E, Lipscombe JM. Adolescent milk, dairy product and fruit consumption and testicular cancer. *Br J Cancer* 1996; **74**: 657-660.

[535] Prior JC. Reversible reproductive changes with endurance training. In: Shephard RJ, Astrand PO eds. *Endurance in Sport*. Oxford: Blackwell Scientific Publications, 1992; 365.

[536] Jones DY, Schatzkin A, Green SB, *et al.* Dietary fat and breast cancer in the National Health and Nutrition Examination Survey. I Epidemiologic follow up study. *J Natl Cancer Inst* 1987; **79**: 465-471.

236

[537] Frisch RE, Wyshak G, Albright NL, Albright TE, Schiff I, Jones KP, Witschi J, Shiang E, Koff E, Marguglio M. Lower prevalence of breast cancer and cancers of the reproductive system among former college athletes compared to non-athletes. *Br J Cancer* 1985; **52**: 885-891.

[538] Frisch RE, Wyshak G, Albright NL, Albright TE, Schiff I, Witschi J, Marguglio M. Lower lifetime occurrence of breast cancer and cancers of the reproductive system among former college athletes. *Am J Clin Nutr* 1987; **45**: 328-335.

[539] Vena JE, Graham S, Zielezny M, Brasure J, Swanson MK. Occupational exercise and risk of cancer. *Am J Clin Nutr* 1987; **45**: 318-327.

[540] Paffenbarger RS Jr, Hyde RT, Wing AL. Physical activity and incidence of cancer in diverse populations: a preliminary report. *Am J Clin Nutr* 1987; **45**: 312-317.

[541] Shepherd RJ. Exercise and cancer: Linkages with obesity? *Crit Rev Fd Sci Nutr* 1996; **36**: 321-339.

[542] Lee IM. Exercise and physical health: Cancer and immune function. *Research Quarterly for Exercise and Sport* 1995; **66 (4)**: 286-291.

[543] Mayberry RM. Age-specific patterns of association between breast cancer and risk factors in black women ages 20 to 39 and 40 to 54. *Ann Epidemiol* 1994; **4**: 205-213.

[544] Mirra AP, Cole P, MacMahon B. Breast cancer in an area of high parity: Sao Paolo, Brazil. *Cancer Res* 1971; **31**: 77-83.

[545] Toti A, Agugiaro S, Amadori D, *et al*. Breast cancer risk factors in Italian women: a multicentric case-control study. *Tumori* 1986; **72**: 241-249.

[546] Schatzkin A, Palmer JR, Rosenbert L, Helmrich SP, Miller DR, Kaufman DW, Leska SM, Shapiro S. Risk factors for breast cancer in black women. *J Natl Cancer Inst* 1987; **78**: 213-217.

[547] Ewertz M. Influence of non-contraceptive exogenous and endogenous sex hormones on breast cancer risk in Denmark. *Int J Cancer* 1988; **42**: 832-838.

[548] Chu SY, Lee NC, Wingo PA, Senie RT, Greenberg RS, Peterson HB. Relationship between body mass and breast cancer among women enrolled in the cancer and steroid hormone study. *J Clin Epidemiol* 1991; **44**: 1197-1206.

[549] Staszewski J. Breast cancer and body build. *Prev Med*, 1977; **6**: 410-4155.

[550] Swanson CA, Brinton LA, Taylor PR, *et al*. Body size and breast cancer risk assessed in women participating in the Breast Cancer Detection Demonstration Project. *Am J Epidemiol* 1989; **130**: 1133-1141.

[551] Franceschi S, *et al*. Breast cancer & history of selected medical conditions linked with female hormones. *Eur J Cancer* 1990; **26**: 781-785.

[552] Hsieh C-C, Tricholpoulos D, Katsouyanni K, Yuasa S. Age at menarche, age of menopause, height and obesity as risk factors for breast cancer: associations and interactions in an international case-control study. *Int J Cancer* 1990; **46**: 796-800.

[553] Segala C, Gerber M, Richardson S. Pattern of risk factors for breast cancer in a Southern France population. Interest for a stratified analysis by age at diagnosis. *Br J Cancer* 1991; **64**: 919-925.

[554] Stavraky K, Emmons S. Breast cancer in premenopausal and postmenopausal women. *J Natl Cancer Inst* 1974; **853**: 647-655.

[555] Paffenbarger RS Jr, Kampert JB, Hwa-Gan C. Characteristics that predict risk of breast cancer before and after the menopause. *Am J Epidemiol* 1980; **112**: 258-268.

[556] Hislop TG, Coldman AJ, Elwood JM. Relationship between risk factors for breast cancer and hormonal status. *Int J Cancer* 1986; **15**: 469-476.

[557] Rosenberg L, Palmer JR, Miller DR, Clarke EA, Shapiro S. A case-control study of alcoholic beverage consumption and breast cancer. *Am J Epidemiol* 1990; **131**: 6-14.

237

[558] Harris RE, Namboodiri KK, Wynder EL. Breast cancer risk: effects of estrogen replacement therapy and body mass. *J Natl Cancer Inst* 1992; **84**: 1575-1582.

[559] Radimer K, Siskind V, Bain C, Schofield F. Relation between anthropometric indicators and risk of breast cancer among Australian women. *Am J Epidemiol*, 1993; **138**: 77-89.

[560] Helmrich SP, Shapiro S, Rosenberg L, Kaufman DW, Stone D, Bain C, Miettiron OS, Stolley PD, Rosenhein NB, Knapp RC, Leavitt Jr T, Schottenfeld D, Engle Jr RL, Levy M. Risk factors for breast cancer. *Am J Epidemiol* 1983; **117**: 35-45.

[561] Kampert JB, Whittemore AS, Paffenbarger Jr RS. Combined effect of childbearing, menstrual events and body size on age-specific breast cancer risk. *Am J Epidemiol* 1988; **128**: 962-979.

[562] Bruning PF, Bonfrer JMG, Hart AAM, van Noord PAH, van der Hoeven H, Collette HJA, Battermann JJ, de Jong-bakker M, Nooijen WJ, de Waard F. Body measurements, estrogen availability and the risk of human breast cancer: a case-control study. *Int J Cancer* 1992; **51**: 14-19.

[563] Zang EA, Wynder EL. The association between body mass index and the relative frequencies of diseases in a sample of hospitalized patients. *Nutr Cancer* 1994; **21**: 247-261.

[564] de Stavola BL, Wang DY, Allen DS, Gioconi J, Fentiman IS, Reed MJ, Bulbrook RD, Hayward JL. Association of height, weight, menstrual and reproductive events with breast cancer: results from two prospective studies on the island of Guernsey (United Kingdom). *Cancer Causes and Control* 1993; **4**: 331-340.

[565] Le Marchand L, Kolonel LN, Earle ME, Mi MP. Body size at different periods of life and breast cancer risk. *Am J Epidemiol* 1988; **128**: 137-152.

[566] Törnberg SA, Holm LE, Carstensen JM. Breast cancer risk in relation to serum cholesterol, serum beta-lipoprotein, height, weight and blood pressure. *Acta Oncol* 1988; **27**: 31-37.

[567] London SJ, Colditz GA, Stampfer MJ, Willet WC, Rasner B, Speizer FE. Prospective study of relative weight, height and risk of breast cancer. *J Am Med Ass* 1989; **262**: 2853-2858.

[568] Vatten LJ, Kvinnsland S. Prospective study of height, BMI and risk of breast cancer. *Acta Oncol* 1992; **31**: 195-200.

[569] Moller H, Mellemgaard A, Lindvig K, Olsen JH. Obesity and cancer risk: a Danish record-linkage study. *Eur J Cancer* 1994; **30A**: 344-350.

[570] Törnberg SA, Carstensen JM. Relationship between Quetelet's Index and cancer of the breast and female genital tract in 47,000 women followed for 25 years. *Br J Cancer* 1994; **69**: 358-361.

[571] den Tonkelaar J, Seidell JC, Colette JA, de Waard F. Obesity and subcutaneous fat patterning in relation to breast cancer in postmenopausal women participating in the Diagnostic Investigation of Mammary Cancer Project. *Cancer* 1992; **69**: 2663-2667.

[572] Sherman B, Wallace R, Bean J. Estrogen use and breast cancer. *Cancer* 1983; **51**: 1527-1531.

[573] Kolonel LN, Nomura AMY, Lee J, Horohata T. Anthropometric indicators of breast cancer risk in post-menopausal women in Hawaii. *Nutr Cancer*, 1986; **8**: 247-256.

[574] Kyogoku S, Hirohata T, Takeshita S, Hirota Y, Shigmatsu T. Anthropometric indicators of breast cancer risk in Japanese women in Fukuoka. *Jpn J Cancer Res* 1990; **81**: 731-737.

[575] Moller H, Mellemgaard A, Lindvig K, Olsen JH. Obesity and cancer risk: a Danish record-linkage study. *Eur J Cancer* 1994; **30A**: 344-350.

[576] de Waard F, Baanders-van Halewijn EA. A prospective study in general practice on breast cancer risk in postmenopausal women. *Int J Cancer* 1974; **14**: 153-160.

[577] Tretli S. Height and weight in relation to breast cancer morbidity and mortality: a prospective study of 570,000 women in Norway. *Int J Cancer* 1989; **44**: 23-30.

238

[578] Folsom AR, Kaye SA, Prineas RJ, Potter ID, Gapshir SM, Wallace RB. Increased incidence of carcinoma of the breast associated with abdominal adiposity in menopausal women. *Am J Epidemiol* 1990; **131**: 794-803.

[579] den Tonkelaar I, Seidell JC, Collette JA, de Waard F. A prospective study on obesity and subcutaneous fat patterning in relation to breast cancer in post-menopausal women participating in the DOM project. *Br J Cancer* 1994; **69**: 352-357.

[580] Schapira DV, Kumar NB, Lyman GH, Cox CE. Abdominal obesity and breast cancer risk. *Ann Int Med*, 1990; **112**: 182-186.

[581] Schapira DV, Clark RA, Wolff PA, Jarrett AR, Kumar NB, Aziz NM. Visceral obesity and breast cancer risk. *Cancer* 1994; **74**: 632-639.

[582] Ballard-Barbash PR, Schatzkin A, Carter CL, Kannel WB, Kreger BE, D'Agoshno RB, Splansky L, Anderson KM, Helsel WC. Body fat distribution and breast cancer in the Framingham Study. *J Natl Cancer Inst* 1990; **82**: 286-290.

[583] Sellers TA, Kushi LH, Potter JD, Kaye SA, Nelson CL, McGovern PG, Folsom AR. Effect of family history, body fat distribution and reproductive factors on the risk of postmenopausal breast cancer. *New Engl J Med* 1992; **326**: 1323-1329.

[584] Sönnischen AC, Lindlacher AC, Richter WO, Schwandt P. Adipositas, körperfettverteilung und inzidenz von mamma-, zerviz-, endometrium- und ovarialkarzinomen (in German). *Deutsche Medizinische Wochenshrift* 1990; **115**: 1906-1910.

[585] Petrek JA, Peters M, Cirrincione C, Rhodes D, Bajorunas D. Is body fat topography a risk factor for breast cancer? *Ann Int Med* 1993; **118**: 356-362.

[586] Lapidus L, Helgesson O, Merck C, Björntorp P. Adipose tissue distribution and female carcinoma - a 12 year follow-up of participants in the population study of women in Gothenburg, Sweden. *Int J Obesity* 1988; **12**: 361-368.

[587] Murayama Y. Plasma sex hormone-binding globulin (SHBG) and obesity in breast cancer patients. *Cancer Detect Prev* 1983; **6**: 425-433.

[588] Sulkes A, Fuks Z, Gordon A, Gross J. Sex hormone binding globulin (SHBG) in breast cancer: a correlation with obesity but not with estrogen receptor status. *Eur J Cancer Clin Oncol* 1984; **20**: 19-23.

[589] Ota DM, Jones LA, Jackson GL, Jackson PM, Kamp K, Bauman D. Obesity, non-protein bound oestradiol levels and distribution of oestradiol in the sera of breast cancer patients. *Cancer* 1986; **51**: 558-567.

[590] Ingram DM, Nottage EM, Willcox DL, Roberts A. Oestrogen binding and risk factors for breast cancer. *Br J Cancer* 1990; **61**: 303-307.

[591] Schapira DV, Dumar NG, Lyman GH. Obesity, body fat distribution and sex hormones in breast cancer. *Cancer* 1991; **67**: 2215-2218.

[592] Kuno F, Fukami A, Hon M, Kasumo F. Hormone receptors and obesity in Japanese women with breast cancer. *Breast Cancer Res Treat* 1981; **1**: 135-139.

[593] Leser ML, Rosen PP, Senie RT. Oestrogen and progesterone receptors in breast carcinoma: correlations with epidemiology and pathology. *Cancer* 1981; **48**: 299-309.

[594] de Waard F, Poortman J, Collette BA. Relationship of weight to the promotion of breast cancer after the menopause. *Nutr Cancer* 1982; **2**: 237-240.

[595] Pascual MR, Lazo R, Fernandez L, Lage A. Clinical factors related to the presence of estrogen receptors in breast cancer: a prognostic stratification analysis. *Neoplasma* 1982; **29**: 453-461.

[596] Donegan WL, Johnstone MF, Biedrzycki L. Obesity, estrogen production, and tumor estrogen receptors in women with carcinoma of the breast. *Am J Clin Oncol* 1983; **6**: 19-24.

[597] Nomura A, Heilbrun LK, Stemmerman GN, Judd HL. Prediagnostic serum hormones and the risk of prostate cancer. *Cancer Res* 1988; **48**: 3515-3517.

[598] Tsyrlina EV, Semiglazov VP, Moiseenko VM, Bornoeva TP. Study of the role of steroid receptors in human breast cancer. *Neoplasma* 1985; **32**: 463-467.

[599] Guiffrida D, Lupo L, La Porta GA, La Rosa GL, Padova G, Foti E, Marchese V, Belfiore A. Relation between steroid receptor status and body weight in breast cancer patients. *Eur J Cancer* 1992; **28**: 112-115.

[600] Little J, Logan R, Hawtin P, Hardcastle JD, Turner ID. Colorectal adenomas and dietary fat, protein, fibre and calcium. *Gastroenterology* 1991;**100**:A380.

[601] Papatestas AE, Panveliwalla D, Pertsemlidis D, Mulvihill M, Aufses AH Jr. Association between estrogen receptors and weight in women with breast cancer. *J Surg Oncol* 1980; **13**: 117-180.

[602] Mason B, Holdaway IM, Yee L, Kay RG. Lack of association between weight and oestrogen receptors in women with breast cancer. *J Surg Oncol* 1982; **19**: 62-64.

[603] Ballard-Barbash R, Griffin MR, Fisher DL. Estrogen receptors in breast cancer. Association with epidemiologic risk factors. *Am J Epidemiol* 1986; **124**: 77-84.

[604] McTiernan A, Thomas DB, Lois K, Roseman D. Risk factors for estrogen receptor-rich and estrogen receptor-poor breast cancers. *J Natl Cancer Inst* 1986; **77**: 849-854.

[605] Lubin F, Ruder AM, Wax Y, Modan B. Overweight and changes in weight throughout adult life in breast cancer etiology. *Am J Epidemiol* 1985; **122**: 579-588.

[606] Whittemore AS, Paffenbarger Jr RS, Anderson K, Lee JE. Early precursors of site-specific cancers in College men and women. *J Natl Cancer Inst* 1985; **74**: 43-51.

[607] Barnes-Josiah D, Potter JD, Sellers TA, Himes JH. Early body size and subsequent weight gain as predictors of breast cancer incidence (Iowa, United States). *Cancer Causes Control* 1995; **6**: 112-118.

[608] Valaoras VG, MacMahon B, Trichopoulos D. Lactation and reproductive histories of breast cancer patients in greater Athens 1965. *Int J Cancer* 1969; **4**: 350-363.

[609] Lin TH, Dhen KP, MacMahon B. Epidemiologic characteristics of cancer of the breast in Taiwan. *Cancer* 1971; **27**: 1497-1504.

[610] de Waard F, Cornelis JP, Aoki K, Yoshida M. Breast cancer incidence according to weight and height in two cities of the Netherlands and in Aichi prefecture, Japan. *Cancer* 1977; **40**: 1269-1275.

[611] Brinton LA, Williams RR, Hoover RN, Stengens NL, Feinlieb M, Fraumeni JFJ. Breast cancer risk factors among screening program participants. *J Natl Cancer Inst* 1979; **62**: 37-43.

[612] Ross RK, Paganini S, Hill A. A case-control study of postmenopausal estrogen therapy and breast cancer. *J Am Med Ass* 1980; **243**: 1635-1639.

[613] Whitehead J, Carlile T, Kopecky KJ, Thompson DJ, Gilbert FI, Present AJ, Threatt BA, Krook P, Hadaway E. The relationship between Wolfe's classification of mammograms, accepted breast cancer risk factors, and the incidence of breast cancer. *Am J Epidemiol* 1985; **122**: 994-1006.

[614] Swanson CA, Coates RJ, Schoenberg JB, Malone KE, Gammon MD, Stanford JL, Shorr IJ, Portischman NA, Brinton LA. Body size and breast cancer risk among women under age 45 years. *Am J Epidemiol* 1996; **143**: 698-706.

[615] Adami HO, Rimsten A, Stenkvist B, Vegelius J. Influence of height, weight and obesity on risk of breast cancer in an unselected Swedish population. *Cancer* 1977; **36**: 787-792.

[616] Kelsey JL, Fischer DB, Holford TR, Livolso VA, Mostow ED, Goldenberg IS, White C. Exogenous estrogens and other factors in the epidemiology of breast cancer. *J Natl Cancer Inst* 1981; **676**: 327-333.

240

[617] Bouchardy C, Le MG, Hill C. Risk factors for breast cancer according to age at diagnosis in a French case-control study. *J Clin Epidemiol* 1990; **42**: 267-275.

[618] Barker DJP, Osmond C, Golding J. Height and mortality in the countries of England and Wales. *Ann Hum Biol* 1990; **17**: 1-6.

[619] van den Brandt PA, Dirx JM, Ronckers CM, van den Hoogen P, Goldbohm A. Height, weight, weight change, and post-menopausal breast cancer risk: the Netherlands Cohort Study. *Cancer Causes Control* 1997; **8**: 39-47.

[620] Willett WC, Stampfer MJ, Colditz GA, Rosner BA, Speizer FE. A prospective study of diet and colon cancer in women. *Am J Epidemiol* 1989; **130**: 820.

[621] Graham S, Marshall J, Haughey B, Mittelman A, Swanson MK, Zielezny M, Byers T, Wilkinson G, West D. Dietary epidemiology of cancer of the colon in Western New York. *Am J Epidemiol* 1988; **128**: 490-503.

[622] Gerhardssen de Verdier M, Hagman U, Steineck G, Rieger A, Norell SE. Diet, body mass and colorectal cancer: a case-referent study in Stockholm. *Int J Cancer* 1990; **46**: 832-838.

[623] Kune GA, Kune S, Watson LF. Body weight and physical activity as predictors of colorectal cancer risk. *Nutr Cancer* 1990; **13**: 9-17.

[624] Williams-Pickle L, Greene MH, Ziegler RG, Toledo A, Hoover R, Lynch R, Fraumani LFJ. Colorectal cancer in rural Nebraska. *Cancer Res* 1984; **44**: 363-369.

[625] Whittemore AS, Wu-Williams AH, Lee M, Shu Z, Gallagher RP, Deng-ao J, Lun Z, Xianghui W, Kun C, Jung D, Teh C, Chengde L, Yao XJ, Paffenbarger Jr RS, Henderson BE. Diet, physical activity and colorectal cancer among Chinese in North America and China. *J Natl Cancer Inst* 1990; **82**: 915-926.

[626] Lew EA, Garfinkel L. Variations in mortality by weight among 750 000 men and women. *J Chron Dis* 1979; **32**: 563-576.

[627] Kreger BE, Anderson KM, Schatzkin A, Splansky GL. Serum cholesterol level, body mass index and risk of colon cancer. *Cancer* 1992; **70**: 1038-1043.

[628] Lee IM, Paffenbarger RS. Quetelet's index and risk of colon cancer in college allumni. *J Natl Cancer Inst* 1992; **84**: 1326-1331.

[629] Chyou PH, Nomura AMY, Stemmermann GN. A prospective study of weight, body mass index and other anthropometric measurements in relation to site-specific cancers. *Int J Cancer* 1994; **57**: 313-317.

[630] Giovannucci E, Ascherio A, Rimm EB, Colditz GA, Stampfer MJ, Willett WC. Physical activity, obesity and risk for colon cancer and adenoma in men. *Ann Internal Medicine* 1995; **122**: 327-334.

[631] Tulinius H, Sigfusson N, Sigvaldason H, Day NE. Can anthropometric and biochemical measurements illustrate the diet-cancer connection? *Näringsforskning* 1985; **29**: 17-22.

[632] Suadichani P, Hein HO, Gyntelberg. Height, weight and risk of colorectal cancer. *Scand J Gastroent* 1993; **28**: 285-288.

[633] Potter JD, McMichael AJ. Large bowel cancer in women in relation to reproductive and hormonal factors. *J Natl Cancer Inst* 1983; **71**: 703-709.

[634] Chute CG, Willett WC, Colditz GA, Stampfer MJ, Baron JA, Rosner B, Spezier FE. A prospective study of body mass, height, and smoking on the risk of colorectal cancer in women. *Cancer Causes Control* 1991; **2**: 117-124.

[635] Bingham SA, Cummings JH. Effect of exercise and physical fitness on large intestinal function. *Gastroent* 1989; **97**: 1389-1399.

[636] Talamini R, La Vecchia C, Decarli A. Nutrition, social factors and prostatic cancer in a Northern Italian population. *Br J Cancer* 1986; **53**: 817-821.

241

[637] Hayes RB, De Jong FH, Raatgever J, Bogdanovicz J, Schroeder FH, Van Der Mass P, Oishi K, Yoshida O. Physical characteristics and factors related to sexual development and behaviour and the risk for prostatic cancer. *Eur J Cancer Prev* 1991; **1**: 239-245.

[638] Honda GD, Bernstein L, Ross RK, Greenland S, Gerkins V, Henderson BE. Vasectomy, cigarette smoking and age at first sexual intercourse as risk factors for prostate cancer in middle aged men. *Br J Cancer* 1988; **57**: 326-331.

[639] Denmark-Wahnfried W, Paulson DF, Robertson CN, Anderson EE, Conaway MR, Rimer BK. Body dimension differences in men with or without prostate cancer. *J Natl Cancer Inst* 1992; **84**: 1363-1364.

[640] Severson RK, Grove JS, Nomura AMY. Body mass and prostatic cancer: a prospective study. *BMJ* 1988; **297**: 713-715.

[641] Zeil HK, Funkle WD. Increased risk of endometrial carcinoma among users of conjugated estrogens. *New Engl J Med* 1975; **293**: 1167-1170.

[642] Elwood JH, Cole P, Rothman KJ, Kaplan DS. Epidemiology of endometrial cancer. *J Natl Cancer Inst* 1977; **59**: 1055-1060.

[643] MacDonald TW, Annegers JF, O'Fallon WM, Dockerty HB, Malkasian GD, Kurtland LT. Exogenous estrogens and carcinoma of the endometrium: case-control and incidence study. *Am J of Obstetrics and Gynecology* 1977; **27**: 572-580.

[644] La Vecchia C, Franceschi S, Gallus C, Decarli A, Colombo E. Oestrogens and obesity as risk factors for endometrial cancer in Italy. *Int J Epidemiol* 1982; **11**: 120-126.

[645] La Vecchia C, Franceschi S, Decarli A, Gallus C, Tigoni G. Risk factors for endometrial cancer at different ages. *J Natl Cancer Inst* 1984; **73**: 667-671.

[646] La Vecchia C, Parazzini F, Negri E, Fasoli M, Gentile A, Franceschi S. Anthropometric indicators of endometrial cancer risk. *Eur J Cancer* 1991; **27**: 487-490.

[647] Shu XO, Brinton LA, Zheng W. Gao YT, Fan J, Fraumeni JFJ. A population based case-control study of endometrial cancer in Shanghai, China. *Int J Cancer* 1991; **49**: 38-43.

[648] Brinton LA, Berman ML, Mortel R, Twiggs LB, Barrett RJ, Wilbanks GD, Lannom L, Hoover RN. Reproductive, menstrual and medical risk factors for endometrial cancer: results from a case-control study. *Am J of Obstetrics and Gynecology* 1992; **167**: 1317-1325.

[649] Levi F, La Vecchia C, Negri E, Parazzini F, Franceschi S. Body mass index at different ages and subsequent endometrial cancer risk. *Int J Cancer* 1992; **50**: 567-571.

[650] Shu XO, Brinton LA, Zheng W, Swanson CA, Hatch MC, Gan Y, Fraumani JFJ. Relation of obesity and body fat distribution to endometrial cancer in Shanghai, China. *Cancer Res* 1992; **52**: 3865-3870.

[651] Olson SH, Trevisan M, Marshall JR, Graham S, Zielezny M, Vena JE, Hellman R, Freudenheim JL. Body mass index, weight gain and risk of endometrial cancer. *Nutr Cancer* 1995; **23**: 141-149.

[652] Folsom AR, Kaye SA, Potter JD, Prineas RJ. Association of incident carcinoma of the endometrium with body weight and fat distribution in older women: early findings of the Iowa Women's Health Study. *Cancer Res* 1989; **49**: 6828-6831.

[653] Tretli S, Magnus K. Height and weight in relation to uterine corpus cancer and morbidity and mortality. A follow-up study of 570,000 women in Norway. *Int J Cancer* 1990; **46**: 165-172.

[654] Farrow DC, Weiss NS, Lyon JL, Daling. Association of obesity and ovarian cancer in a case-control study. *Am J Epidemiol* 1989; **129**: 1300-1304.

[655] Byers TE, Marshall J, Graham S, Mettlin C, Swanson MK. A case-control study of dietary and non-dietary factors in ovarian cancer. *J Natl Cancer Inst* 1983; **71**: 681-686.

242

[656] Cramer DW, Welch WR, Hutchinson GB, Willett WC, Scully RF. Dietary animal fat in relation to ovarian cancer risk. *Am J Obs Gyne* 1984; **63**: 833-838.

[657] La Vecchia C, Negri E, Parazzini F, Boyle P, D'Avanzo B, Levi F, Gentile A, Franceschi S. Height and cancer risk in a network of case-control studies from Northern Italy. *Int J Cancer* 1990; **45**: 275-279.

[658] Palli D, Bianchi S, Decarli A, *et al.* A case-control study of cancers of the gastric cardia in Italy. *Br J Cancer* 1992; **65**: 263-266.

[659] Yarnold JR, Stratton MR, McMillan TJ eds. *Molecular Biology for Oncologists.* London: Chapman and Hall, 1996.

[660] Lawley PD. Basic concepts of carcinogenesis. In: Cohen RD, Lewis B, Alberti KGMM, Denman AM, eds. *The Metabolic and Molecular Basis of Acquired Disease. Volume 1.* London: Bailliere Tindall, 1990; 44-73.

[661] Barrett JC. Mechanisms of multistep carcinogenesis and carcinogen risk assessment. *Environ Hlth Pers* 1993; **100**: 9-20.

[662] Renan MJ. How many mutations are required for tumorigenesis? Implications from human cancer data. *Molec Carcinogen* 1993; **7:** 139-146.

[663] Vogelstein B, Kinzler KW. The multistep nature of cancer. *Trends Genet* 1993; **9**: 138-141.

[664] Foulds L. *Neoplastic Development Volume 1.* London: Academic Press, 1969; 439.

[665] Lawley PD. Historical origins of current concepts of carcinogenesis. *Adv Cancer Res* 1994; **65**: 17-111.

[666] Venitt S. Mechanisms of spontaneous human cancers. *Environ Hlth Pers* 1996; **104(suppl 3)**: 633-637.

[667] Cavanee K, White RL. The genetic basis of cancer. *Scientific American* 1995; **272**: 50-57.

[668] Tomlinson IPM, Novelli MR, Bodmer WF. The mutation rate and cancer. *Proc Natl Acad Sci USA* 1996; **93**: 14800-14803.

[669] Carbone DP. Oncogenes and tumour suppressor genes. *Hospital Practice* 1993; **28**: 145-161.

[670] Tahara E. Molecular mechanism of stomach carcinogenesis. *J Cancer Res Clin Oncol* 1993; **119**: 265-272.

[671] Nishimura S, Sekiya T. Human cancer and cellular oncogenes. *Biochem J* 1987; **243**: 313-327.

[672] Bishop JM. The molecular genetics of cancer. *Science* 1987; **235**: 305-311.

[673] Varmus H. An historical overview of oncogenes. In: Weinberg RA, ed. *Oncogenes and the Molecular Origins of Cancer.* New York: Cold Spring Harbor Laboratory Press, 1989, 3-44.

[674] Hall M, Grover PL. Polycyclic aromatic hydrocarbons: metabolism, activation and tumour initiation. In: Cooper CS, Grover PL, eds. *Chemical Carcinogenesis and Mutagenesis I. Handbook of Experimental Pharmacology Volume 94/1.* Berlin: Springer-Verlag, 1990, 327-372.

[675] Weinberg RA. Oncogenes, antioncogenes, and the molecular bases of multistep carcinogenesis. *Cancer Res* 1989; **49**: 3713-3721.

[676] Bishop JM. Molecular themes in oncogenesis. *Cell* 1991; **64**: 235-248.

[677] Barrett JC. Mechanisms of action of known human carcinogens. In: Vainio H Magee PN, McGregor DB, McMichael AJ, eds. *Mechanisms of Carcinogenesis in Risk Identification.* Lyon: International Agency for Research on Cancer, 1992, 115-134.

[678] Marshall CH. Tumor suppressor genes. *Cell* 1991; **64**: 313-326.

[679] Smith G, Dale Smith CA, Wolf CR. Pharmacogenetic polymorphisms. In: Phillips DH, Venitt S eds. *Environmental Mutagenesis:* Oxford Bios Scientific Publishers, 1995, 83-106.

243

[680] Lindahl T. Instability and decay of the primary structure of DNA. *Nature* 1993; **362**: 709-715.

[681] Adams RLP. DNA methylation. The effect of minor bases on DNA-protein interactions. *Biochem J* 1990; **265**: 309-320.

[682] Kumar S, Cheng X, Klimauskas S, Mi S, Posfai J, Roberts RJ, Wilson GG. The DNA (cytosine) methyltranferases. *Nucl Acids Res* 1994; **22**: 1-10.

[683] Verdine GL. The flip side of DNA methylation. *Cell* 1994; **76(2)**: 197-200.

[684] Baylin SB, Makos M, Wu J, Yen R-WC, de Buystros A, Vertino A, Nelkin BD. Abnormal patterns of DNA methylation in human neoplasia: potential consequences for tumor progression. *Cancer Cells* 1991; **3**: 383-389.

[685] Bird A. The essentials of DNA methylation. *Cell* 1992; **70**: 5-8.

[686] Meehan RR, Lewis JD, Bird AP. Characterization of MeCP2, a vertebrate DNA binding protein with affinity for methylated DNA. *Nucl Acid Res* 1992; **20**: 5085-5092.

[687] Meehan RR, Lewis J, Cross S, Nan X, Jeppesen P, Bird A. Transcriptional repressions by methylation of CpG. *J Cell Sci* 1992; **Suppl 16**: 9-14.

[688] Tate PH, Bird AP. Effects of DNA methylation on DNA-binding proteins and gene expression. *Curr Opin Genet Develop* 1993; **3**: 226-231.

[689] Cooper DN, Krawczak M. *Human Gene Mutation.* Oxford: Bios Scientific Publishers, 1993; 402.

[690] Biggs PJ, Warren W, Venitt S, Stratton MR. Does a genotoxic carcinogen contribute to human breast cancer? The value of mutational spectra in unravelling the aetiology of cancer. *Mutagenesis* 1993; **8**: 275-283.

[691] Frisch RE, McArthur JW. Menstrual cycles: fatness as a determinant of minimum weight for height necessary for their maintenance or onset. *Science* 1985; **185**: 949-951.

[692] Tornaletti S, Pfeifer GP. Complete and tissue-independent methylation of CpG sites in the p53 gene: implications for mutations in human cancers. *Oncogene* 1995; **10**: 1493-1499.

[693] Michalowsky LA, Jones PA. DNA methylation and differentiation. *Environ Hlth Pers* 1989; **80**: 189-197.

[694] Jones PA. DNA methylation and cancer. *Cancer Res* 1986; **46**: 461-466.

[695] Jones PA, Wolkowicz MJ, Rideout WM, Gonzales FA, Marziasz CM, Coetzee GA, Tapscott SJ. De novo methylation of the MyoD1 CpG island during the establishment of immortal cell lines. *Proc Natl Acad Sci USA* 1990; **87**: 6117-6121.

[696] Feinberg AP, Gehrke CW, Kuo KC, Ehrlich M. Reduced Genomic 5-methylcytosine content in human colonic neoplasia. *Cancer Res* 1988; **48**: 1159-1161.

[697] Ames BN, Saul RL, Schwiers E, Adelman R, Cattcart R. Oxidative DNA damage as related to cancer and ageing. The assay of thymine glycol, thymidine glycol and hydroxymethyl uracil in human and rat urine. In: *Proceedings of the Symposium on Molecular Biology of Ageing: Gene stability and gene expression.* New York: Raven Press, 1984.

[698] Breimer L. Repair of DNA damage induced by reactive oxygen species. *Free Radic Res Commun* 1991; **14**: 159-71.

[699] Cattcart R, Cattcart R, Schwiers E, Saul RL, Ames BN. Thymine glycol and thymidine glycol in human and rat urine: a possible assay for oxidative DNA damage. *Proc Natl Acad Sci USA* 1984; **81**: 5633-5637.

[700] Shigenaga HF, Ames BN. Oxidants and mitogenesis as causes of mutation and cancer: the influence of diet. In: Bronzetti G *et al* eds. *Antimutagenesis and Anticarcinogenesis. Mechanisms III.* New York: Plenum Press, 1993.

244

[701] Reid TM, Loeb LA. Mutagenic specificity of oxygen radicals produced by human leukaemia cells. *Cancer Res* 1992; **52**: 1082-1086.

[702] Kasai H, Okada Y, Nishimura S, Rao MS, Reddy JK. Formation of 8-hydroxydeoxyguanosine in liver DNA of rats following long-term exposure to peroxisome proliferator. *Cancer Res* 1989; **49**: 2603-2605.

[703] Nishikimi M. Oxidation of ascorbic acid with superoxide anion generated by xanthine-xanthine oxidase system. *Biochem Biophys Res Commun* 1975; **63**: 463-468.

[704] Anderson R, Lukey PT. A biological role for ascorbate in the selective neutralisation of extra-cellular phagocyte-derived oxidants. *Ann NY Acad Sci* 1987; **498**: 229-246.

[705] Delange RJ, Glazer AN. Phycoerythrin flourescence-based assay for peroxy radicals: a screen for biologically relevant protective agents. *Anal Biochem* 1989; **177**: 300-306.

[706] McCoy PB. Vitamin E: interactions with free radicals and ascorbate. *Ann Rev Nutr* 1985; **5**: 323-340.

[707] Mirvish SS. Effects of vitamins C and E on N-nitroso compound formation, carcinogenesis and cancer. *Cancer* 1986; **58**: 1842-1850.

[708] Burton GW. Antioxidant action of carotenoids. *J Nutr* 1989; **119**: 109-111.

[709] Krinsky NI. Mechanisms of inactivation of oxygen species by carotenoids. In: Cerutti PA, Nygaard OF, Simie MG eds. 1987. p41-46.

[710] Rock CL, Jacob RA, Bowen P. Update on the biological characteristics of the antioxidant micronutrients: vitamin C, vitamin E and carotenoids. *J Am Diet Ass* 1996; **96**: 693-702.

[711] Al-Sheikhly M, Simic MG. Inhibition of auto-oxidation by vitamin E and bilirubin. In: Cerutti PA, Nygaard OF, Simie MG eds. 1987. p47-50.

[712] Gorman AA, Rodgers MAJ, Singlet molecular oxygen. *Chem Soc Rev* 1981; **10**: 205-231.

[713] Nishikimi M, Yamada H, Yagi K. Oxidation by superoxide of tocopherols dispersed in aqueous media with deoxycholate. *Biochem Biophys Res Commun* 1980; **627:** 101-108.

[714] Foye WD. Radiation protective agents in mammals. *J Pharmac Sci* 1969; **58**: 283-300.

[715] Pratt DE. Natural antioxidants from plant material. In: Huang MT, Ho CT, Lee CY eds. *Phenolic compounds in foods and their effect on health.* Volume II, ACS Symposium series 507, Washington DC: American Chemical Society, 1992; 54-71.

[716] Aruoma OI, Halliwell B, Aeschbach R, Loligers J. Antioxidant and pro-oxidant properties of active rosemary constituents - carnosol and carnosic acid. *Xenobiotica* 1992;**22**:257-268.

[717] Shi X, Dalal NS, Jain AC. Antioxidant behaviour of caffeine: efficient scavenging of hydroxyl radicals. *Food Chem Toxicol* 1991; **29**: 1-6.

[718] Liu J K, Mori A. Antioxidant and pro-oxidant activities of p-hydroxybenzyl alcohol and vanillin-Effects on free radicals, brain peroxidation and degradation of benzoate, deoxyribose, amino acids and DNA. *Neuropharmacol* 1993; **32**: 659-669.

[719] Horie T, Awazu S, Itakura Y, Fuwa T. Identified diallyl polysulphides from an aged garlic extract which protects the membranes from lipid peroxidation. *Planta Medica* 1992; **58**: 468-469.

[720] Singer B, Grunberger D. *Molecular Biology of Mutagens and Carcinogens.* New York: Plenum Press, 1983; 348.

[721] Osborne MR. DNA interactions of reactive intermediates derived from carcinogens. In: Searle CE, ed. *Chemical Carcinogens. Second Edition, Vol. 1. ACS Monograph 182.* Washington DC: American Chemical Society, 1984; 485-575.

245

[722] Beland FA, Kadlubar FF. Metabolic activation and DNA adducts of aromatic amines and nitroaromatic hydrocarbons. In: Cooper CS, Grover PL, eds. *Chemical Carcinogenesis and Mutagenesis I. Handbook of Experimental Pharmacology Volume 94/1*. Berlin: Springer-Verlag, 1990; 267-325.

[723] Groopman JD, Cain LG. Interactions of fungal and plant toxins with DNA: aflatoxins, sterigmatocystin, safrole, cycasin, and pyrrolizidine alkaloids. In: Cooper CS, Grover PL, eds. *Chemical Carcinogenesis and Mutagenesis I. Handbook of Experimental Pharmacology Volume 94/1*. Berlin: Springer-Verlag, 1990; 373-407.

[724] Turtletaub KW, Mauthe RJ, Dingley KH, Vogel JS, Frantz CE, Garner RC, Shen N. MeIQx-DNA adduct formation in rodent and human tissue at low doses. *Mutat Res* 1997; **376**: 243-252.

[725] Coles B, Ketterer B. The role of glutathione and glutathione transferases in chemical carcinogenesis. *Crit Rev Biochem Molec Biol* 1990; **25**: 47-70.

[726] Nebert DW. Role of genetics and drug metabolism in human cancer risk. *Mutat Res* 1991; **247**: 267-281.

[727] Bigger CAH, Flickinger DJ, St John J, Harvey RG, Dipple A. Preferential mutagenesis at G:C base pairs by the anti 3,4-dihydrodiol 1,2-epoxide of 7-methylbenz[a]anthracene. *Molec Carcinog* 1991; **4**: 176-179.

[728] Horsfall MJ, Zeilmaker MJ, Mohn GR, Glickman BW. Mutational specificities of environmental carcinogens in the lac 1 gene of *Escherichia coli*. II: A host-mediated approach to N-nitroso-N,N-dimethylamine and endogenous mutagenesis in vivo. *Molec Carcinog* 1989; **2**: 107-115.

[729] Zeilmaker MJ, van Teylingen CMM, van Helten JBM, Mohn GR. The use of EDTA-permeabilized *Escherichia Coli* cells as indicators of aflatoxin B1-induced differential lethality in the DNA repair host-mediated assay. *Mutat Res* 1991; **263**: 137-142.

[730] Friedberg EC. *DNA Repair*. New York: WH Freeman & Co, 1984; 614.

[731] Harnden DG. Inherited susceptibility to mutation. In: *Environmental Mutagenesis*. Phillips DH, Venitt S eds. Bios Scientific Publishers: Oxford, 1995; 61-81.

[732] Weisburger JH, Williams GM. Bioassay of carcinogens: in vitro and in vivo tests. In: Searle CE ed. *Chemical Carcinogens. Second Edition*, Vol.2. ACS Monograph 182. Washington D.C: American Chemical Society, 1984; 1323-1373.

[733] Ames BN, Gold LS. Too many rodent carcinogens: mitogenesis increases mutagenesis. *Science* 1990; **249**: 970-971.

[734] Preston-Martin S, Pike MC, Ross RK, Jones PA, Henderson BE. Increased cell division as a cause of human cancer. *Cancer Res* 1990; **50**: 7415-7421.

[735] Dietrich DR, Swenberg JA. Preneoplastic lesions in rodent kidney induced spontaneously or by non-genotoxic agents: predictive nature and comparison to lesions induced by genotoxic carcinogens. *Mutat Res* 1991; **248**: 239-260.

[736] Anderson RL. Early indicators of bladder carcinogenesis produced by non-genotoxic agents. *Mutat Res* 1991; **248**: 261-270.

[737] Grasso P, Hinton RH. Evidence for and possible mechanisms of non-genotoxic carcinogenesis in rodent liver. *Mutat Res* 1991; **248**: 271-290.

[738] Woutersen RA, van Garderen-Hoetmer A, Lamers CBHW, Scherer E. Early indicators of exocrine pancreas carcinogenesis produced by non-genotoxic agents. *Mutat Res* 1991; **248**: 291-302.

[739] Poynter D, Selway SAM. Neuroendocrine cell hyperplasis and neuroendocrine carcinoma of the rodent fundic stomach. *Mutat Res* 1991; **248**: 303-319.

[740] Clayson DB, Iverson F, Nera EA, Lok E. Early indicators of potential neoplasia produced in the rat forestomach by non-genotoxic agents: the importance of induced cellular proliferation. *Mutat Res* 1991; **248**: 321-331.

[741] Thomas GA, Williams ED. Evidence for and possible mechanisms of non-genotoxic carcinogenesis in the rodent thyroid. *Mutat Res* 1991; **248**: 357-370.

[742] Green S. The search for molecular mechanisms of non-genotoxic carcinogens. *Mutat Res* 1991; **248**: 371-374.

[743] Wattenberg LW. Inhibition of carcinogenesis by minor dietary constituents. *Cancer Res* 1992; **52**: 2085s-2091s.

[744] Dragsted LO, Strube M, Larsen JC. Cancer-protective factors in fruits and vegetables: biochemical and biological background. *Pharmacol Toxicol* 1993; **72**: 117s-135s.

[745] La Vecchia C, Ferraroni M, D'Avanzo B, Decarli A, Franceshi S. Selected micronutrient intake and the risk of gastric cancer. *Cancer Epid Biomarkers Prev* 1994; **3**: 393-398.

[746] Verhoeven DTH, Verhagen H, Goldbohm RA, van den Brandt PA, van Poppel G. A review of mechanisms underlying anticarcinogenecity by brassica vegetables. *Chemico-Biological Interactions* 1997; **103**: 79-129.

[747] Nijhoff AM, Groen GM, Peters WHM. Induction of rat hepatic and intestinal glutathione S-transferases and glutathione by dietary naturally occurring anticarcinogens. *Int J Oncol* 1993; **3**: 1131-1139.

[748] Finkelstein JD. Methionine metabolism in mammals. *J Nutr Biochem* 1990; **1**: 228-237.

[749] Wainfan D, Dizik M, Stender M, Christman JK. Rapid appearance of hypomethylated DNA in livers of rats fed cancer-promoting, methyl-deficient diets. *Cancer Res* 1989; **49**: 4094-4097.

[750] Christman JK, Sheikhnejad G, Dizik M, Abileah S, Wainfan E. Reversibility of changes in nucleic acid methylation and gene expression induced in rat liver by severe dietary methyl deficiency. *Carcinogenesis* 1993; **14**: 551-557.

[751] Balaghi M, Wagner C. DNA methylation in folate deficiency: use of CpG methylase. *Biochem Biophys Res Commun* 1993; **193**: 1184-1190.

[752] Cravo ML, Mason JB, Dayal Y, Hutchinson M, Smith D, Selhub J, Rosenberg IH. Folate deficiency enhances the development of colonic neoplasia in dimethylhydrazine-treated rats. *Cancer Res* 1992; **52**: 5002-5006.

[753] Kunz BA. Mutagenesis and deoxyribonucleotide pool imbalance. *Mutat Res* 1988; **200**: 133-147.

[754] MacGregor JT, Schlegel R, Wehr CM, Alperin P, Ames BN. Cytogenetic damage induced by folate deficiency in mice is enhanced by caffeine. *Proc Natl Acad Sci USA* 1990; **87**: 9962-9965.

[755] Rogers AE, Zeisel SH, Groopman J. Diet and carcinogenesis. *Carcinogenesis* 1993; **14**: 2205-2217.

[756] Shamsuddin A M, Ullah A. Insitol hexaphosphate inhibits large intestinal cancer in F344 rats 5 months following induction by azoxymethane. *Carcinogenesis*, 1989; **10**: 625-626.

[757] Reddy B S, Simi B, Englea A. Effects of types of fibre on colonic DAG in women. *Gastroenter* 1994; **106**: 883-889.

[758] Nishino H. Antitumor-promoting activity of glycyrrhetinic acid and its related compounds. In: Wattenberg L, Lipkin M, Boone CW, Kelloff GJ eds. *Cancer Chemoprevention.* Boca Raton: CRC Press, 1992: pp 457-467.

[759] Leighton T, Ginther C, Fluss L, Harter WK, Cansado J, Notario V. Molecular characterisation of quercetin and quercetin glycosides in Allium vegetables their effects on malignant cell transformation. In: Huang MT, Ho CT, Lee CY eds. *Phenolic compounds in food and their effects on health II. Antioxidants and cancer prevention.* American Chemical Society Symposium Series Vol 507. Washington: ACS 1992.

[760] Reddy B S, Burill C, Rigotty J. Effects of diets high in w3 and w6 fatty acids on initiation and postinitiation stages of colon carcinogenesis. *Cancer Res* 1991; **51**: 487-491.

247

[761] Lai PBS, Ross JA, Fearon KCH, Anderson JD, Carter DC. Cell cycle arrest and induction of apoptosis in pancreatic cancer cells exposed to eicosapentaenoic acid in vitro. *Br J Cancer* 1996; **74**: 1375-1383.

[762] Caygill CPJ, Charlett A, Hill MJ. Fat, fish, fish oil and cancer. *Br J Cancer* 1996; **74**: 159-164.

[763] Hussey HJ, Tisdale MJ. Inhibition of tumour growth by lipoxygenase inhibitors. *Br J Cancer* 1996; **74**: 683-687.

[764] Leaf A, Webber PC. Cardiovascular effects on n3 fatty acids. *New Engl J Med* 1988; **318**: 549-557.

[765] Marnett LJ. Aspirin and the potential role of prostaglandins in colon cancer. *Cancer Res* 1992; **52**: 5575-5589.

[766] Nakadate T, Yamamoto S, Aizu E, Kata R. Effects of flavonoids and antioxidants on 12-O-tetradecanoylphorbol-13-acetate-caused epidermal ornithine decarboxylase induction and tumour promotion in relation to lipoxygenase inhibition by these compounds. *Gann* 1984; **75**: 214-222.

[767] British Nutrition Foundation Task Force. Trans Fatty Acids. London: BNF, 1995.

[768] Tucker MJ. The effect of long-term food restriction on tumours in rodents. *Int J Cancer* 1979; **23**: 803-807.

[769] Coneybeare G. Effect of quality and quantity of diet on survival and tumour incidence in outbred Swiss mice. *Fd Cosmet Toxicol* 1980; **18**:65-75.

[770] Roe FJC. 1200-rat Biosure Study: Design and Overview of Results. In: L Fishbein ed. *Biological Effects of Dietary Restriction*. ILSI Monograph. Springer-Verlag, Berlin. 1991; 287-304.

[771] Roe FJC. Are nutritionists worried about the epidemic of tumours in laboratory animals? *Proc Nutr Soc* 1981; **4**: 57-65.

[772] Shimokawa I, Yu BP, Masoro EJ. Influence of diet on fatal neoplastic disease in male fischer F344 rats. *J Gerontol*, 1991; **46**: B228-232.

[773] Keenan KP, Smith PF, Hertzog P, *et al*. The effects of overfeeding and dietary restriction on Sprague-Dawley rat survival and early pathologic biomarkers of aging. *Toxicol Pathol*, 1994; **22**: 3300-3315.

[774] Fishbein L ed. *Biological Effects of Dietary Restriction*. Berlin: Springer-Verlag, 1991; 1-354.

[775] Turturro A, Haft RW. Calorie restriction and its effects on molecular parameters, especially DNA repair. 1991; 1185-1190. *In: Fishbein L, loc. cit.*

[776] Kono S, Imanishi K, Shinchi K, Yanai F. Relationship of diet to small and large adenomas of the sigmoid colon. *Jpn J Cancer Res* 1993; **84**: 13-19.

[777] Love JM, Gudas LJ. Vitamin A, differentiation and cancer. *Current Op Cell Biol* 1994; **6**: 825-831.

[778] Moore JW, Clarke GMG, Takatano Q, Wakabayashi Y, Hayward JL, Bulbrook RD. Distribution of 17-oestradiol in the sera of normal British & Japanese women. *J Natl Cancer Inst* 1983; **71**: 749-750.

[779] Ip C, Chin SF, Scimeca JA, Pariza MW. Mammary cancer prevention by conjugated dienoic derivative of linoleic. *Cancer Res* 1991; **51**: 6118-6124.

[780] Chin SF, Liu W, Storkson JM, Ha YL, Pariza MW. Dietary sources of conjugated dienoic isomers of linoleic a newly recognised class of anticarcinogens. *J Food Compos Anal* 1992; **5**: 185-197.

[781] Goldin BR, Adlercreutz H, Gorbach SL. Relationship between oestrogen levels and diets of Caucasian American and Oriental immigrant women. *Am J Clin Nutr* 1986; **44**: 945-953.

[782] Key TJA, Chen J, Wang DY, Pike MC. Sex hormones in women in rural China and in Britain. *Br J Cancer* 1990; **62**: 631-636.

[783] Shimizu H, Ross RIC, Bernstein L, Pike MC, Hendersen BE. Serum oestrogen levels in postmenopausal women: comparison of American whites and Japanese in Japan. *Br J Cancer* 1990; **62**: 451-453.

[784] Bernstein L, Ross RK, Pike MC, *et al*. Hormone levels in older women: a study of post menopausal breast cancer cases and healthy population controls. *Br J Cancer* 1990; **61**: 298-302.

[785] Wang DY, Key TA, Pike MC, Boreham J, Chen J. Serum hormone levels in British and rural Chinese females. *Breast Cancer Res Treat* 1991; **18**: S41-S45.

[786] Bulbrook RD, Swain MC, Wang DY, Hayward JL, Kumaoka S. Breast cancer in Britain and Japan: plasma oestradiol-M, oestrone and progesterone, and their urinary metabolites in normal British and Japanese women. *Eur J Cancer* 1976; **12**: 725-735.

[787] Rose DP, Cohen LA, Berke B, Boyar AP. Effect of a low-fat diet on hormone levels in women with cystic breast disease. II. Serum radioimmunoassayable prolactin and growth hormone and bioactive lactogenic hormones. *J Natl Can Inst* 1987; **78**: 627-631.

[788] Rose DP, Boyar AP, Cohen C, Strong LE. Effect of a low-fat diet on hormone levels in women with cystic breast disease. I. Serum steroids and gonadotropins. *J Natl Can Inst* 1987; **78**: 623-626.

[789] Williams CM, Maunder K, Teale D. Effect of a low fat diet on luteal phase prolactin & oestradiol concentrations and RBI phospholipids in normal premenopausal women. *Br J Nutr* 1989; **61**: 651-661.

[790] Bhathena SJ, Berlin E, Judd J, Nair PP, Kennedy BW, Jones H, Smith PM, Jones Y, Taylor PR, Campbell, WS. Hormones regulating lipid and carbohydrate metabolism in premenopausal women: modulation by dietary lipids. *Am J Clin Nutr* 1989; **49**: 752-757.

[791] Goldin BR, Gorbach SL. Hormone studies and the diet and breast cancer connection. *Adv Exp Med Biol* 1994; **364**: 35-46.

[792] Longcope C, Gorbach S, Goldin B, *et al*. The effect of a low fat diet on estrogen metabolism. *J Clin Endocrinol Metab* 1987; **64**: 1246-1250.

[793] Hill P, Garbaczewski L, Helman P, Huskisson J, Sporangisa E, Wynder EL. Diet, lifestyle, and menstrual activity. *Am J Clin Nutr* 1980; **33**: 1192-1198.

[794] Boyd NF, McGuire V, Shannon P, Cousins M, Kriukov V, Mahoney L, Fish E, Lickley L, Lockwood G, Tritchler D. Effect of a low-fat high-carbohydrate diet on symptoms of cyclical mastopathy. *Lancet* 1988; **ii**: 128-132.

[795] Hagerty MA, Howie BJ, Tan S, Shultz TD. Effect of low and high-fat intakes on the hormonal milieu of premenopausal women. *Am J Clin Nutr* 1988; **47**: 653-659.

[796] Crighton IL, Dowsett M, Hunter M, Shaw C, Smith IE. The effect of a low fat diet on hormone levels in healthy pre- and postmenopausal women: relevance for breast cancer. *Eur J Cancer* 1992; **28A**: 2024-2027.

[797] Boyar AP, Rose DP, Loughridge JR, Engle A, Palgi A, Laakso, K, Kinne D, Wynder EL. Response to a diet low in total fat in women with postmenopausal breast cancer: a pilot study. *Nutr Cancer* 1988; **11**: 93-99.

[798] Prentice R, Thompson D, Clifford C, Gorbach S, Goldin B, Byar D. Dietary fat reduction and plasma estradiol concentration in healthy postmenopausal women. *J Natl Cancer Inst* 1990; **82**: 129-134.

[799] Rose DP, Chlebowski RT, Connolly JM, Jones LA, Wynder EL. Effects of tamoxifen adjuvant therapy and a low fat diet on serum binding proteins and estradiol bioavailability in postmenopausal breast cancer patients. *Cancer Res* 1992; **52**: 5386-5390.

[800] Woods MN, Gorbach SL, Longcope C, Goldin BR, Dwyer JT, Morril-La Brode A. Low-fat, high-fiber diet and serum estrone sulfate in premenopausal women. *Am J Clin Nutr* 1989; **49**: 1179-1183.

[801] Ingram DM, Bennett FC, Willcox D, de Klerk N. Effect of low-fat diet on female sex hormone levels. *J Natl Cancer Inst* 1987; **79**: 1225-1229.

[802] Bennett FC, Ingram DM. Diet and female sex hormone concentrations: an intervention study for the type of fat consumed. *Am J Clin Nutr* 1990; **52**: 808-812.

[803] Rose DP, Goldman M, Connolly JM, Strong LE. High-fibre diet reduces serum estrogen concentrations in premenopausal women. *Am J Clin Nutr* 1991; **54**: 520.

[804] Barnes S, Grubbs C, Setchell KDR, Carlson J. Soyabeans inhibit mammary tumor growth in models of breast cancer. In: Pariza, MW, eds. *Mutagens and carcinogens in the diet*. New York: Wiley-Liss, 1990: 239-253.

[805] Cassidy A, Bingham S, Setchell K. Biological effects of isoflavones present in soy in premenopausal women: Implications for the prevention of breast cancer. *Am J Clin Nutr* 1994; **60**: 333-340.

[806] Phipps WR, Martini MC, Lampe JW, Slavin JL, Kurzer MS. Effect of flaxseed ingestion on the menstrual cycle. *J Clin Endocrinol Metab* 1993; **77**: 1215-1219.

[807] Bruning PF, Bonfrer JMG, van Noord PAH, Hart AAM, de Jong-Bakker M. Insulin resistance and breast cancer risk. *Int J Cancer* 1992; **52**: 511-516.

[808] de Waard F, Trichopoulos D. A unifying concept of the aetiology of breast cancer. *Int J Cancer* 1988; **41**: 666-669.

[809] Garn S.M. The secular trend in size and maturational timing and its implication for nutritional assessment. *J Nutr* 1987; **117**: 817-823.

[810] Kissinger DG, Sanchez A. The association of dietary factors with age of menarche. *Nutr Res* 1987; **7**: 471-479.

[811] Cameron JL. Nutritional Determinants of Puberty. *Nutr Revs* 1996; **54**: 517-522.

[812] Arts CJM, Govers CARL, Van den Berg H, Thijssen JHH. Effects of wheat bran and energy restriction on onset of puberty, cell proliferation and development of mammary tissue in famale rats. *Acta Endocrinologica* 1992; **126(5)**; 451-459.

[813] Hughes RE, Jones E. Intake of dietary fibre and age of menarche. *Ann Hum Biol* 1985; **12**: 325-332.

[814] Ridder CM, Thijssen JHH, Van't Veer P, Van Duuren R, Bruning PF, Zonderland MI, Erich WBM. Dietary habits, sexual maturation and plasma hormones in pubertal girls: a longitudinal study. *Am J Clin Nutr* 1991; **54**: 805-813.

[815] Sandstead HH. Growth, sexual maturation and dietary fibre in pubertal girls. *Am J Clin Nutr* 1992; **55**: 1186-1189.

[816] Snyderwine EG. Some perspectives on the nutritional aspects of breast cancer research. *Cancer* 1994; **74**: 1070-1077.

[817] Bingham S, Pignatelli B, Pollock, JH, Ellul A, Mallaveille C, Gross G, Runswick S, Cummings J.H, O'Neill J.K. Does increased formation of endogenous N Nitroso compounds in the human colon explain the association between red meat and colon cancer? *Carcinogenesis* 1996; **17**: 515-523.

[818] Ziegler RG. Mayne ST, Swanson CA. Nutrition and lung cancer. *Cancer Causes Control* 1996; **7**: 157-177.

[819] Cummings J H. Dietary fibre and large bowel cancer. *Proc Nut Soc* 1981; **40**: 7-14.

[820] Phillips J, Muir G, Birkett A, Zhong XL, Jones GP, O'Dea K, Young GP. Effect of resistant starch on fecal bulk and fermentation dependent events in humans. *Am J Clin Nutr* 1995; **61**: 121-130.

[821] Cummings JH, Bingham SA, Heaton KW, Eastwood MA. Faecal weight, colon cancer and dietary intake of NSP (dietary fibre). *Gastroenterol* 1992; **103**: 1783-1789.

[822] Sonnenberg A, Muller A. Constipation and cathartics as risk factors in colorectal cancer. *Pharmacol* 1993; **4**: 224-233.

[823] Scheppach W, Burghart W, Bartgram P, *et al*. Addition of dietary fibre to liquid formula diets. *J Par Ent Nutr* 1990; **14**: 204-209.

[824] Roediger WEW. Role of anaerobic bacteria in the metabolic welfare of the colonic mucosa in man. *Gut* 1980; **21**: 793-798.

[825] Cummings JH, Pomare EW, Branch WJ, Naylor CPE, Macfarlane GT. SCFA in human and large intestine, portal, hepatic and venous blood. *Gut* 1987; **28**: 1221-1227.

[826] Kruh J, Defer N, Tichonicky L. Effects of butyrate on cell proliferation and gene expression. In: Cummings JH *et al* eds. *Physiological and Clinical Aspects of SCFA*. Cambridge: University Press, 1994.

[827] Smith PJ. Butyrate alters chromatin accessibility to DNA repair enzyme. *Carcinogenesis* 1986; **7**: 423-429.

[828] Kim YS, Gum JR, Ho SB, Deng G. In: Binder, HJ, Cummings J, Soergel KH, eds. '*Short Chain Fatty Acids' Falk symposium 73 1993, Strasburg*. Lancaster: Kluwer Academic, 1994.

[829] Hague A, Manning AM, Hanlon KA, Hueschtchav L, Hart D, Paraskeva C. Sodium butyrate induces apoptosis in human colonic tumour cell lines. *Int J Cancer* 1993; **55**: 498-505.

[830] Boffa LC, Luption JR, Mariana MR, Ceppi M, Newmark H, Scalmati A, Lipkin M. Modulation of colonic cell proliferation, histone acetylation and luminal short chain fatty acids by variation of dietary fibre (wheat bran) in rats. *Cancer Res* 1992; **52**: 5906-5912.

[831] Caderni G, Bianchini F, Dolora P, Kreibel D. Proliferative Activity in the Colon of the Mouse and its Modulation by Dietary Starch, Fat and Cellulose. *Cancer Res* 1989; **49**: 1655-1659.

[832] Van Munster IP, Nagengast EF, Tangerman A. The effect of resistant starch on colonic fermentation, bile acid metabolism, and mucosal proliferation. *Dig Dis Sci* 1994; **39**: 834-842.

[833] Cummings JH, Wiggins H, Jenkins D, Houston H, Drasar B, Hill M, Jivraj T. Influence of diets high and low in animal fat on bowel habit, gastrointestinal transit time, fecal microflora, bile acid and fat excretion. *J Clin Invest* 1978; **61**: 953-963.

[834] Narisawa T, Magadia NE, Weisburger JH, Wynder EL. Promoting effects of bile acids on colon carcinogenesis after NMNG in rats. *J Natl Cancer Inst* 1974; **53**: 1093-1095.

[835] Morotomi M, Giullem JG, Logerfo PL, Weistein B. Production of DAG by human intestinal microflora. *Cancer Res* 1990; **50**: 3595-3599.

[836] Midvedt T, Norman AM. Parameters in 7 alpha dehydroxylation of bile acids by anaerobic bacteria. *Acta Micobiol Pathol Scand* 1968; **72**: 313-329.

[837] Van Munster IP, Nagengast EF, Tangerman A. The effect of resistant starch on fecal bile acids, cytoxicity and colonic mucosal proliferation. *Gastroenterol* 1993; **104**: A460.

[838] Rafter JJ, Eng VW, Furrer R, Medline A, Bruce WR. Effects of calcium and pH on the mucosal damage produced by deoxycholic acid in the rat colon. *Gut* 1986; **27**: 1320-1329.

[839] Zimmerman J. Does dietary calcium supplementation reduce the risk of cancer? *Nutr Rev* 1993; **51**: 109-112.

[840] Weisgerber UM, Boeing H, Owen RW, Waldherr R, Raedsch R, Wahrendorf J. Effect of long term placebo controlled calcium supplementation on sigmoidal cell proliferation in patients with sporadic adenomatous polyps. *Gut* 1996; **38(3)**: 396-402.

[841] Bostick RM, Fosdick L, Wood JR, Grambsch P, Grandits GA, Lillemoe TJ, Louis TA, Potter JD. Calcium and colorectal epithelial cell proliferation in sporadic adenoma patients: a randomized, double-blinded, placebo-controlled clinical trial. *J Natl Cancer Inst* 1995; **87**: 1307-1315.

842 Graf E, Eaton JW. Suppression of colonic cancer by dietary phytic acid. *Nutr Cancer* 1993; **19**: 11-19.

843 Nelson RL, Yoo SJ, Tanure JC, Andrainopoulos G, Misumi A. The effect of iron on experimental colorectal carcinogenesis. *Anticancer Res* 1989; **9**: 1477-1482.

844 Ullah A, Shamsuddin AM. Dose dependent inhibition of large intestinal cancer by inositol, hexa-phosphate in F344 rats. *Carcinogenesis* 1990; **11**: 2219-2222.

845 Kuratko C, Pence BC. Dietary lipid and iron modify normal colonic mucosa without affecting phospholipase A2 activity. *Cancer Letters* 1995; **95**: 181-187.

846 Nair PP, Shami S, Sainz E, *et al.* Influence of dietary fat on fecal mutagenicity in premenopausal women. *Int J Cancer* 1990; **46**: 374-377.

847 Venitt S, Bosworth D, Aldrick AJ. Pilot study of the effect of diet on the mutagenicity of human faeces. *Mutagenesis* 1986; **1** : 353-358.

848 Vahter M, Johansson G, Akesson A, Rahnster B. Faecal elimination of lead and cadmium in sub-jects on a mixed and a lactovegetarian diet. *Food Chem Toxicol* 1992; **30**: 281-287.

849 Gupta I, Suzuki K, Bruce WR, Krepinsky JJ, Yates P. A model study of fecapentaenes. *Science* 1984; **225**: 521-523.

850 Van Tassell RL, Piccariello T, Kingston DGI, Wilkins TD. The precursors of fecapentaenes. *Lipids* 1989; **24**: 454-459.

851 Garg ML, Haerdi JC. The biosynthesis and functions of plasmalogens. *J Clin Biochem Nutr* 1993; **14**: 71-82.

852 Schiffmann M H, Van Tassell R L, Robinson A, Smith L, *et al.* Case-control study of colorectal cancer and fecapentaene excretion. *Cancer Res* 1989; **49**: 1322-1326.

853 De Kok TMCM, Pachen D, Van Iersel MLPS, Baeten CGMI, Engles LGJB, Ten Hoor F, Kleinjans JCS. Case control study on fecapentaene excretion in adenomatous polyps in the colon and rectum. *J Natl Can Inst* 1993; **85**: 1241-1244.

854 MacFarlane G, Cummings J H. The colonic flora fermentation, and large bowel digestive function pp51-92. In: Phillips S, Pemberton JH, Shorter RG eds. *The large intestine: physiology, patho-physiology and Disease.* New York: Raven, 1991.

855 Tsujii M, Kawao S, Tsuji S, Nagano K, Ito T, Hyaashi N, Fusamoto H, Kamada T, Tamura K. Ammonia - a possible promoter in *Helicobacter-pylori* related gastric carcinogenesis. *Cancer Letters* 1992; **65**: 15-18.

856 Tsujii M, Kawano S, Tsuji S, Ito T, Nagano K, Sasaki Y, Hayashi N, Fusamoto H, Kamada T. Cell kinetics of mucosal atrophy in rat stomach induced by long term administration of ammonia. *Gastroenterol* 1993; **104**; 796-810.

857 Visek WJ. Diet and cell growth modulation by ammonia. *Am J Clin Nutr* 1978; **31**: S216-S220.

858 Cooper DP, O Connor PJ, Povey AC, Rafferty JA. Cell and molecular mechanisms in chemical carcinogenesis. In: Peckham M, Pinedo B, Veronesi U eds. *Oxford Textbook of Oncology. Vol 1.* Oxford: Oxford University Press, 1995.

859 Hall CN, Badawi AF, O'Connor PL, Saffhill R. The detection of DNA damage in the DNA of human GI tissues. *Br J Cancer* 1991; **64**: 59-63.

860 Buiatti E, Palli D, Decarli A, *et al.* A case-control study of gastric cancer and diet in Italy. II. Association with nutrients. *Int J Can*cer 1990; **45**: 896-901.

861 Bingham S. Epidemiology and Mechanisms relating diet to risk of colorectal cancer. *Nutr Res Revs* 1996; **9**: 197-239.

862 Sugimura T. Past, present and future of mutagens in cooked foods. *Environ Hlth Pers* 1986; **67**: 5-10.

[863] Weisburger JH. Heterocyclic amines in foods. *Cancer Res* 1993; **53**: 2422-2424.

[864] Canzian F, Ushijima T, Serikawa T, Wakabayashi K, Sugimara T, Nagao M. Instability of microsatellites in rat colon tumours induced by heterocyclic amines. *Cancer Res* 1994; **54**: 6315-6317.

[865] Layton DW, Bogen KT, Knise MG, Hatch FT, Johnson VM, Felton JS. Cancer risk of heterocyclic amines in cooked foods. *Carcinogenesis* 1995; **16**: 39-62.

[866] Friesen MD, Kaderlik K, Lin DX, Garren L, Bartsch H, Lang NP, Kadlubar FF. Analysis of DNA adducts of 2-amino-1methyl-6-phenylimidazo[4,5-b]pyridine in rat and human tissues by alkaline hydrolysis and gas chromatography electron capture mass spectrometry: validation by comparison with ^{32}P postlabelling. *Chemical Res Toxicol* 1994; **7**: 733-739.

[867] Steinbach G, Kumar SP, Reddy BS, Lipkin M, Holt PR. Effects of caloric restriction and dietary fat on epithelial cell proliferation in the rat. *Cancer Res* 1993; **53**: 2745-2749.

[868] Takahashi M, Minamoto T, Yamashita N, Yazawa T, Sugimura T, Esumi H. Reduction in formation and growth of DMH aberrant crypt foci in rat colon by docosohexanoic acid. *Cancer Res* 1993; **53**: 2786-2789.

[869] Bartram HP, Gostner A, Scheppach W, Reddy B, Rao C, Dusel GR, Fichter F, Kasper H. Effects of fish oil on rectal cell proliferation, mucosal fatty acids and PGE2 release in healthy subjects. *Gastroenter* 1993; **105**: 1317-1322.

[870] Anti M, Mara G, Armelo F, *et al.* Effects of w3 fatty acids on rectal mucosal proliferation in subjects at risk for colon cancer. *Gastroenter* 1992; **103**: 883-891.

[871] Anti M, Armelao F, Marra G, Percesepe A, Bartoli GM, Palozza P, *et al.* Effect of different levels of w3 fatty acids on rectal cell proliferation in patients at high risk for colorectal cancer. *Gastroenter* 1994; **107**: 1709-1718.

[872] Hsing AW, Comstock GW. Serological precursors of cancer: serum hormones and risk of subsequent prostate cancer. *Cancer Epid Biomarkers Prev* 1993; **2**: 27-32.

[873] Nomura A, Heilbrun LK, Stemmerman GN, Judd HL. Prediagnostic serum hormones and the risk of prostate cancer. *Cancer Res* 1988; **48**: 3515-3517.

[874] Shultz TD, Bonorden WR, Seaman WR. Effect of short term flaxseed consumption on lignan and sex hormone metabolism in men. *Nutr Res* 1991; **11**: 1089.

[875] Hughes R, Cassidy A, Bingham S. Hormonal effects of lignans in a group of men. *Proc Nutr Soc* 1994; **53**; 3: 230A.

[876] Cassidy A, Bingham S, Setchell K. Hormonal effects of phytoestrogens in postmenopausal women and elderly men. (Submitted for publication).

[877] Correa P. Human gastric carcinogenesis: a multistep and multifactorial process-first. American cancer society award lecture on cancer epidemiology and prevention. *Cancer Res* 1992; **52**: 6735-6740.

[878] Hill MJ. Mechanisms of gastric carcinogenesis. *Eur J Cancer Prev* 1994; **3**: S25-S29.

[879] Forman D. The etiology of gastric cancer. In: O'Neill, IK, Chen J and Bartsch H eds. *"Relevance to Human Cancer of N-Nitroso Compounds, Tobacco Smoke and Mycotoxins"*. Lyon: IARC, 1991; 22-32.

[880] Caygill CPJ, Hill MJ, Knowles RL *et al.* Occupational and socio-economic factors associated with peptic ulcer and with cancers following subsequent gastric surgery. *Ann Occup Hyg* 1990; **34**: 19-27.

[881] Thomason H, Burke V, Gracey M. Impaired gastric function in experimental malnutrition. *Am J Clin Nutr*, 1981; **34**: 1278-1280.

[882] Joosens J, Kesteloot H. Salt and stomach cancer. In: Reed PI and Hill MJ eds. *Gastric Carcinogenesis*. Excerpta Medica, Amsterdam 1988; 105-126.

[883] Gledhill T, Buck M, Paul A. Epidemic hypochlorhydria. *Gut* 1982; **23**: A888.

[884] Siurala M, Isokoski M, Varis K, Kekki M. Prevalence of gastritis in rural population. Bioptic study of subjects selected at random. *Scand J Gastroenterol* 1968; **3**: 211-223.

[885] Davies GR, Rampton DS. *Helicobacter pylori*, free radicals and gastroduodenal disease. *Eur J Gastroent Hepatol* 1994; **6**: 1-10.

[886] Sobala GM, Schorah CJ, Shires S, Lynch DAF, Gallacher B, Dixon MF. Effect of eradication of *Helicobacter pylori* on gastric juice ascorbic acid concentration. *Gut* 1993; **34**: 1038-1041.

[887] Banerjee S, Hawksby C, Miller S, Dahill S, Beattie AD and McColl KEL. Effect of *Helicobacter pylori* and its eradication on gastric juice ascorbic acid. *Gut* 1994; **35**: 317-322.

[888] Rokkas T, Papaptheodorou G, Karameris A, Mavrogeorgis A, Kalogeropoulos N, Giannikos N. *Helicobacter pylori* infection and gastric juice vitamin C levels. Impact of eradication. *Dig Dis Sci* 1995; **40**: 615-621.

[889] Cross CE, Halliwell B, Borish ET, *et al*. Oxygen radicals and human disease. *Ann Intern Med* 1987; **107**: 526-545.

[890] Drake I M, Wazrland D, Carswell N, Schorah C J, Mapstone N, *et al*. Reactive oxygen species (ROS) activity and damage in *Helicobacter pylori* associated gastritis - effect of eradication therapy. *Gut*, 1995; **36(suppl 1)**: A10.

[891] Xu GP, Song PJ, Reed PI. Effects of fruit juices, processed vegetable juice, orange peel and green tea on endogenous formation of N-nitrosoproline in subjects from a high risk area for gastric cancer in Moping County, China. *Eur J Cancer Prev* 1993; **2**: 325-335.

[892] Reed PI. The ECP-IM Intervention Study. *Eur J Cancer Prev* 1994; **3**: S99-S104.

[893] Wattenberg LW. Chemoprevention of cancer. *Cancer Res* 1985; **45**: 1-8.

[894] Huang MT, Ferraro T. Phenolic compounds in food and cancer prevention. In: Huang, MT, Ho, CT, Lee CY, eds. *Phenolic Compounds in Food and Their Effects on Health II* Washington: American Chemical Society Symposium Series, 1992.

[895] Hertog MGL, Kromhout D, Aravanis C. *et al*, Flavonoid intake and long-term risk of coronary heart disease and cancer in Seven Countries Study. *Arch Intern Med* 1995; **155**: 381-386.

[896] Hertog MGL, Feskens EJM, Hollman PCH, *et al*. Dietary antioxidant flavonoids and cancer risk in the Zutphen Elderly Study. *Nutr Cancer* 1994; **22**: 175-184.

[897] Price KR, Fenwick GR. Naturally occurring oestrogens in foods - A review. *Food Add Contam* 1985; **2**, 73-106.

[898] Jones AE, Price KR, Fenwick GR. Development and application of a high-performance liquid chromatographic method for the analysis of phytoestrogens. *J Sci Food Agric* 1989; **46**: 357-364.

[899] Messina M. "Isoflavone intakes by Japanese were overestimated". *Am J Clin Nutr* 1995; **62**: 645.

[900] Juniewicz PE, Pallante Morell S, Moser A, Ewing LL. Identification of phytoestrogens in the urine of male dogs. *J Steroid Biochem* 1988; **31**: 987-944.

[901] Jordan VC. The only true antiestrogen is a non estrogen. *Mol Cell Endocrinol* 1990; **74**: C91.

[902] Fenwick GR, Heaney RK & Mawson R. Glucosinolates. In: *Cheeke PR*, ed. *Toxicants of Plant Origin Vol II, glycosides*. Boca Raton, USA: CRC Press, 1989: 1-41.

[903] Nugon-Baudon L *et al*. Production of toxic glucosinolate derivatives from rapeseed meal by intestinal microflora of rat and chicken. *J Sci Fd Agri* 1988; **43**, 299-308.

[904] Rabot S, Nugon-Baudon L, Raibaud P, Szylit O. Rapeseed meal toxicity in gnotobiotic rats; influence of a whole human faecal flora or single human strains of *Escherichia coli* and *Bacteroides vulgatus*. *Br J Nutr* 1993; **70**: 323-331.

254

[905] Steinmetz KA, Potter JD. Vegetables, fruit and cancer. I. Epidemiology. *Cancer Causes Control* 1991; **2**: 325-357.

[906] Whitty JP, Bjeldanes LF. The effects of dietary cabbage on xenobiotic-metabolising enzymes and the binding of aflatoxin B1 to hepatic DNA in rats. *Food Chem Toxicol*, 1987; **25**: 581-587.

[907] Ramsdell HS, Eaton DL. Modification of aflatoxin B1 biotransformations in vitro and DNA binding in vivo by dietary broccoli in rats. *J Toxicol Environ Hlth* 1988; **25**: 269.

[908] Wattenberg LW. Inhibition of carcinogenesis by nonnutrient constituents of the diet. In: Waldron KW, Johnson IT, Fenwick GR, eds. *Food and Cancer Prevention: Chemical and Biological Aspects*. Cambridge: Royal Society of Chemistry, 1993; 12-23.

[909] Stoewsand GS, Anderson JL, Munson L, Lisk DJ. Effect of dietary brussels sprouts with increased selenium content on mammary carcinogenesis in the rat. *Cancer Letters* 1989; **45**: 43-48.

[910] Scholar EM, Wolterman K, Birt DF, Bresnick E. The effect of diets enriched in cabbage and collards on murine pulmonary metastasis. *Nutr Cancer* 1989; **12**: 121-126.

[911] Stoner GD, Morrissey DT, Heur YH, Daniel EM, Galati AJ, Wagner SA. Inhibitory effect of phenethyl isothiocyanate on N-nitrosobenzyl methylamine carcinongenesis in the rat oesophagus. *Cancer Res* 1991; **51**: 2063-2068.

[912] Morse MA, Eklind KA, Amin SG, Chung FL. Effect of frequency of isothiocyanate administration on inhibition of 4-(methylnitrosamino)-1-(3-pyridyl)-1-butanone-induced pulmonary adenoma formation in A/J mice. *Cancer Letters* 1992; **62**: 778-781.

[913] Tanaka T, Mori Y, Morishita Y, Hara A, Ohno T, Kojima T, Mori H. Inhibitory effect of snigrin and indole-3-carbinol on diethylnitrosamine-induced hepatocarcinogenesis in male ACI/N rats. *Carcinogenesis* 1990; **11**: 1403-1406.

[914] Sugie S, Okumura A, Tanaka T, Mori H. Inhibitory Effects of Benzyl Isothiocyanate and Benzyl Thiocyanate on Diethylnitrosamine-Induced Hepatocarcinogenesis in Rats. *Jap J Cancer Res* 1993; **84**: 865-870.

[915] Loub WD, Wattenberg LW, Davis DW. Aryl hydrocarbons hydroxylase induction in rat tissues by naturally occurring indoles of cruciferous plants. *J Natl Cancer Inst* 1975; **54**: 985-988.

[916] Pence BC, Buddingh F, Yang SP. Multiple dietary factors in the enhancement of DMH carcinogenesis: main effect of indole 3 carbinol. *J Natl Cancer Inst* 1986; **77**: 269-276.

[917] Vistisen K, Loft S, Poulsen HE. Cytochrome P450 1A2 activity in man measured by caffeine metabolism: effect of smoking, broccoli and exercise. In: Witmer CM *et al*, ed. *Advances in experimental medicine and biology: Biological reactive intermediates IV*. New York: 9 Plenum Press, 1990, 407-411.

[918] Pantuck EJ, Pantuck CB, Garland WA, Min BH, Wattenberg LW, Anderson KE, Kappas A, Conney AH. Stimulatory effect of brussels sprouts and cabbage on human drug metabolism. *Clin Pharmacol Therapy* 1979; **25**: 88-95.

[919] Bogaards JJP, Verhagen H, Willems MI, van Poppel GV, van Bladeren PJ. Consumption of Brussels sprouts results in elevated alpha-class glutathione s-transferase levels in human blood plasma. *Carcinogenesis* 1994; **15**: 1073-1075.

[920] Verhagen H, Poulsen HE, Loft S, van Poppel GV, Willems MI, van Bladeren, PJ. Reduction of oxidative damage in humans by brussels sprouts. *Carcinogenesis* 1995; **16**: 969-970.

[921] Fenwick GR, Hanley AB. The genus allium. *CRC Crit Revs Fd Sci Nutr* 1985; **22**: 199-377.

[922] You WC, Blot WJ, Chang YS, *et al*. Allium vegetables and reduced risk of stomach cancer. *J Natl Cancer Inst* 1989; **81**: 162-164.

[923] Liu J, Lin RI, Milner JA. Inhibition of 7,12-dimethylbenz(a)anthracene-induced mammary tumors and DNA adducts by garlic powder. *Carcinogenesis* 1992; **13**: 1847-1851.

255

[924] Arnagase H, Milner JA. Impact of various sources of garlic and their constituents on 7, 12-dimethylbenzene(a)anthracene binding to mammary cell DNA. *Carcinogenesis* 1993; **14**: 1627-1631.

[925] Lin X-Y, Liu J-Z, Milner JA. Dietary garlic suppresses DNA adducts caused by N-nitroso compounds. *Carcinogenesis* 1994; **15**: 349-352.

[926] Lai CN, Dabney BJ, Shaw CR. Inhibition of in vitro metabolic activation of carcinogens by wheat sprout extracts. *Nutr Cancer* 1978; **1**: 27-30.

[927] Lai CN. Chlorophyll: the active factor in wheat sprout extract inhibiting the metabolic activation of carcinogens in vitro. *Nutr Cancer* 1979; **1**: 19-21.

[928] Lai CN, Butler MA, Matney TS. Antimutagenic activities of common vegetables and their chlorophyll content. *Mutat Res* 1980; **77**: 245-250.

[929] Dashwood RH, Breinholt V, Bailey GS. Chemopreventive properties of chlorophyllin: inhibition of aflatoxin B1(AFB)-DNA binding in vivo and anti-mutagenic activity against AGBI and 2 heterocyclic amines in the Salmonella mutagenicity Assay. *Carcinogenesis* 1991; **12**: 939-942.

[930] Arimoto S, Fukuoka S, Itome H, *et al*. Binding of polycyclic planar mutagens to chlorophyllins resulting in inhibition of the mutagenic activity. *Mutat Res* 1993; **287**: 297-305.

[931] Sarkar D, Sharma A, Talukder G. Chlorophyll and chlorophyllin as modifiers of genotoxic effect. *Mutat Res* 1994; **318**: 239-247.

[932] González CA, Riboli E, Badosa J, *et al*. Nutritional factors and gastric cancer in Spain. *Am J Epidemiol* 1994; **139**: 466-473.

[933] Ministry of Agriculture, Fisheries and Food. *The Dietary and Nutritional Survey of British Adults – Further Analysis*. London: HMSO, 1994.

[934] Yang CS, Brady JF, Hong J. Dietary effects on cytochromes-P450, xenobiotic metabolism and toxicity. *FASEB Journal*, 1992; **6**: 737-744.

[935] Crowell PL, Chang RR, Ren Z, Elson CE, Gould MN. Selective inhibition of isoprenylation of 21-26 kDa proteins by the anticarcinogen d-limonene and its metabolities. *J Bio Chem* 1991; **266**: 17679-17685.

[936] Newmark HL, Wargovitch MJ, Bruce WR. Colon cancer and dietary fat, phosphate, and calcium, a hypothesis. *J Natl Cancer Inst* 1984; **72**: 1323-1325.

[937] Fenwick GR, Heaney RK & Mullin WJ. Glucosinolates and their breakdown products in foods and food plants. *CRC Crit Rev Fd Sci Nutr* 1983; **18**: 123-201.

12.　Glossary

Absolute risk: the observed or calculated likelihood of the occurrence of an event in a population under study, over a specified period of time, as contrasted with the relative risk (qv)

Adduct: a chemical moiety which is covalently bound to a large molecule such as DNA or protein

Adenocarcinoma: a malignant epithelial tumour derived from glandular tissue or where the tumour cells form recognisable glandular structures

Adenoma: a benign epithelial tumour derived from glandular tissue or exhibits clearly defined glandular structures. Some adenomas can progress to become malignant

Aetiology: the cause or causes of a disease

Aflatoxin: a family of closely related toxic and carcinogenic substances produced by the spores of the fungus *Aspergillus flavus*, which can infect most dietary staples, particularly nuts

Age-standardised: an adjustment of the values of a variable to take account of differences in the age distribution of the populations being compared

Alkylating agent: chemicals which are electrophilic reactants that, without the need for metabolic activation, leave the alkyl group covalently bound to a nucleophilic centre (mainly sulphur, nitrogen and oxygen atoms) in biologically important macromolecules such as proteins and nucleic acids. Many alkylating agents are mutagenic, carcinogenic and immunosuppressive

Allium: a plant genus which includes onions, garlic and leeks

Anti-carcinogen: a chemical which inhibits the development of cancer or the growth of tumours (qv)

Anticlastogenic: acting against agents which produce chromosome breaks and other structural aberrations such as translocations which play an important part in the development of some tumours

Antioxidant: a substance that inhibits oxidation

257

Apoptosis:	an active process of cell death in which DNA degradation and nuclear destruction precede loss of plasma membrane integrity and cell necrosis
Atrophic gastritis:	inflammation of the gastric mucosa with loss of the characteristic microscopic architecture, e.g. in pernicious anaemia, infection with *Helicobacter pylori* can be precancerous
Benign tumour:	a tumour which is usually slow growing, retaining many of the structural and functional features of its tissue of origin and not invading surrounding tissue or metastasising to distant organs.
Bias:	a characteristic of a study which tends systematically to produce results that depart from the true values (to be distinguished from random error). Any trend in the collection, analysis, interpretation, publication or review of data that can lead systematically to conclusions that are different from the truth.
Biomarkers:	parameters measurable in biological samples which indicate either the extent of exposure to an environmental factor, or the status of an individual in respect to a particular metabolic function
Biomethylation:	the enzyme-mediated attachment of methyl groups to specific sites on biologically-active molecules, such as DNA or protein, with consequent changes in structure and/or function
Body Mass Index:	an indirect measure of body fatness; BMI = weight (kg) $\div$ height (m)^2
Brassicas:	a plant genus which includes broccoli, cabbage, cauliflower, Brussels sprouts, kale and mustard
Cancer:	any malignancy either solid tumour or more diffuse myelo or lympho proliferative disorders. The term cancer encompasses all neoplastic diseases in which normal cells are transformed into malignant ones
Cancer incidence data:	registered data on the incidence of specific cancers in the population
Carcinogenesis:	the origin, causation and development of tumours
Carcinogenicity:	the degree to which a given substance is carcinogenic
Carcinogens:	the causal agents which induce tumours. They include exogenous factors (chemicals, physical agents, viruses) and endogenous factors such as hormones.
Carcinoma:	a malignant tumour derived from epithelial tissue

258

Cardiovascular disease: disease of the heart and blood vessels

Carotenoids: a group of about 100 red and yellow pigments derived from and found principally in plants, comprising carotenes, many of which e.g. β-carotene are precursors for retinol, and xanthines e.g. lycopene, which are not. They may act as antioxidants.

Case-control studies: a study that starts with the identification of persons with a condition of interest and a matched control group of persons without the disease. The extent of past exposure to known or suspected risk factors is measured in each group and the risk associated with each factor is estimated.

Chemotherapy: the treatment of disease with chemical compounds or drugs

Cisplatin: a cytotoxic drug with an alkylating action, used particularly in the treatment of solid tumours of the ovary and testes, which impedes cell division by damaging DNA

Clastogenic: producing chromosome breaks and other structural aberrations such as translocations. Clastogens may be viruses or physical agents as well as chemicals. Clastogenic events play an important part in the development of some tumours

Cohort or prospective study: study of a population whose exposure to a factor or factors hypothesised to influence the probability of occurrence of a given disease is measured at recruitment. The participants are followed over time and development of disease ascertained. Such a sample identified at one period of time, is called a cohort

Confidence interval: the range around a measured value, e.g. the mean, within which the true value of a parameter can be predicted, with the specified level of confidence, to lie

Confounding variable: a factor that distorts the observed relationship between two other variables. It must be controlled for in order to obtain an undistorted estimate of the true relationship

Contaminant: a substance, in foods, that is not a natural component or intentionally added

Connective tissue: the tissue that supports, binds or separates more specialised tissues. It comprises a matrix in which is embedded a variety of specialised tissues and cells e.g. bone, cartilage, tendons

Cross-sectional study:	a study which examines the relationships between different variables within time
Cruciferous:	a family of plants which includes the genus *brassica* (*qv*)
Cryptorchidism:	the condition in which the testes fail to descend into the scrotum and are retained in the abdomen or inguinal canal
Differentiation:	a term that denotes the degree of morphological and functional sophistication or organisation within the cells and organs
Dysplasia:	abnormal development of cells, which may be predisposed to form tumours
Ecological studies:	epidemiological investigations in which various measures of the characteristics of a whole population are associated with measures of disease occurrence. These paired observations are contrasted over differing circumstances (geographical, social).
Epigenetic carcinogens:	substances that lead to the development of cancer without directly affecting cellular DNA
Epithelial tissue:	tissue which covers the external surface of the body and lines hollow structures (except blood and lymphatic vessels)
Familial adenomatous polyposis:	a hereditary disease characterised by the presence of large numbers of polypoid tumours in the large bowel one or more of which inevitably undergoes cancerous change
Fecapentaene:	an alkylating mutagen produced by *Bacteroides spp* found in the human colon
Flavonoids:	a generic term for a group of aromatic compounds found in tea, plants, fruits and vegetables which may have antioxidant properties
Free radical:	atoms or molecules that contain an unpaired electron and that seek out another electron to attain a more stable and less reactive state and that by doing so can damage molecules such as DNA, lipids or proteins
Genotoxic:	the ability of a substance to cause DNA damage, either directly, or after metabolic activation
Glucosinolates:	bioactive compounds derived from *brassica* vegetables which may act as anticarcinogens
Haemopoietic system:	the system which produces all cellular components of the blood

Human papilloma virus:	viruses containing a closed circular DNA molecule of about 8000 base pairs, and which cause non-malignant and malignant tumours in man
Hyperplasia:	an increase in the number of cells in a tissue or organ caused by stimulation of mitosis
IARC:	International Agency for Research on Cancer
ICD Codes:	International Classification of Disease Codes
Incidence:	the number of new cases of a disease occurring in a given size of population during a specific period of time, usually a year
Induction period:	the interval from causal action of a factor to the initiation of the disease
Initiation:	the first step in the development of cancer (often caused by a mutation)
Intervention studies (experimental studies):	an investigation involving intentional change in some aspect of the status of the subjects. The intervention can be at the individual or community/population level.
Ionising radiation:	radiation which causes ionisation (loss of electrons from atoms) in the medium through which it passes
Isoflavones:	colourless, crystalline ketones occurring in many plants, generally in the form of a hydroxy derivative which may have anticarcinogenic properties
Latent period:	the interval between the first exposure to a carcinogenic stimulus and the appearance of a clinically diagnosable tumour. For a disease like cancer, which usually involves a sequence of steps over a long period, the term "latent period" may be unhelpful.
Leukaemia:	cancers of the blood-forming organs, characterised by abnormal proliferation and development of leucocytes (white blood cells) and their precursors in the bone marrow, blood, lymph and lymph glands
Lycopene:	the red carotenoid (qv) pigment of tomatoes, various berries and fruits
Lymphoma:	a cancer of cells of the immune system (e.g. lymphocytes) confined to lymph glands and related tissues, such as the spleen
Malignant melanoma:	tumour of the skin cells that produce the pigment melanin

261

Malignant neoplasm or tumour:	a tumour with the potential for invading neighbouring tissue and/or metastasising to distant body sites, or one that has already done so
Metaplasia:	a change of cellular morphology in one kind of tissue into that characteristic of another
Metastasis:	the spread of malignant cells from a primary neoplasm via the blood, lymphatic system or body cavities to distant sites where they form secondary or metastatic tumours
Mitogenesis:	the stimulus for cells to undergo mitosis
Monounsaturated fatty acids (MUFA):	fatty acids with one double (unsaturated) bond
Mortality rate:	the number of deaths from a disease in a given size of population during a specified period of time
Mutagenesis:	process of generating mutations. It may occur spontaneously or be induced by mutagens
Mutagenic:	the property of an agent to produce mutation
Mutagenicity:	the degree by which an agent increases the rate of mutation
Mutation:	a permanent change in the amount or structure of the genetic material in an organism, which may result in a change in the phenotypic characteristics of the organism. The alterations may involve a single gene, or block of genes, or a whole chromosome
Neoplasia:	new abnormal growth of tissue. Malignant neoplasms show a greater degree of anaplasia and have the properties of invasion and metastasis, compared with benign neoplasms
Non-starch polysaccharides (NSPs):	a precisely measurable and major component of dietary fibre
Nulliparous:	never having given birth
Obesity:	BMI over 30kg/m^2
Odds Ratio:	the ratio of odds of exposure to non-exposure among the diseased (cases) compared to the non-diseased (controls) in case-control studies. The odds ratios derived in case-control studies are approximately equivalent to the relative risks (qv) determined in cohort studies
Oesophagitis:	inflammation of the oesophagus

Oncogenes:	genes which can potentially induce neoplastic transformation. They include genes for growth factors, growth factor receptors, protein kinases, signal transducers, nuclear phosphoproteins, and transcription factors. When these genes are constitutively expressed after structural and/or regulatory changes, uncontrolled cell proliferation may result.
Overweight:	BMI 25-30kg/m^2
Papilloma:	a benign or malignant tumour composed of papillae growing from the surface of the skin or mucous membrane
Phytoestrogens:	compounds found in plants which may have variable degrees of oestrogenic activity
Polymorphism:	the occurrence in a population of two or more genetically determined alleles in such frequency that the rarest of them could not be maintained by mutation alone
Polyphenols:	compounds made up of a number of conjoined, hydroxylated benzene rings e.g. flavonoids (qv)
Polyunsaturated fatty acids (PUFA):	fatty acids with more than one double (unsaturated) bond
PRR (Proportional Registration Ratios):	the ratio of the proportion of registrations from each cancer in a population subgroup to the proportion of registrations in the general population, expressed as a percentage
Prevalence:	the number of cases observed in a given size of population at a designated time
Primary site:	the site of an initial neoplastic growth
Progression:	a complex process which describes the development of a benign tumour into a malignancy which has the potential to invade and disseminate
Promotion:	events in a multistage process of cancer formation where initiated cells undergo clonal expansion to form overt tumours
Prospective studies:	see cohort studies
P/S ratio:	the ratio of the polyunsaturated fatty acid content divided by the saturated fatty acid content of the diet
Randomised controlled trials:	intervention studies in which groups are randomly allocated to receive specific interventions
Relative risk:	the ratio of the risk of event among those exposed to a factor to that of those unexposed

263

Risk:	a technical term which is said to indicate the probability of an adverse health effect such as cancer developing in a human population within a defined set of circumstances
Risk factor:	any exposure or lifestyle factor which increases the risk of developing a given disease
Saturated fatty acid (SFA):	a fatty acid with no double (unsaturated) bonds
Sarcoma:	a tumour, often highly malignant, developing in the connective tissue of bones, muscles, blood vessels, cartilage etc.
Secular trend:	changes in a population over time, generally measured over years or decades
Standardised Mortality Ratio:	the percentage of the number of deaths observed in the study population to the number of deaths expected if it had the same age structure as the standard population
Superoxide radical:	a molecule of oxygen with an extra unpaired electron
Threshold effect:	the lowest dose which will produce an effect, below which no effect is observed
Tumorigenesis:	the formation of a tumour
Tumour:	literally means any swelling but usually taken as referring to a mass of abnormal, disorganised cells, arising from pre-existing tissue, which are characterised by excessive and uncoordinated proliferation and by abnormal differentiation; may be benign or malignant

Annex 1

Reports

Development of a Scoring System to Judge the Scientific Quality of Information From Case-Control and Cohort Studies of Nutrition and Disease

Barrie M. Margetts, Rachel L. Thompson, Tim Key, Stephen Duffy,
Michael Nelson, Sheila Bingham, and Martin Wiseman

Abstract

A scoring system was developed to help judge the scientific quality of observational epidemiologic studies linking diet with risk of cancer. The scoring system was developed from key headings used in developing research protocols and included questions under headings: three for case-control studies (dietary assessment, recruitment of subjects, and analysis) and four for cohort studies (dietary assessment, definition of cohort, ascertainment, and analysis). Points were awarded for questions in each section, and a total score was derived.

Interobserver variation was assessed for five case-control and five cohort studies for 13 observers; 1 observer repeated the assessment of each paper. Absolute scores and ranking within observer were assessed. There was good agreement between observers in the ranking of studies. Papers that scored higher presented sufficient detail to enable the questions in the scoring system to be answered more easily. For some studies, the information required was either not collected or, if it was collected, not presented. In either case, the frequent lack of information available to judge papers raises questions about the editorial policy and review process of journals publishing dietary studies as much as it does about the scoring system.

Applying the scoring system to a review of meat and cancer risk suggested that, taking the score into account, from what seemed like a large literature, there were relatively few studies that scored well (defined as a score >65%), but these studies tended to provide more consistent information.

*(Nutr Cancer **24**, 231–239, 1995)*

B. M. Margetts and R. L. Thompson are affiliated with the Wessex Institute of Public Health Medicine, University of Southampton, Southampton, UK. T. Key is affiliated with the Imperial Cancer Research Fund Cancer Epidemiology Unit, University of Oxford, Oxford, UK. S. Duffy is affiliated with the Medical Research Council Biostatistics Unit, University of Cambridge, Cambridge, UK. M. Nelson is affiliated with the Department of Nutrition and Dietetics, Kings College, London, UK. S. Bingham is affiliated with the Dunn Clinical Nutrition Centre, Cambridge, UK. M. Wiseman is affiliated with the Nutrition Unit, Department of Health, London, UK.

Introduction

There has been considerable interest over the last 10 years in developing critical appraisal skills for reviewing the medical literature to help policy makers judge whether one treatment or approach may be more effective than another (1). By and large, the methodology for critical appraisal has been developed to assess the quality of reviews of randomized controlled trials. The Cochrane collaboration has been a major international initiative to pull together all the randomized controlled trials to enable reviewers to be more systematic. Experimental studies provide the best evidence for drawing causal inferences about the effect of an exposure on an outcome. However, for most major public health problems, there are relatively few experimental studies available, and the reviewer has to make judgments about the strength of causal inference that can be drawn about associations between exposure and outcomes on the basis of observational studies. This is particularly the case for cancer epidemiology, where there are few experimental studies with cancer as an outcome and where the applicability of studies with surrogate endpoints may be limited.

Many reviews of the epidemiologic literature linking diet to cancer have been published, but few have used a systematic approach to judge the impact of the scientific quality of the information included on the conclusions that may be drawn from the review. While reviewers have increasingly differentiated results among ecological, case-control, and cohort studies, few have systematically assessed whether the inconsistencies among studies relate to the design and conduct of the studies (2–4). Whereas for experimental studies there are generally agreed criteria for including studies in reviews, mainly related to whether subjects were properly randomized, few such criteria have been used when reviewing case-control and cohort studies.

The Nutritional Epidemiology Group, an informal group of researchers from across the United Kingdom, was asked to provide a systematic review of the epidemiologic literature linking diet with cancer. A systematic review of sources of papers revealed that about 800 papers had been published for nine major cancer sites. From a superficial review of these papers, it was clear that not all studies were conducted in the same way, and we therefore felt that they should not be judged in the same way. We did not want to exclude any studies from the review, so we developed a scoring system to enable us to judge the relative merits of different studies and to assess whether taking the scoring system into account influenced our interpretation of the relationships reported. From our collective experience of designing studies, we drew up a checklist of questions that should be addressed in a good study; broadly this list looked like a study protocol. The answers to questions were scored to enable a quantitative comparison to be made across studies. Here we set out the detail of the scoring system, a review of the between-observer reliability of the score, and an example of a review where the scoring system was used to help in the interpretation of the results. We have published elsewhere the summary of the review(5).

Objective of the Scoring System

The objective of the scoring system was to codify in an objective way commonly expressed subjective judgments on the quality of information on diet in relation to cancer development derived from epidemiologic studies. More weight could then be given to better information in drawing conclusions. The emphasis was on evaluating the quality of information available from the study with respect to diet.

Method: Development of the Scoring System

The scoring system was intended to reflect the quality and quantity of information yielded by each study on diet and cancer risk. Thus a study primarily aimed at nondietary factors, but with a very small dietary component, will tend to have a low score, regardless of the

232

effectiveness of the study in researching its primary target. The score assigned to a study should not therefore be interpreted as a judgment of the overall quality of that study but as a reflection of the amount and reliability of information on diet and cancer.

Separate scoring systems were used for case-control and cohort studies, because some markers of reliability (e.g., control selection) apply to only one type of study. For this reason, case-control and cohort studies were reviewed separately, and their scores should not be directly compared.

The detailed criteria for scoring are given in **Appendixes A** and **B.**

Case-control studies were scored in three broad areas: quality of dietary assessment, recruitment of subjects, and analysis of results. The three areas potentially contribute 28%, 49%, and 23% to the total score. Within each category, some aspects have more weight than others. For example, 30% of the dietary assessment score is assigned to appropriateness of the methods, whereas description of the usage of the method is assigned only 10% of the score.

Cohort studies were scored in four broad areas: dietary assessment, definition of the cohort, ascertainment of disease cases, and analysis of results. These potentially contribute 36%, 7%, 38%, and 19% to the overall score. Within the broad areas, the weight assigned to individual aspects varies.

In assigning the scores, there is a subjective element, and an interobserver variation study was conducted to judge the robustness of the approach (described below). The proportion of the potential score assigned to different areas of study design, execution, and analysis reflects the relative importance of these areas in the opinion of the Steering Group: other epidemiologists might assign these proportions differently.

Results

Between- and Within-Observer Variation in the Application of the Scoring System

All the papers included in the original review were scored by the same reviewer, and the distribution of scores is therefore not biased by interobserver variation. To establish whether different reviewers would score the same papers in the same way, we sent papers describing five case-control and five cohort studies to 20 members of the Nutritional Epidemiology Group and asked them to score each paper using the scoring system. Eleven completed scores for each paper were returned. One of us (RT) scored each paper on two separate occasions, and with the original reviewer there were 13 completed scores for each paper. The scores have been tabulated (Tables 1 and 2). We considered that the main benefit of the scoring system would be to rank papers, and to make presentation simple, we have summarized the overall score and rank for each paper for each reviewer for the case-control and cohort studies separately.

Table 1 summarizes the main results for the overall scores and ranks for case-control studies. There was a reasonable spread of scores between papers; across reviewers within papers, the scores tended to be quite consistent. Overall there was reasonable agreement across reviewers in the ranking of the papers. Paper 3 was ranked either best or second best by all reviewers and Paper 4 was judged to be the worst by 8 of 13 reviewers. For each paper, Reviewer M repeated the assessment, and the repeat result is presented as N*; there was exact agreement in the ranking for the first and repeat measures, and the overall scores were very similar.

For each paper, we also tabulated the scores allocated for each question in Sections A (dietary assessment), B (recruitment of subjects), and C (analysis) to see if we could identify any areas were there seemed to be greatest disagreement between reviewers (these are not presented here). Under the section on dietary assessment, reviewers were not very consistent for some papers in the way they answered the questions about the validation of the dietary assessment (Question A4), particularly "Is the validation appropriate?" and "How have the

Table 1. Results From Interobserver Study: Summary of Case-Control Studies[a]

Reviewer	Paper 1		Paper 2		Paper 3		Paper 4		Paper 5	
	Score	Rank	Score	Rank	Score	Rank	Score	Rank	Score	Rank
A	80.2	1	68.4	3	73.8	2	39.8	5	65.9	4
B	68.2	2	65.9	3	84.4	1	52.1	5	63.6	4
C	75.7	1	60.4	4	70.7	2	49.3	5	61.8	3
D	75.7	2	69.2	3	76.7	1	57.2	5	63.0	4
E	67.3	2	66.9	3	74.4	1	52.1	5	55.1	4
F	73.0	2	68.1	3	75.8	1	63.2	4	61.8	5
G	64.5	4	69.6	3	82.3	1	70.0	2	62.7	5
H	53.7	3	72.7	2	79.0	1	44.7	4	41.2	5
I	52.5	3	63.4	1	55.4	2	42.8	5	46.7	4
J	67.1	2	65.7	4	79.0	1	66.0	3	56.0	5
K	50.1	3	61.0	1	60.4	2	39.1	5	43.5	4
L	48.3	5	75.0	2	76.2	1	52.6	4	60.8	3
M	66.7	3	69.2	2	79.0	1	56.7	5	58.0	4
N[b]	65.6	3	69.2	2	76.2	1	51.2	5	58.0	4
Average	64.8	2.5	67.3	2.6	74.4	1.3	52.7	4.4	56.9	4.2

a: Score, total score (%); rank, 1 (highest) to 5 (lowest).
b: Repeat measure for Reviewer M (not included in average).

Table 2. Interobserver Study: Summary of Cohort Studies[a]

Reviewer	Paper 6		Paper 7		Paper 8		Paper 9		Paper 10	
	Score	Rank	Score	Rank	Score	Rank	Score	Rank	Score	Rank
A	46.9	2	44.4	3	36.4	4	33.9	5	59.3	1
B	40.7	3	70.4	2	28.6	5	32.7	4	77.8	1
C	46.3	3	54.3	2	34.4	5	39.7	4	74.1	1
D	48.1	3	54.7	2	32.5	5	33.9	4	77.8	1
E	40.7	3	54.1	2	30.5	5	38.9	4	75.9	1
F	58.8	2	56.0	3	42.4	4	31.7	5	81.5	1
G	52.9	3	66.3	2	41.2	4	36.0	5	67.3	1
H	57.0	3	69.1	2	28.0	5	45.3	4	83.7	1
I	45.7	3	49.6	2	13.8	5	25.3	4	83.7	1
J	56.6	2	52.1	3	32.5	4	25.5	5	77.8	1
K	48.4		46.9				41.1		83.9	
L	52.7	3	81.1	1	38.5	5	51.2	4	71.0	2
M	44.9	3	50.2	2	36.8	5	40.8	4	71.8	1
N[b]	42.8	4	55.6	2	36.8	5	43.6	3	69.8	1
Average	49.2	2.8	57.6	2.2	33.0	4.7	36.6	4.3	75.8	1.1

a: Score, total score (%); rank, 1 (highest) to 5 (lowest).
b: Repeat measure for Reviewer M (not included in average).

validation results been used in analysis?" It was also apparent that several reviewers confused validity and repeatability and so incorrectly scored some papers. For the best and worst papers, the scores were quite consistent, but for the intermediate papers, the scores ranged from 0 to the maximum 3. There were also a wide range of scores given for the questions on the number of cases in the study and the response rate.

For each of the above questions where there was greatest between-reviewer variability, part of the problem could be explained by the way the paper presented the relevant data and part

234

by the care required in reading the paper to find the information. The questions on the validity of the dietary assessment also required the reviewer to exercise considerable judgment.

Table 2 presents the results for the cohort studies. For both the scores and the ranking, there was good agreement across reviewers. For the papers that were, on average, ranked first or last, there was very little disagreement between reviewers; Paper 10 was judged to be the best by all but one reviewer, and Paper 8 was judged to be either worst or second worst by all reviewers. There was also good agreement between repeat measures by the same reviewer (M, N*). We again looked at scores allocated for individual questions for each reviewer for each paper. As in case-control studies, the greatest between-reviewer variability was seen for the questions relating to the validity of the dietary assessment, the response rate, number of cases, and completeness of follow-up.

Intraclass correlations (6), which are a rough estimate of agreement among scores, were 0.71 for the case-control studies and 0.92 for the cohort study papers. This suggests good agreement.

General Comments From Reviewers About Using the Scoring System

Most reviewers offered some comments. A number of reviewers felt that it might be difficult to answer certain questions without some familiarity with the disease under study or with epidemiologic studies in general. Others commented that the relevant information required to answer all the questions was hard to find in some papers. Here our original reviewer was at a considerable advantage, because she also had access to other papers from the same researchers to enable her to check certain details (like the actual numbers included in the analysis). Two issues are raised: 1) the layout of papers to draw relevant information together in a format that is easier to follow and 2) editorial guidelines on what information should be considered essential in the methods section of a paper.

Guidelines have been produced for the description of the dietary assessment (7), but perhaps more detailed guidance is also required for the epidemiologic methods, particularly for nonepidemiologic journals.

Application of the Scoring System to a Review of Meat and Cancer Risk

A test of the usefulness of the scoring system, having demonstrated that it is reasonably robust, is whether taking the scores of studies into account in a review alters the conclusions reached. To test this, we reviewed the scores and results for all the studies in our data base with information on meat consumption and risk of cancer. The summary of the number of studies involved is presented in Table 3. When studies scoring >65% (judged to be "good" studies) were reviewed separately, two observations were made: 1) that there were few good studies and 2) that the good studies were more consistent in showing a positive relationship between meat and risk of cancer than if all studies were reviewed without consideration of the score. It is not intended to discuss here the implications of the findings in this area; the aim is to use these data as an example to illustrate the method. It is worth pointing out, however, that part of the difficulty of judging the evidence linking meat to risk of cancer related to clarifying what was meant by meat; few studies looked at the effects of different types of meat on cancer risk.

Validity of the Scoring System

The above has demonstrated that the score can be used reliably to rank studies, but it does not say whether the score is valid, in the sense of describing the truth. To establish the validity of the scoring system would require some external standard against which to compare the

Table 3. Use of the Scoring System to Judge the Epidemiologic Literature Linking Meat Consumption to Risk of Cancer

	No. of Studies	No. of Studies Showing Increased Risk	No. of Studies Showing Statistically Significant Increased Risk
Case-control studies			
(total)	106	85 (80%)	35 (33%)
Score >65	34		16 (47%)
Cohort studies			
(total)	41	30 (73%)	12 (29%)
Score >65	10		5 (50%)
Total no. of studies	147	115 (78%)	47 (32%)

scoring system. It is difficult to imagine how this could be done, because the whole process of judging the scientific quality of information is subjective. The best that we can offer in support of the scoring system is that it appears to be reliable and that it produces a range of scores that allow papers to be ranked. If all papers scored high or low, the score would not have been a useful tool to differentiate study information. Whether the ranking represents the important differences between "good" and "bad" information is less certain.

Greenland (8), and more recently Doll (9), discussed the requirements for an appropriate review of observational studies. A review of the literature requires a systematic approach to the collection of all available studies (to minimize potential publication bias) and the avoidance of a priori hypotheses about the outcome of the review that may prejudice the interpretation of the studies included. Whereas meta-analyses can provide a pooled quantitative summary of the studies reviewed, a purely statistical approach does not describe the shortcomings of the studies included in the review. Whereas it may be possible in a quantitative meta-analysis to adjust for some of the biases present in the studies included, it cannot take into account all potential problems.

Several authors developed criteria for judging the quality of studies included in reviews. Friedenreich and co-workers (4) published criteria for case-control studies that included 13 questions on study design and 16 on dietary data collection methods. Longnecker and colleagues (2) awarded up to 100 points to studies based on whether they were cohort or case-control studies and other subject characteristics. Boyd and others (3) developed a simple score and ranked studies according to the percentage of standards met. Steinberg and co-workers (10), in a review of estrogen replacement therapy and breast cancer, developed criteria for case-control and cohort studies separately, pooled scores across three reviewers, and assessed whether the ranking altered study conclusions. Friedenreich and colleagues cautiously concluded that the score is not a direct measure of validity or of precision and must be interpreted as a guide to aid the reviewers' judgment.

Conclusions

The scoring system introduces an objective element to judging the usefulness of the information presented in papers being reviewed. Considerable effort has gone into developing a quality review of randomized controlled trials but much less into judging observational studies, which provide most of the evidence in many areas of nutrition and health.

In our opinion, the prototype scoring system reported here aided our description of the epidemiologic data on diet and cancer (5) and highlights the need for authors and editors to design and describe studies appropriately.

Appendix A

Scoring System for Case-Control Studies

Section A. Dietary assessment:
Studies without dietary data and only biochemical data were not included in the review.
1) Is the method appropriate for the question being asked? (3,2,1,0)
2) Is the description of the method sufficient to judge whether the method is likely to be used correctly? (1,0)
3) Does the assessment cover an appropriate time frame? (1,0)
4) Has the method been validated? (1,0); Is the validation appropriate (e.g., same population)? (1,0); How have the validation results been used in analysis? (1,0)
5) For studies where nutrient intakes are presented, Have foods been translated to nutrient intakes appropriately (enough information, e.g., on portion sizes)? (1,0); Has an appropriate database been used? (1,0)
The maximum score for this section is 10; if the study does not present nutrient data (food or alcohol only), the maximum score is 8 and therefore needs to be weighted to scale up to a maximum score of 10 (score out of 8 * 10/8).

Section B. Recruitment of subjects:
1) Number of cases: Allocated points depending on number of cases in the study as follows: 0–49 = 0, 50–99 = 1.0, 100–199 = 2.0, 200–299 = 2.8, 300–399 = 3.4, 400–499 = 4.0, 500–599 = 4.4, 600–699 = 4.8, 700–799 = 5.2, 800–899 = 5.6, 900–999 = 6.0, ≥1,000 = 6.4
2) Response rate: (cases and controls scored separately for each) percentage of eligible sample, excluding deaths: ≥80%, 5 points; 65–79%, 3 points; 50–64%, 2 points; <50%, 1 point; not stated or not able to be calculated, 0 points
3) Source of information: interview with subject, 3 points; self-completed by subject, but checked by interviewer, 2.5 points; self-completed, not checked, 2 points; proxy data-spouse, 1 point; other relative, 0.5 points
(Divide by 2 if source is different for cases and controls. If different methods are mixed, add points for each method and divide by number of methods.)
4) Source of controls: Community, if random sample, 2 points; if uncertain, 1 point. Hospital, if appropriate, 1 point; if uncertain, 0.5 points. Hospital and community, if analyzed separately (add points above); Family controls, 0.5 points
5) Has diagnosis been confirmed: by histology/cytology/radiology, 3 points; by reference to clinical notes, 2 points; from death certificates, 1 point; unconfirmed, from subjects only, 0 points
6) Have unconfirmed cases been excluded? (1,0)
Maximum score for this section is 26.4 points.

Section C. Analysis:
1) Consideration of other factors: Have data been collected on other factors? (1,0); Have these factors been assessed appropriately? (1,0); Does the study adjust for age and gender by 1) matching on controls of these variables (1,0) and using matched analysis (1,0) or 2) adjusting for these variables in the analysis? (2,0) (note for breast and cervical cancer adjusted for pre/postmenopausal instead of gender)
2) Presentation of results: Have unadjusted results been presented? (1,0); Have means or some indication of levels of dietary exposure been presented? (1,0); Have odds ratios been calculated across levels of intake (thirds, e.g., rather than simple presentation of means for groups)? (1,0); Have results been adjusted for energy? (1,0); What method has been used? (1 point for description); Have results been adjusted for other factors (if relevant)? (1,0)
Maximum score for this section is 10 points.

To derive total score

[(score in Section A + score in Section B/1.5 + score in Section C/1.2) / 35.9] * 100

Scores in Sections B and C have been downweighted to reflect the greater importance of Section A.

Appendix B

Scoring System for Cohort Studies

Section A. Dietary assessment:
1) As per case-control study, score out of 10 (note weighting as appropriate) plus score the following items.
2) Has more than one method been used? (1,0)
3) Does the study include diet and biologic samples? (1,0)
4) Are the biologic samples appropriate? (2,1,0)
5) Has the assessment (including biologic sample) been repeated during study? (1,0)
6) Is the repeat measure appropriate? (2,0)
7) Has the repeat measure been used in the analysis? (2,0)
Maximum score in this section is 19 points. If there are no dietary data, score 0 for this section and divide total score by 34.4, not 53.4.

Section B. Definition of cohort:
1) Is the reference population clearly defined? (1,0)
2) Is it clear how the sample relates to the reference population and what inclusion criteria have been used? (1,0)
3) What is the response rate in those asked to participate? ≥60%, 2 points; <60%, 1 point; not mentioned, 0 points
Maximum score in this section is 4 points.

Section C. Ascertainment:
1) How complete is the follow-up of subjects? ≥95%, 4 points; 90–94%, 2 points; <90%, 0 points; not stated, 0 points
2) For how long have subjects been followed up? >15 years, 3 points; 10–15 years, 2 points; <10 years, 1 point
3) Has the way in which outcome was assessed been clearly described? (2,1,0)
4) Has diagnosis been confirmed? by histology/cytology/radiology, 3 points; by reference to clinical notes, 2 points; from death certificates, 1 point; unconfirmed, from subjects only, 0 points
5) Have unconfirmed cases been excluded? (1,0)
6) Has the statistical power of the study been assessed a priori? (1,0)
7) Number of subjects (cases): 0–49 = 0, 50–99 = 1.0, 100–199 = 2.0, 200–299 = 2.8, 300–399 = 3.4, 400–499 = 4.0, 500–599 = 4.4, 600–699 = 4.8, 700–799 = 5.2, 800–899 = 5.6, 900–999 = 6.0, ≥1,000 = 6.4
Maximum score in this section is 20.4 points.

Section D. Analysis and results:
1) Consideration of other factors: Have data been collected on other factors? (1,0); Have these factors been assessed appropriately? (1,0)
2) Presentation of results: Have unadjusted results been presented? (1,0); Have relative risks been calculated across levels of intake (thirds, e.g., rather than simple presentation of means for groups)? (1,0); Have means or some indication of levels of dietary exposure been presented? (1,0); Have incident cases been excluded from the analysis: first year of follow-up only? (1,0), in first five years of follow-up? (1,0); Have results been adjusted for energy? (1,0), what method has been used? (1 point for description); Have results been adjusted for other factors? (1,0)
Maximum score in this section 10 points.

To derive total score

[(score in Section A + score in Section B + score in Section C + score in Section D)/53.4] * 100

With no dietary data score

[(B + C + D)/34.4] * 100

238

Acknowledgments and Notes

The work presented here was directed by a steering group of scientists from across the United Kingdom meeting under the umbrella of the United Kingdom Nutritional Epidemiology Group. The authors thank members of the Nutritional Epidemiology group for helpful comments in drafts of the scoring system and also for participating in the assessment of between-observer variation. This work was in part funded by a grant from The Department of Health and a grant to The Institute of Human Nutrition, University of Southampton from The Rank Prize Funds. Address reprint requests to Dr. B. M. Margetts, Wessex Institute of Public Health Medicine, University of Southampton, Southampton General Hospital, B Level South Academic Block, Southampton, SO16 6YD United Kingdom.

Submitted 2 June 1995; accepted in final form 20 July 1995.

References

1. Petitti, DB: *Meta-Analysis, Decision Analysis, and Cost-Effectiveness Analysis.* New York: Oxford Univ Press, 1994.
2. Longnecker, MP, Orza, MJ, Adams, ME, Vioque, J, and Chalmers, TC: "A Meta-Analysis of Alcoholic Beverage Consumption in Relation to Risk of Colorectal Cancer." *Cancer Causes Control* 1, 59–68, 1990.
3. Boyd, NF, Martin, LJ, Noffel, M, Luckwood, G, and Ritchler, DL: "A Meta-Analysis of Studies of Dietary Fat and Breast Cancer Risk." *Br J Cancer* 68, 627–636, 1993.
4. Friedenreich, C, Brant, RF, and Riboli, E: "Influence of Methodologic Factors in a Pooled Analysis of 13 Case-Control Studies of Colorectal Cancer and Dietary Fiber." *Epidemiology* 5, 56–79, 1994.
5. The Nutrition Society: *Diet and Cancer. A Review of the Epidemiological Literature.* London: Nutr Soc, 1993.
6. Snedecor, GW, and Cochran, WG: *Statistical Methods.* Ames, IA: Iowa State Univ Press, 1980.
7. Nelson, M, Margetts, BM, and Black, AS: "Checklist for the Methods Section of Dietary Investigations." *Br J Nutr* 69, 935–940, 1993.
8. Greenland, S: "Quantitative Methods in the Review of Epidemiologic Literature." *Epidemiol Rev* 9, 1–30, 1987.
9. Doll, R: "The Use of Meta-Analysis in Epidemiology. Diet and Cancers of the Breast and Colon." *Nutr Rev* 52, 233–237, 1994.
10. Steinberg, KK, Thacker, SB, Smith, J, Stroup, DF, Zack, MM, et al.: "A Meta-Analysis of the Effect of Oestrogen Replacement Therapy on the Risk of Breast Cancer." *J Am Med Assoc* 265, 1985–1989, 1991.

273

Annex 2

Terminology

The evidence was broken down into broad categories, for which different terms were applied, as follows:

Epidemiology data	– none/few/some/many studies – insufficient – inconsistent – weakly consistent – moderately consistent – strongly consistent
Extent of evidence for mechanism	– no/little/some/substantial evidence – evidence exists in animals/*in vitro* – evidence that operates in humans exists
Strength of evidence for mechanism	– the Working Group was convinced – evidence is equivocal – evidence is unconvincing – evidence is lacking/no evidence
Overall evidence for link	– not enough evidence – evidence is weak – evidence is moderate – evidence is strong